S.
——FOR A——
BILLION

TO, Sarah.

With best wishes

Basil Hetzel

cpandu —

London
10th May 1996

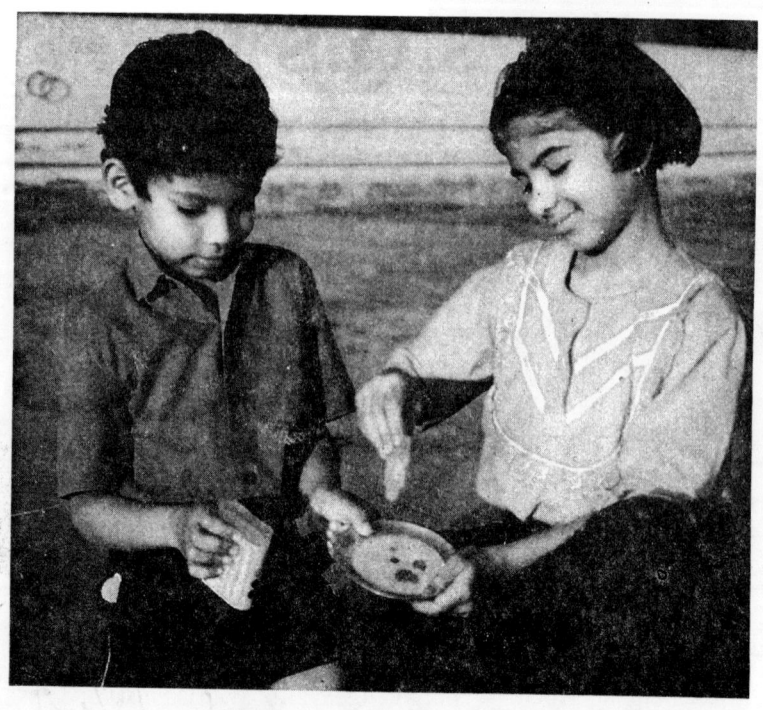

Monitoring of iodine content of salt—an important aspect of the conquest of Iodine Deficiency Disorders.

S.O.S. FOR A BILLION

The Conquest of Iodine Deficiency Disorders

Edited by
BASIL S HETZEL
Chairman
International Council for Control of
Iodine Deficiency Disorders

AND

CHANDRAKANT S PANDAV
Regional Coordinator for South Asia & Pacific
International Council for Control of
Iodine Deficiency Disorders

DELHI
OXFORD UNIVERSITY PRESS
CALCUTTA CHENNAI MUMBAI
1997

Oxford University Press, Walton Street, Oxford OX2 6DP

*Oxford New York
Athens Auckland Bangkok Calcutta
Cape Town Chennai Dar es Salaam Delhi
Florence Hong Kong Istanbul Karachi
Kuala Lumpur Madrid Melbourne Mexico City
Mumbai Nairobi Paris Singapore
Taipei Tokyo Toronto*

and associates in

Berlin Ibadan

© *B. S. Hetzel and C. S. Pandav 1996*

First published 1994
Second edition 1996
Second impression 1997

ISBN 0 19 564002 0

**This book is published in collaboration with the
International Council for Control of
Iodine Deficiency Disorders**

Cover picture: Conquest of Iodine Deficiency Disorders is
necessary for the well-being of many millions of
mothers and children throughout the world.

Printed at Gopsons Papers Ltd., Noida 201301
and published by Manzar Khan, Oxford University Press
YMCA Library Building, Jai Singh Road, New Delhi 110001

TO THE GLOBAL PARTNERSHIP DEDICATED TO THE ELIMINATION OF IODINE DEFICIENCY DISORDERS

An Ancient Scourge of Mankind

The People of the affected countries
The Governments of the affected countries
The Salt Producers of each country

The International Agencies-especially
The World Health Organization
The United Nations Children's Fund
The World Bank
The Micronutrient Initiative
Kiwanis International
Program Against Micronutrient Malnutrition

The International Expert Network of
International Council for Control of
Iodine Deficiency Disorders
(ICCIDD)

The Bilateral Agencies especially
The Australian Agency for International Development
The Canadian International Development Agency
The Netherlands Ministry for Development Cooperation
The Swedish International Development Agency
The United States Agency for International Development

The International Council for the Control of Iodine Deficiency Disorders (ICCIDD) is a non-profit non-governmental organization dedicated to the sustainable elimination of iodine deficiency disorders (IDD) throughout the world. The ICCIDD was granted an offical status as an International NGO at the 47th World Health Assembly held in Geneva in 1994. Its activites are supported by donations/grants from the Australian Agency for International Development (AusAID), the Canadian International Development Agency (CIDA), the Micronutrient Initiative (MI), the Netherlands Ministry for Development Cooperation, the Swedish International Development Agency (SIDA), the United Nations Children's Fund (UNICEF), the United States Agency for International Development (USAID), The World Bank, the World Health Organisation (WHO) and others.

PREFACE TO FIRST EDITION

This book aims to 'Spread the word' to a global audience of the great opportunity presented for the elimination of the ancient scourge of the iodine deficiency disorders (IDD) by the year 2000. Iodine deficiency is recognized as the most common preventable cause of mental defect in the world today.

This book follows 'The Story of Iodine Deficiency' (1989) which gives the full historical and scientific background of the problem. In the present book, written five years later, remarkable progress is recorded which encourages confidence that the elimination of IDD may be achieved by the year 2000.

The International Council for Control of Iodine Deficiency Disorders (ICCIDD), founded in 1985-86, has been in the forefront of this development. In close collaboration with the World Health Organization, UNICEF and with the support and participation of the bilateral agencies especially the Australian International Development Assistance Bureau (AIDAB), and the Canadian International Development Agency (CIDA) and more recently the salt industry and Kiwanis International, a global partnership has been established which gives hope that an ancient scourge of mankind can and will be eliminated.

We express thanks to our colleagues in the ICCIDD who have so willingly contributed to this book.

One of us (BSH) was very fortunate to be a Resident Scholar at the Bellagio Conference and Study Centre, Italy, as a guest of the Rockefeller Foundation which enabled him to work fulltime on the book for a period of three weeks in April 1993.

We are indebted to Lyn Giehl and Barbara McNamara of the ICCIDD Secretariat in Adelaide, Australia for expert secretarial support, Smita Pandav, K. Anand and Shankar Nene at ICCIDD (SEARO) office for technical and editorial assistance and our colleagues at Oxford University Press in New Delhi, India for assistance with the final publication.

BSH
CSP

PREFACE TO SECOND EDITION

The First Edition of this book was launched by the late Mr James P. Grant, Executive Director of UNICEF on the 9th April 1994 in Quito, Ecuador.

This was the occasion of the Regional Meeting for Universal Salt Iodization Towards the Elimination of Iodine Deficiency Disorders, which attracted representation from 26 Latin American countries.

Mr Grant was a great champion of the goal of elimination of IDD and was particularly impressed with the title 'The Conquest of Iodine Deficiency Disorders.'

As he pointed out we have moved from 'The Story of Iodine Deficiency' (the previous book published in 1989) to 'SOS for a Billion: the conquest of Iodine Deficiency Disorders' (1994).

It is a remarkable story of increasing impact since 1990 when the UN World Summit for Children included the goal of elimination of IDD as one of the goals. This goal is now seen as the summit goal most likely to be achieved by the year 2000.

Distribution of the First Edition (4,500 copies) was completed earlier this year. The rapidity of developments towards the elimination of IDD throughout the world has led to this Second Edition appearing a little over a year since the First Edition.

There is an update on recent developments in Europe, Latin America and Central Asia, the problem of the translation of knowledge to policy into practice as well as new sections on IDD in animals, new alliances in IDD elimination, WHO statements on safety of iodized salt in non-deficient populations and ICCIDD statement on iodized oil in pregnancy.

Spanish and French translations will be available shortly.

We are indebted again to our colleagues in the International Council for Control of Iodine Deficiency Disorders for their cooperation.

In Delhi, Smita Pandav, K. Anand, Rajesh Pandav and our colleagues at Oxford University Press have worked very efficiently once again and so ensured rapid production of this Second Edition.

We invite all readers to discuss this great programme with their friends and colleagues and to assist realisation of the conquest of an ancient massive scourge of mankind.

B S H
C S P

CONTENTS

List of Authors xv

Introduction xvii

Glossary xix

Part I THE CONQUEST OF IODINE DEFICIENCY DISORDERS – THE GLOBAL PICTURE

1. S.O.S for a Billion – The Nature and Magnitude of the Iodine Deficiency Disorders 3
   B.S. HETZEL

2. Recent Progress in the Elimination of Iodine Deficiency Disorders 31
   B.S. HETZEL

3. The Conquest of Iodine Deficiency through a Global Partnership of People, Governments, International Agencies, the Salt Industry, Kiwanis International and Micronutrient Initiative 57
   B.S. HETZEL

Part II NATIONAL PROGRAMMES FOR THE ELIMINATION OF IODINE DEFICIENCY DISORDERS

4. Measurement of Iodine Deficiency Disorders 81
   J.B. STANBURY and A. PINCHERA

5.	The Iodization of Salt for the Elimination of Iodine Deficiency Disorders M.G. VENKATESH MANNAR	99
6.	The Use of Iodized Oil and Other Alternatives for the Elimination of Iodine Deficiency Disorders J.T. DUNN	119
7.	The Economic Benefits of the Elimination of IDD C.S. PANDAV	129
8.	From Knowledge to Policy to Practice DAVID P. HAXTON	147
9.	The Process of Communicating the Message DAVID P. HAXTON	165
10.	Planning and Managing National Programmes for Elimination of Iodine Deficiency Disorders Africa K.V. BAILEY	177
	Asia C.S. PANDAV	
	Latin America MAURO RIVADENEIRA	
11.	The Role of the International Agencies UNICEF J.P. GREAVES and D. ALNWICK	205
	WHO G.A. CLUGSTON and K.V. BAILEY	

12.	The Role of Kiwanis International W. BLECHMAN	229

Part III STORIES FROM THE COUNTRIES

13.	**IDD in Africa**	235
	IDD in Eastern and Southern Africa F.P. KAVISHE	
	IDD in Western and Central Africa M. BENMILOUD and D.N. LANTUM	
	IDD in Nigeria O.L. EKPECHI	
14.	**IDD in Central Asia** GREGORY GERASIMOV and DAVID P. HAXTON	257
15.	**IDD in South-East Asia** C.S. PANDAV	271
16.	**IDD in China** T. MA and T.Z. LU	293
17.	**IDD in Europe** F. DELANGE	303
18.	**IDD in Latin America** E.A. PRETELL and J.T. DUNN	325
19.	**IDD in the Middle East** K. BAGCHI and A. VERSTER	337

Part IV SUSTAINING ELIMINATION OF IODINE DEFICIENCY DISORDERS

20. Monitoring and Verification of Progress towards the Elimination of IDD by the Year 2000 and beyond   347
    J.T. DUNN, C.S. PANDAV and B.S. HETZEL

Part V STATEMENT ON SAFETY OF IODIZED SALT AND IODIZED OIL

21. Statement on Safety of Iodized Salt and Iodized Oil   357

Part VI NEW ALLIANCES AND PROGRESS TOWARDS ELIMINATION OF IDD

22. IDD in Livestock Populations   375
    C.S. PANDAV and M.G. VENKATESH MANNAR

23. Patnership to End Hidden Hunger - Collaboration of Stakeholders in Sustaining the Elimination of Iodine Deficiency Disorders   399
    C.S. PANDAV, DAVID P. HAXTON and HEMA VISWANATHAN

24. Progress Towards Elimination of IDD   429
    - Excerpts from Publications of International Agencies (UNICEF, WHO, World Bank) and International conference on Nutrition (ICN)

Index   459

LIST OF AUTHORS

Mr David Alnwick
Senior Nutrition Adviser,
(Micronutrients),
UNICEF
New York   USA

Dr F. Delange
Executive Director, ICCIDD
Avenue de la Fauconnerie 153
B-1170
Brussels   Belgium

Dr D.N. Lantum
University Centre for Health Sciences
CUSS BP 1364
Younde Cameroon

Dr John T. Dunn
Secretary, ICCIDD
Department of Medicine,
University of Virginia,
Health Sciences Centre,
PO Box 511,
Charlottesville VA 22908,
USA

Dr Gregory Gerasimov
Head of Therapy Department
Russian Endocrinology Research Centre
Dm. Uljanavo
11 Moscow 117036
Russia

Dr O.L. Ekpechi
Professor of Medicine,
College of Medicine,
University of Nigeria,
ENUGU   Nigeria

Dr Kalyan Bagchi
WHO Consultant,
World Health Organization,
Egypt

Dr Peter Greaves
Senior Adviser, ICCIDD
2 The Plantation,
London SE3 OAB

Dr K.V. Bailey
WHO Consultant,
World Health Organization,
Switzerland

Mr David P. Haxton
Senior Adviser, ICCIDD
909 Elizabethan drive,
Greensboro NC 27410,
USA

Dr Moulay Benmiloud
ICCIDD Regional Co-ordinator for Africa,
University of Algiers,
Service d' Endocrinologie,
Centre Pierre et Marie Curie,
Avenue Battandier,
Algiers 16005,
Algeria

Dr Basil S. Hetzel
Chairman ICCIDD
C/-Health Development Foundation,
Women's and Children's Hospital,
72 King William Road,
North Adelaide 5006 SA,
Australia

Dr W. Blechman
Kiwanis International Foundation,
5250 SW 84th Street,
Miami 33143-8434,
Florida   USA

Dr Festo Kavishe
Managing Director,
Tanzania Food and Nutrition
Centre, PO Box 977
(Ocean Road No 22),
Dar es Salaam   Tanzania

Dr Graeme Clugston
Chief, Nutrition Section,
World Health Organization,
1211 Geneva,
27 Switzerland

Dr T.Z. Lu
Institute of Endocrinology,
Tianjin Medical University,
Tianjin 300070,
Peoples Republic of China

Dr Tai-Ma
132 Chong-Quing Road
Tianjim 300050
People's Republic of China

Dr Eduardo A. Pretell
ICCIDD Regional Co-ordinator
for Latin America,
AV Cuba 532,
Apartado Postal 110388,
Lima 11   Peru

Mr M.G. Venkatesh Mannar
Executive Director
The Micronutrient Initiative
C/- IDRC
Ottawa K1G 3H9
Canada

Dr Mauro Rivadeneira
Project Officer IDD,
UNICEF,
Casilla: 0134 CEQ16,
Av. Republica 481 y Almagro,
Quito   Ecuador

Dr C.S. Pandav
ICCIDD Regional Co-ordinator
for South Asia and Pacific
Centre for Community
Medicine, All India Institute of
Medical Sciences,
Ansari Nagar,
New Delhi 110 029   India

Dr John Stanbury
Emeritus Chairman, ICCIDD
43 Circuit Road,
Chestnut Hill, Mass 02167,
USA

Dr Aldo Pinchera
Institute of Endocrinologia,
Actolologia Clinca E Medicina
de Lavoro,
Universita Degli Studi di Pisa,
Viale del Tirreno 64,
56018 Tirrenia, PISA   Italy

Ms Hema Viswanathan
Sr. Vice President and Managing
Director
Social & Rural Research Institute
201 Ansal Chambers II,
Bhikaji Cama Place
New Delhi - 110066, India

Dr Anna Verster
Regional Adviser NUT/EMRO,
World Health Organization,
PO Box 1517,
Alexandria 21511   Egypt

INTRODUCTION

This book sets forth the exciting opportunity we have in the current decade to eliminate an ancient scourge of mankind. This scourge, the iodine deficiency disorders (IDD) constitutes the most common preventable cause of mental defect in the world today. At least 20 million people are suffering a mental handicap that could easily be prevented at very modest cost.
Great progress has been made in the last five years so that there is increasing confidence that the conquest of IDD can be achieved.
The book is divided into four parts:

Part I Outlines the global challenge of eliminating IDD as a public health problem by the year 2000, and describes the global partnership that has now come together to meet the challenge.

Part II Presents the national programme strategy that is now being implemented to achieve the elimination of IDD at country level. The major proven technology is that of iodized salt within a multisectoral programme including community education, the social mobilization of the salt industry and monitoring of the programme. One of the great advantages of iodized salt is that it can be readily financed through the salt industry at very modest cost to the consumer.

Part III Describes progress at country level towards the goal of elimination by the year 2000. Detailed stories of success and failure are described and lessons drawn.

Part IV Describes the monitoring and verification process required to ensure sustainability of the elimination of IDD for the year 2000 and into the next century.

Part V Reproduces the statement on safety of iodized salt by WHO and of ICCIDD on safety of iodised oil in pregnany & iodine induced thyrotoxicosis

Part VI Describes the new alliances in Iodine Deficiency Disorders elimination and progress towards elimination of IDD

'With the ever-growing development of national control programmes, supported by regional working groups and the remarkable global collaborative network of the International Council for Control of Iodine Deficiency Disorders, the essential infrastructure for global elimination is already in place. Now required are the resources to reinforce the national programmes which will drive this global support system. If these resources are forthcoming, I am certain we shall see the virtual elimination of iodine deficiency disorders by the year 2000'.

Dr Hiroshi Nakajima
Director-General
World Health Organization

'Micronutrient deficiency does not produce hunger as we know it: it gnaws at the core of health, but not in the belly. Most of its consequences are not readily perceived; like the iceberg, its bulk lies beneath the surface. Even its most apparent effects such as blindness and cretinism seem to most people to be unrelated to diet. That is why we call it "hidden hunger" and why such an extraordinary effort must be made through every available channel to drag it into the open, make it visible as an issue at the political level, and empower families with the prevention knowledge they need'.

Mr James P. Grant
Executive Director
UNICEF

From:
Ending Hidden Hunger
(A Policy Conference on Micronutrient Malnutrition)
Montreal, Quebec, Canada
October 1991

Glossary

ACC/SCN	Administrative Committee on Coordination - Subcommittee on Nutrition of the United Nations System
ASEAN	Association of South East Asian Nations
AusAID	Australian Agency for International Development
CIDA	Canadian International Development Agency
DNA content	DNA is the basic material within a cell which stores the genetic code and is responsible for cellular growth.
Dulberg model	A statistical model for estimating prevalence of all the manifestations of IDD from prevalence of goitre and other demographic variables.
ECO	European Cooperation Organization
ECSA	Eastern, Central and Southern Africa
ECSS	European Committee for the Study of Salt
EEC	European Economic Community
EMCOSAL	A semi-autonomous Corporation in Bolivia for building salt iodization plants.

Endemia	An area where a disease is endemic.
Endemic	Occurrence of a disease confined to a community.
Endemic Cretinism	A state resulting from the loss of function of the thyroid gland characterized by mental defect, deaf-mutism, spastic paralysis.
Endocrinologists	People who study endocrine glands i.e. glands that secrete hormones. Thyroid gland is one such gland.
EPI 30 Cluster	A sampling method initially proposed under Expanded Programme of Immunization for estimating immunization coverage levels of a community, now being used for other purposes including estimating the prevalence of IDD.
Global Verification Commission	Proposed by the ICCIDD to WHO and UNICEF be jointly responsible to these agencies-to provide an independent verification of progress towards the goals of elimination of IDD by the year 2000.
Goitre	An enlarged thyroid gland.
Goitrogens	A chemical, capable of causing goitre by inhibiting iodine uptake by thyroid.
Hypothyroidism	The result of a lowered level of circulating thyroid hormone with slowing of mental and physical functions.

ICCIDD	International Council for Control of Iodine Deficiency Disorders
IDD	Iodine Deficiency Disorders-the spectrum of the effects of iodine deficiency at various stages in life.
IEC	Information, Education and Communication
IIT	Iodine Induced Thyrotoxicosis
INACG	International Nutritional Anaemia Consultative Group
Iodization	The general term covering iodization programmes using various agents (iodine, iodate) or technology (salt, oil, bread and water).
Iodized Oil	Iodine in poppy seed oil-lipiodol formerly extensively used in radiology as a radio contrast medium. Available both by injections (lipiodol) and by mouth (oridol).
Iodized Salt	Salt to which potassium iodate or potassium iodide has been added.
IVACG	International Vitamin A Consultative Group
IWGIDD	International Working Group on Iodine Deficiency Disorders in China

Kiwanis	A world service group with 9,000 club and 330,000 members who have agreed to raise US$ 50 million over the next five years for the elimination of IDD.
MDIS	Micronutrient Deficiency Information System developed by WHO with ICCIDD and UNICEF to provide data for governments and agencies on progress in elimination of IDD.
Median UIC	If the urinary iodine concentrations in a community survey of individuals are arranged in ascending order, median UIC refers to the one which occurs at the centre (i.e. equal number of observation on either side of it).
MI	Micronutrient Initiative
MNM	Micronutrient Malnutrition
Myxedematous	An oedema (swelling) which occurs due to poor thyroid functioning.
NGOs	Non-Government Organizations
NRDC	Nutrition Research Development Centre in BOGOR Indonesia
OAU	Organization for African Unity
PAMM	Program Against Micronutrient Malnutrition, Atlanta, USA

PAHO	Pan American Health Organization
PEG	Program for Eradication of Goitre
Phalanx	Digital bone of a finger
Prophylaxis	An intervention aimed at preventing the occurrence of a disease.
Radio-immune assay	A technique of estimating the level of a hormone in the serum by using a radioactive (eg. I^{131}) element which the hormone utilizes.
SAARC	South Asian Association for Regional Cooperation
SCN	Subcommittee on Nutrition of the UN system
SIDA	Swedish International Development Agency
TFNC	Tanzania Food and Nutrition Centre
Thiocyanate	Chemicals known to have goitrogenic potential
TGR	Total Goitre Rate
Thyroid size	Measured by ultrasonography-a much more sensitive and reproducible measurement than is possible by palpation.
Thyroxine	Thyroid Hormone

Triiodothyronine	One of the thyroid hormones which utlises 3 iodine molecules
TSH	Thyroid Stimulating Hormones-which controls thyroid activity.
UIC	Urinary Iodine Concentration
UNDP	United Nations Development Programme
UNICEF	United Nations Children's Fund
USAID	United States Agency for International Development
USI	Universal Salt Iodization
WFP	World Food Program
WHO	World Health Organization.

PART I

The Conquest of Iodine Deficiency Disorders
The Global Picture

1

S.O.S for a Billion – The Nature and Magnitude of the Iodine Deficiency Disorders

B.S. Hetzel

Introduction

The headline 'SOS for a Billion' appeared in a Japanese newspaper reporting an interview I gave on the subject of iodine deficiency when visiting Tokyo in 1991. Such a phrase is useful to denote the task of the elimination of an ancient scourge which affects an estimated one billion people in developing countries. This risk arises from the effect of dietary iodine deficiency on the early development of the brain.

Iodine deficiency is the most common preventable cause of mental deficiency in the world today. The World Health Organization has estimated that the elimination of iodine deficiency would prevent the brain damage that has caused irreversible mental handicap to at least 43 million people in the world today! (Fig 1.1). Remarkable sucess has been

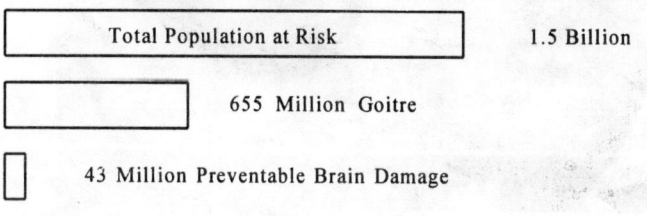

Fig. 1.1 Global population data for the prevalence of IDD in developing countries.
Source: ICCIDD/UNICEF/WHO Indicators for assessing Iodine Deficiency Disorders and their control through salt iodization, WHO/NUT/94.

achieved by the use of iodized salt to correct this deficiency in many industrialized countries since 1920. But a great challenge remains in developing countries, particularly in Asia, Africa and Latin America (Hetzel 1989).

The importance of iodine, as an essential element, arises from the fact that it is a constituent of the thyroid hormones thyroxine (T_4) and triiodothyronine (T_3). The thyroid hormones are essential for normal growth – physical and mental development in man and animals.

The biological importance of the thyroid gland is indicated by the fact that without a thyroid, the tadpole will not metamorphose into a frog. The thyroid hormones increase body warmth by increasing the rate of metabolism so that the transition from the relatively warm aquatic to the relatively cold terrestrial life can be made.

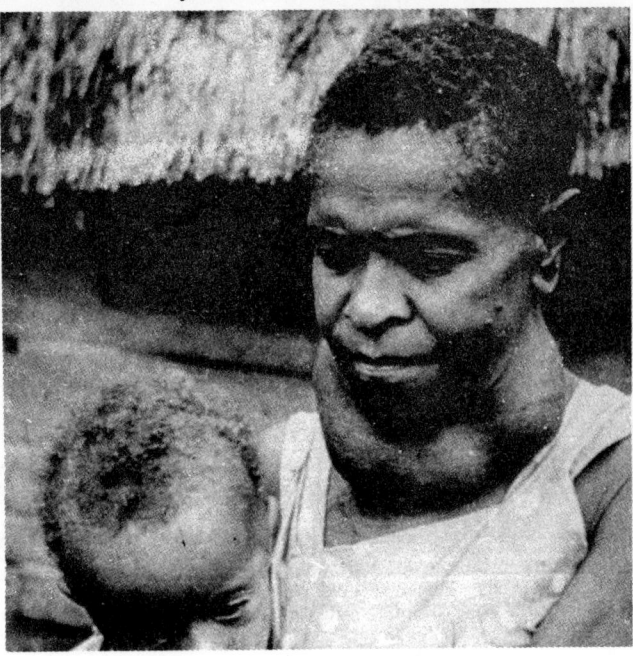

Fig. 1.2 A mother and child from a New Guinea village who are severely iodine deficient. The mother has a large goitre and the child is also affected. The bigger the goitre, the more likely it is that she will have a cretin child. This can be prevented by eliminating the iodine deficiency before the onset of pregnancy.

Iodine, which is the Greek word for violet, was first isolated as a violet vapour during the making of gunpowder at the end of the eighteenth century. The most familiar effect of iodine deficiency is goitre – a swelling of the thyroid gland in the neck (Fig. 1.2). Goitre has been noted and commented on since ancient times. In the Renaissance period, goitre was a common feature of the paintings of the Madonna in Italy. Indeed, Thomas Wharton in 1656 suggested that the larger thyroid in the female served to beautify the neck!

However, our understanding of iodine deficiency has now gone far beyond goitre to all the effects it has on growth and development including brain development, now denoted by the term 'iodine deficiency disorders' (IDD) (Hetzel 1989).

The Ecology of Iodine Deficiency

There is a cycle of iodine in nature (Fig. 1.3). Most of the iodine exists in the ocean. It was present during the primordial development of the earth but large amounts were leached from the surface soil by glaciation, snow, or rain and were carried by the wind, rivers and floods into the sea. Iodine occurs in the deeper layers of the soil and is found in oil-well and natural gas effluents. Water from such deep wells can provide a major source for iodine. In general, the older an exposed soil surface, the more likely it is to be leached of iodine.

But the most likely areas to be leached are the mountainous areas of the world. The most severely deficient areas are those of the Himalayas, the Andes, the European Alps and the vast mountains of China. Iodine deficiency is likely to occur in all elevated regions subject to glaciation, higher rainfall, with run-off into rivers. However, it also occurs in flooded river valleys such as the Ganges in India.

Iodine occurs in the soil and the sea as iodide. Iodide ions are oxidized by sunlight to elemental iodine which is volatile, so that every year some 400,000 tones of iodine escapes from the surface of the sea. The concentration of iodide in the sea water is about 50 µg per litre; in the air it is approximately 0.7 µg per cubic metre. The iodine in the atmosphere is returned to the soil by the rain which has concentrations in the range 1:8-8.5 µg/litre. In this way the cycle is completed.

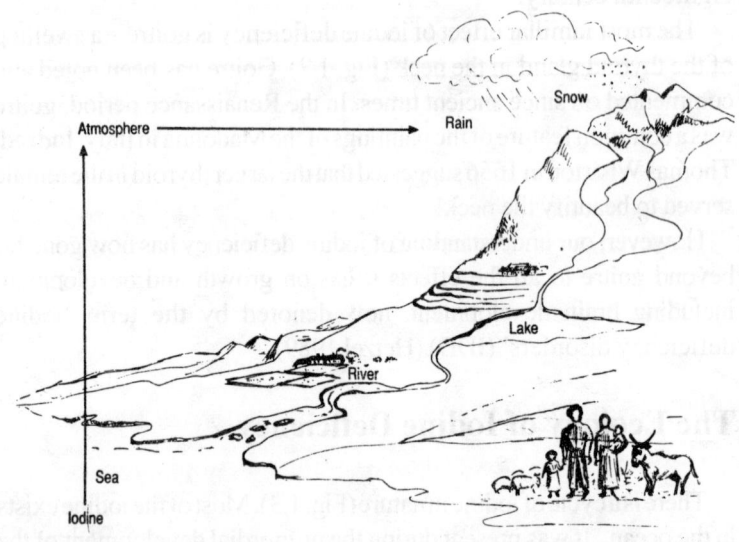

Fig. 1.3 The iodine cycle in nature. The atmosphere absorbs iodine from the sea which then returns through the rain and snow to the mountainous regions. It is then carried by rivers to the lower hills and plains, eventually returning to the sea. High rainfall, snow, and floods increase the loss of soil iodine which has often been already denuded by past glaciation. This causes the low iodine content of food for man and animals (From Hetzel 1989 with permission).

However, the return of the iodine is slow and small in amount compared to the original loss, and subsequent repeated flooding ensures that iodine deficiency in the soil continues. There is no natural correction and iodine deficiency persists in the soil indefinitely. All crops grown in these soils will be iodine deficient. As a result, human and animal populations which are totally dependent on food grown in such soil become iodine deficient. The iodine content of plants grown in iodine deficient soils may be as low as 10 µg/kg compared to 1 mg/kg dry weight in plants in an iodine replete soil. This accounts for the occurrence of severe iodine deficiency in vast populations in Asia that live within systems of subsistence agriculture in flooded river valleys as in India, Bangladesh and Myanmar.

An indication of the iodine content of the soil can be given by iodine levels in the local drinking water. These are below 2 µg per litre as in Nepal and in severe iodine deficient areas of India (0.1-1.2 µg/litre) compared to levels of 9.0 µg/litre in the city of Delhi in India which is only mildly iodine deficient.

Iodine deficiency in affected populations will continue unless there is a supplement provided, or alternatively diversification of the diet occurs, with an increase in iodine intake derived from food sources outside the iodine deficient areas. This has happened progressively in Europe during the nineteenth century. However, substantial areas of iodine deficiency remain in some European countries (Germany, Italy and Spain) as well as more localized areas in other countries (see further below).

Effects of Iodine Deficiency through the Thyroid Gland on Growth and Development

The healthy adult human body contains 15-20 mg of iodine of which about 70-80% is in the thyroid gland. The thyroid weighs only 15-25 g. Thus, the pool of iodine is concentrated mainly in the thyroid.

Iodine is rapidly absorbed through the gut. The normal intake and requirement is 100-150 µg per day. Excess iodine is readily excreted by the kidney. The level of excretion correlates well with the level of intake so that it can be used to assess the level of iodine intake.

The thyroid has to trap about 60 µg of iodine per day to maintain an adequate supply of thyroxine. This is possible because of the very active iodide trapping mechanism which maintains a gradient of 100:1 between the thyroid cell and the blood stream. In iodine deficiency, this gradient may exceed 400:1 in order to maintain the output of thyroxine. The amount of iodine in the gland is closely related to the iodine intake—the content may drop to 1 mg or less in the iodine deficient thyroid gland.

This increased trapping of iodine in iodine deficiency can be well demonstrated using radioiodine namely I^{131}. This was first shown in the field in the Andes in South America by the classical studies carried out by Stanbury and his colleagues in the Andes at Mendoza, Argentina in

1951. The relation found between the progressive fall in urinary iodine excretion as an indication of the severity of iodine deficiency in this region and the rise in uptake of I^{131} in the thyroid gland was clear.

Table 1.1 *Recommended daily intake of iodine*

Age	Intake (µg/day)
0 to 6 months	40
6 to 12 months	50
1 to 10 years	70 - 120
11 years - Adulthood	120 - 150
Pregnancy	175
Lactation	200

Source: World Health Organization. Trace Elements in Human Nutrition. Geneva, WHO, In Press, 1994.

Thyroid function is essential to normal growth and development. A deficiency of the thyroid hormone whether produced by the absence of the thyroid, a severe iodine deficiency or a congenitally defective thyroid, is associated with severe retardation of growth and maturation in almost all organ systems. Body weight does not increase and there is retardation of bone growth. These effects can be shown clearly following removal of the thyroid in the foetal and neonatal periods but are also apparent at later stages. The effects are most apparent in tissues that are rapidly growing. Measurements of weight and cellular growth by estimating the DNA content of the tissues confirms the retardation in the different organs.

The sensitivity of different organs to iodine and thyroid deficiency varies. The brain is particularly susceptible to damage during the foetal and early postnatal period. At birth, the human brain is still at a stage of early maturation as it would have reached less than a third of its mature weight. For this reason, every newborn child in many Western countries is now checked for the level of thyroid hormones soon after birth (usually by a heel prick sample of blood on the 4th or 5th day after birth), so that if there is any deficiency, the level can be made normal by giving replacement therapy with thyroxine. The results of this measure are generally satisfactory although there is evidence of some residual effects even with optimal treatment. The IQ decreases sharply when therapy is delayed after the age of 3 months.

The Development of Goitre

The preceding discussion on the production and regulation of thyroid hormones provides the framework for understanding the occurrence of goitre as a result of iodine deficiency. Although not the only cause, iodine deficiency is the primary cause of goitre. 'Goitrogens' such as thiocyanates can enhance the effect of iodine deficiency by blocking the uptake of iodine by the gland and are referred to as secondary factors.

The basic effect of iodine deficiency is to interfere with the production of thyroid hormones because iodine is an essential constituent of the thyroxine (T_4) and triiodothyronine (T_3) molecules. The lowering of output from the thyroid leads to a fall in the blood levels of T_4 but some increase in T_3 (the less iodinated hormone is produced preferentially in iodine deficiency). This compensatory mechanism may fail in the case of severe iodine deficiency.

The fall in the level of T_4 leads to an increase in the thyroid stimulating hormone (TSH) output from the pituitary and an increase in the uptake of iodide with an increased turnover associated with hyperplasia of the cells of the thyroid follicles. The reserves of colloid containing thyroglobulin are gradually used up so that the gland has a much more cellular appearance than normal. The size of the gland increases with the formation of a goitre—enlargement is regarded as significant in humans when the size of the lateral lobes is greater than the terminal phalanx of the thumb of the person examined. More precise measurements can now be made using ultrasound.

The Iodine Deficiency Disorders

The adoption of the term iodine deficiency disorders (IDD) reflects a new dimension of understanding of the full spectrum of the effects of iodine deficiency – on the foetus, the neonate, the child and adolescent, and the adult in the whole population (Table 1.2) (Hetzel 1983). All these effects can be prevented by correction of the iodine deficiency.

The studies on humans have been complemented by recent studies on animal models. This has established the effects of iodine deficiency on brain development and foetal survival and has confirmed that these effects are mediated through the secretion of the thyroid hormones by the thyroid gland. The definition of the problem of IDD as one concerned with brain development, and not just enlargement of the thyroid gland as 'goitre', and also the recognition of the large populations at risk has led to the acceptance of IDD as a major priority in international health and nutrition.

Foetal Iodine Deficiency

Iodine deficiency in the foetus is the result of iodine deficiency in the mother (Fig. 1.2). The condition is associated with a greater incidence of stillbirths, abortions and congenital abnormalities all of which can be reduced by iodine supplementation. The effects are similar to those observed in thyroid deficiency from other causes which can be reduced by thyroid hormone replacement therapy. Another major effect of foetal iodine deficiency is the condition of endemic cretinism. This condition, which occurs with an iodine intake of below 25 µg per day in contrast to a normal intake of 100-150 µg per day, is still widely prevalent, affecting up to 10 per cent of the populations living in severely iodine deficient areas in India, Indonesia and China. In its most common form, it is characterized by mental deficiency, deaf-mutism and spastic diplegia (Fig. 1.4), which is referred to as the 'nervous' or neurological type in contrast to the less common 'hypothyroid' type characterized by hypothyroidism with dwarfism (Fig. 1.5).

Table 1.2 *The spectrum of iodine deficiency disorders*

Stage in Life	Health Effects
Foetus	Abortions
	Stillbirths
	Congenital Anomalies
	Increased Perinatal Mortality
	Increased Infant Mortality
	Neurological Cretinism:
	- mental deficiency
	- deaf-mutism
	- spastic diplegia
	- squint
	Myxedematous Cretinism:
	- mental deficiency
	- dwarfism
	Psychomotor defects
Neonate	Neonatal goitre
	Neonatal hypothyroidism
Child and Adolescent	Goitre
	Juvenile hypothyroidism
	Impaired mental function
	Retarded physical development
Adult	Goitre with complications
	Hypothyroidism
	Impaired mental function

Apart from its prevalence in Asia and Oceania, cretinism also occurs in Africa and in South America in the Andean region (Ecuador, Peru, Bolivia). In all these situations, with the exception of Zaire, neurological features are predominant.

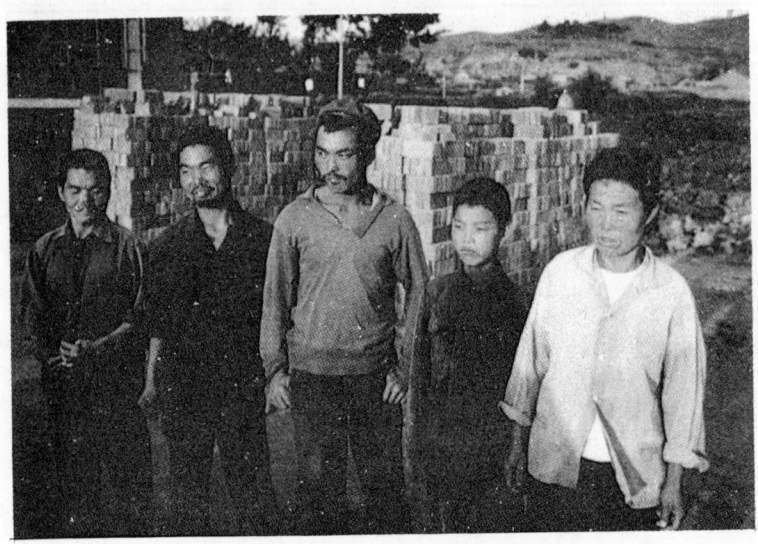

Fig. 1.4 A mother with her four sons three of them (aged 31, 29, 28) are cretins born before iodized salt was introduced and the fourth is normal(aged 14), born after iodized salt became available in Chengde, China.

In Zaire, the myxedematous form is more common with the severe growth retardation probably due to the high intake of the goitrogen derived from the consumption of cassava. (Fig. 1.6).

Although isolated instances of cretinism can still be found in the more remote areas of southern Europe, the apparent spontaneous disappearance of endemic cretinism raised considerable doubts as to whether iodine deficiency was related to the condition.

It was under these circumstances that it was decided in 1966 to set up a controlled trial in the Western Highlands of Papua New Guinea to see whether endemic cretinism could be prevented by the correction of iodine deficiency with an injection of iodized oil which was available at the time. Earlier studies showed the injection could correct iodine deficiency for up to five years.

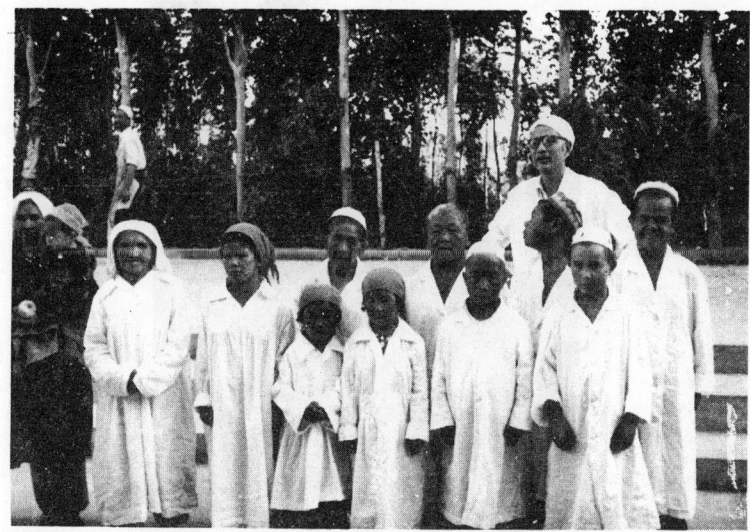

Fig. 1.5 A group of middle-aged myxedematous cretins in Hetian, Singjiang, China, showing dwarfism and mask-like faces. Other evidence of gross hypothyroidism includes mental torpor, dry skin, and skeletal retardation. The photograph also shows Dr Tai Ma who has been a great pioneer in IDD control in China (See Chapter 15) (From Hetzel 1989 with permission).

The 1966 study revealed that the injection of iodized oil given prior to pregnancy would prevent the occurrence of the neurological syndrome of endemic cretinism in the infant. The occurrence of the syndrome in those who were pregnant at the time of the injection indicated that the damage probably occurred during the first half of pregnancy. The controlled trial with iodized oil also revealed a significant reduction in recorded foetal and neonatal deaths in the treated group. This is consistent with other evidence indicating the effect of iodine deficiency on foetal survival. (Pharoah et al 1971)

Further data from Papua New Guinea indicates a relationship between the level of maternal T_4 and the outcome of pregnancies both current and in the recent past, including mortality and the occurrence of cretinism. There were proportionally more perinatal (i.e. still births and neonatal) deaths and cretins, among the offspring of women who showed the lowest levels of serum T_4.

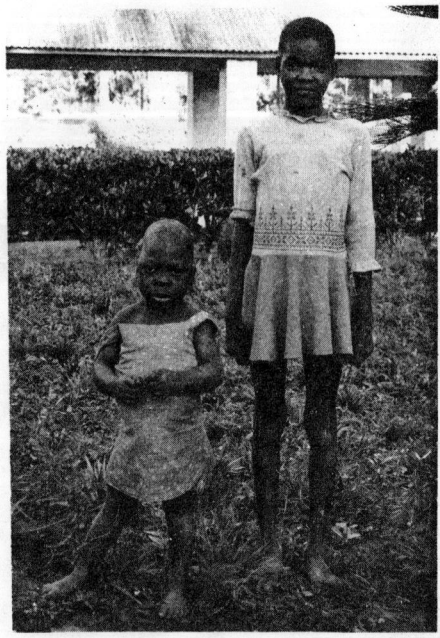

Fig. 1.6 A myxedematous cretin girl from Zaire, aged 9, showing gross dwarfism as compared to a normal girl of 9 years (From Delange 1981 with permission).

These data, indicating the importance of maternal thyroid function for foetal survival and development, are complemented by extensive data on animals. Recent findings from the study of experimental animal models and more recently on human beings, indicate that there is a transfer of maternal T_4 early in pregnancy. It would seem likely, therefore, that the early effects of iodine deficiency on the foetus are mediated by reduced transfer of maternal T_4 before the onset of foetal thyroid function. (Hetzel 1989)

Iodine Deficiency in the Neonate

An increased perinatal mortality due to iodine deficiency has been shown in Zaire from the results of a controlled trial of iodized oil injections given during the latter half of pregnancy, alternatively with a control injection. There was also a substantial fall in infant mortality with improved birth weight following the iodized oil injection. Low birth weight is generally (whatever the cause) associated with a higher rate of congenital anomalies and a higher risk through childhood. This has been demonstrated in the longer term follow-up of the controlled trial in Papua New Guinea.

Apart from the question of mortality, the importance of the state of thyroid function in the neonate relates to the fact that at birth the brain of the human infant has only reached about one-third of its full size and continues to grow rapidly until the end of the second year of life. The thyroid hormones, dependent on an adequate supply of iodine, are essential for normal brain development; as has been confirmed by the studies on animals already cited.

Recently, data on iodine nutrition and neonatal thyroid function in Europe, confirms the continuing presence of severe iodine deficiency affecting neonatal thyroid function and therefore being a threat to early brain development. A series of 1076 urine samples were collected and analysed from 16 centres in 10 different countries in Europe and one additional series from Toronto, Canada; which confirmed the iodine deficiency. Data on neonatal thyroid function was analysed for four cities where enough newborns (30,000-102,000) had been studied. The incidence of permanent sporadic hypothyroidism was very similar in the four cities but the rate of transient hypothyroidism due to iodine deficiency was much greater in Freiberg, associated with the lowest level of urine iodine excretion, than in Stockholm, with intermediate findings from Rome and Brussels. (Delange et al 1986)

In developing countries with more severe iodine deficiency, observations have now been made using blood taken from the umbilical vein just after birth. Neonatal chemical hypothyroidism was defined by a T_4 level less than 3 µg/dl and TSH>50 µu/ml. In the most severely iodine deficient environments in Northern India, where more than 50% have urinary iodine levels below 25 µg per gram creatinine, the incidence of neonatal hypothyroidism was 75 to 115 per thousand births. By contrast in Delhi, where only mild iodine deficiency is present with a low prevalence of goitre and no cretinism, the incidence drops to 6 per thousand. In control areas without goitre, the level was only one per thousand. (Kochupillai and Pandav 1987)

There is similar evidence from neonatal observations on newborns in Zaire in Africa where rates of up to 10% of neonatal hypothyroidism have been found. In Zaire, it has been observed that if the deficiency is not corrected this hypothyroidism persists into infancy and childhood with resultant retardation of physical and mental development.

These observations indicate a much greater risk of mental defects in severely iodine deficient populations than is indicated by the presence of gross cretinism. They provide strong evidence for the need of adequate correction of iodine deficiency in Europe as well as in developing countries.

Iodine Deficiency in Childhood

Studies on school children living in iodine deficient areas from a number of countries, indicate–impaired school performance and IQs, in comparison to similar groups from iodine-replete areas. Recent critical studies in Indonesia and in an iodine deficient area in Spain, using a wide range of psychological tests, have shown that the mental development of children from iodine deficient areas lags behind that of children from iodine-replete areas. The differences in psychomotor development became apparent after the age of two and a half years. In studies in China, lower intelligence quotient scores resulted due to nerve deafness, which was detected by audiometry, and the presence of abnormal neurological signs similar to the pattern observed more obviously in overt neurological cretinism. It was concluded that iodine deficiency results in a shift of the entire population distribution of cognitive skills to a lower level. These studies confirm the large dimension of the brain component in iodine deficiency disorders. (Boyages et al 1989)

The next question is whether these differences can be affected by correction of the iodine deficiency. In a pioneering study initiated in Ecuador in 1966, Fierro Benitez and his colleagues have reported the long term effects of iodized oil injections by comparing two Highland villages one (Tochachi) being treated, the other (La Esperanza) acting as a control. Particular attention was paid to 128 children aged between 8 and 15 years whose mothers had received iodized oil prior to the second trimester of pregnancy and a matched control group of 293 of similar age. All the children were periodically examined from birth at key stages in their development. The results indicate the significant role of iodine deficiency, but other factors were also considered to be important in the performance at school of these Ecuadorean children, such as social deprivation and other nutritional factors. (Fierro Benitez et al 1986).

A controlled trial carried out with oral iodized oil in a small Highland village (Tiquipaya) in Bolivia showed that the IQ of those children who showed a significant reduction of goitre improved considerably. This was particularly evident in girls. It was concluded that the correction of iodine deficiency could improve the mental performance of children of school-going age (Bautista A, et al 1982). These studies are now being followed up in a number of countries. More data are required. However these data do point to significant improvements in the intellectual performance of school children who have benefitted from the correction of iodine deficiency.

The major determinant of brain T_3 (and pituitary T_3) is serum T_4 and not serum T_3 in contrast to the liver, kidney and muscle. Low levels of brain T_3 have been demonstrated in an iodine deficient rat in association with reduced levels of serum T_4 and these have been restored to normal with the correction of iodine deficiency. These studies on animals provide a rationale for suboptimal brain function in subjects with endemic goitre and the commonly lowered serum T_4 levels and its improvement following the correction of iodine deficiency. This is the condition called cerebral hypothyroidism which refers to the condition of mental dullness or lethargy so characteristic of hypothyroidism in children and adults. Such lethargy can be reversed by correcting the iodine deficiency unlike the effects at the foetal and early stage of infant brain development which are not reversible. (For review see Hetzel 1989 and Stanbury 1994).

Iodine Deficiency in the Adult

In Northern India, a high degree of apathy has been noted in populations living in iodine deficient areas. This may even affect domestic animals such as dogs. It is apparent that reduced mental function due to brain hypothyroidism is widely prevalent in iodine deficient communities. This has an effect on their capacity for initiative and decision-making. This indicates that iodine deficiency can be a major obstacle to the human and social development of communities living in an iodine deficient environment. Therefore the correction of the iodine deficiency is indicated as a major contribution to community development.

An instructive example of the possibilities is provided by observations of the effect of an iodized salt programme dating from 1978 in the village of Jixian in Heilongjiang province in Northern China. This village was locally regarded as 'the village of the idiots'. Between 1978 and 1983, productivity, as measured by per capita income, increased by a factor of 10, school performance improved, for the first time recruits were provided for the People's Liberation Army, and girls from neighbouring villages were prepared to marry men from Jixian! (Table 1.3).

Such evidence indicates that although iodine deficiency is a major obstacle to the human and social development of communities living in an iodine deficient environment, correction of the iodine deficiency can bring communities to life in a remarkable way. This is comparable to the effects of the correction of thyroid deficiency by the use of thyroid hormones in individual patients.

Another more subtle effect of iodine deficiency is the increased susceptibility to nuclear radiation. Radioactive iodine I^{131} is one of the major constituents of nuclear radiation. Increased uptake, particularly in childhood, is associated with an increased risk of thyroid cancer. Protection from this increased risk can only be provided by the elimination of iodine deficiency.

Table 1.3 *Effects of iodine deficiency control in Jixian village, China*

	Before (1978)	After (1986)
Goitre Prevalence	80%	4.5%
Cretinism Prevalence	11%	None
School ranking (of 14 schools in the district)	14th	3rd
School failure rate	>50%	2%
Value of farm production (Yuan)	19,000	180,000
Per capita income (Yuan)	43	550

Effects of Iodine Deficiency in Animals

Epidemiological and experimental studies indicate that reproductive, neurological and other defects are important effects of iodine deficiency in animal populations.

Observations on naturally occurring iodine deficiency have been made on farm animals in which reproductive failure and thyroid insufficiency have been fully reported in older literature. In areas of iodine deficiency, development of the foetus has been retarded or arrested at some stage during gestation, resulting in early death or resorption, abortion and still birth, or the birth of weak, hairless offspring associated with prolonged gestation and parturition and the retention of placental membranes. Subnormal thyroid hormone levels in herds of cattle have been accompanied by a high incidence of aborted, still born and weak calves. (Hetzel 1989)

An important new dimension has been provided by recent experimental work with animal models. Severe iodine deficiency has been established prior to and during pregnancy and then the effects on foetal development studied. Iodine deficiency in sheep (5-8 µg/day for sheep weighing 40 kg) is associated with increased incidence of abortions and still births. At the end of the pregnancy, the foetus shows a reduced body weight, complete absence of wool growth, deformation of the skull, and retardation of bone development (Fig. 1.7). There is retardation of brain development as indicated by reduced brain weight and a reduced number of cells (as measured by DNA). Similar effects have been observed in the marmoset monkey. (Hetzel 1994)

The Costs of Iodine Deficiency

The various effects of iodine deficiency impose human, social and economic costs on individuals and communities. The human and social costs arise from the obvious disabilities of mental deficiency and deaf = mutism.

These effects have economic implications in reduced work output in the household and in the labour market, and the costs of medical and institutional care. The more subtle effects on mental status cause poor levels of school performance by children and hence produce long term effects over the whole life span (Table 1.4).

Table 1.4 *Effects of iodine interventions and measurements of economic benefits in human populations*

Effects	Benefits
Reductions in :	
1. Mental Deficiency	1. Value of higher work output in the household and labour market
2. Deaf-mutism	2. Reduced costs of medical and custodial care
3. Hypothyroidism	3. Lower educational costs from reduced absenteeism and grade repetition

Source: Levin et al (1991).

Detailed calculations have been made of the economic costs of medical assessment and the treatment of goitre. In Germany, where there is still much uncontrolled IDD, the costs of diagnosis have been estimated at US$ 250 million per year and the costs of treatment have been estimated at US$ 300 million per year. The cost of hours lost in working time for this medical care was calculated to be US$ 150 million. This makes a total of US$ 700 million (Pfannensteil 1985). These figures have recently been confirmed by data from insurance sources in Germany.

In considering hypothyroidism, the costs of decreased productivity due to reduced mental and physical energy, and the costs of follow-up after neonatal screening tests, are substantial. It is estimated that the screening programme in Canada in the province of Quebec saves the province 3 million dollars per year.

The costs of losses in animal production can be more readily calculated in terms of reduced milk and meat production, and reduced wool production. Effects will be apparent in poultry (egg production) and fish, as well as cattle and sheep (Table 1.5). These add very significantly to the benefits of IDD elimination programmes.

Table 1.5 *Effects of iodine interventions and measurements of economic benefits in livestock populations*

Effects	Benefits
Increase in :	
1. Live births	1. Value of higher output of meat and other animal products
2. Weight	
3. Strength	
4. Health (less deformity)	2. Value of higher animal work output
5. Wool coat in sheep	

Source: Levin et al (1991).

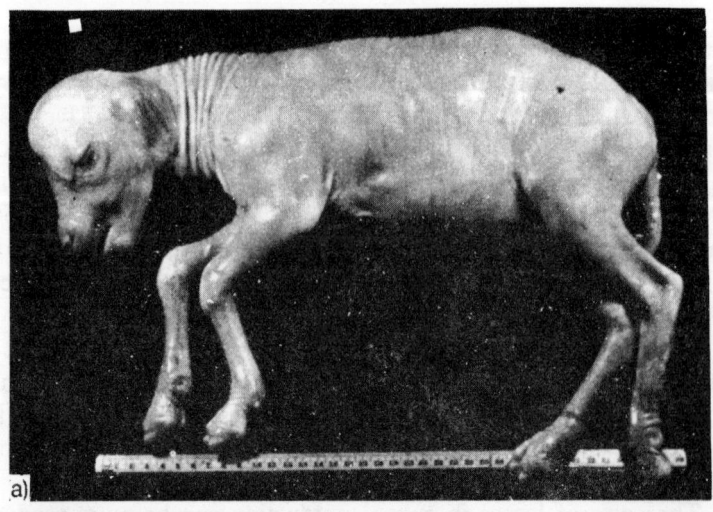
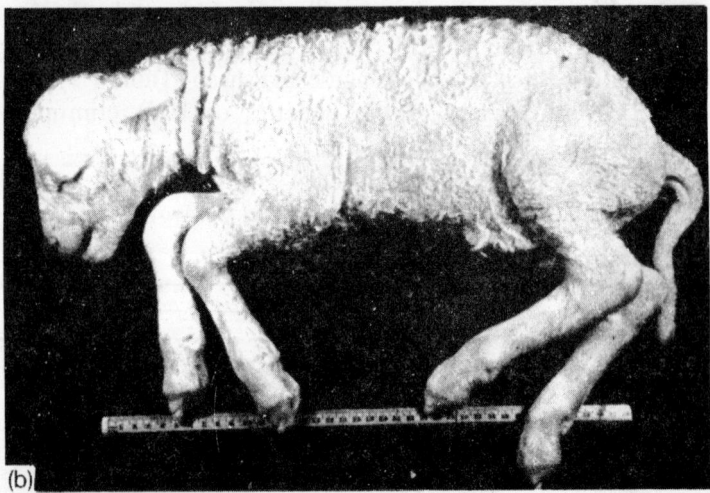

Fig. 1.7 Effect of severe iodine deficiency during pregnancy on the development of lamb. A 140-day-old lamb foetus (a) was subjected to severe iodine deficiency by feeding the mother an iodine deficient diet for 6 months prior to and during pregnancy (full term 150 days), compared to a control lamb (b) of the same age fed the same diet but with the addition of an iodine supplement. The iodine deficient lamb showed an absence of a woolly coat, dislocation of the leg joints, with a smaller brain. The figure illustrates that iodine is essential for animal development and is important to the animal industry (From Hetzel 1989 with permission).

Nature and Magnitude of the IDD

The elimination of iodine deficiency disorders is readily achievable at a very modest cost. The details are described in Chapter 7 of this book.

The major technology that has been successful in industrialized countries has been iodized salt. This technology is described in detail in Chapter 5 of this book.

However, the cost of iodizing salt only adds 5% to the retail price of salt (see Chapter 5). In most countries such a modest increment can well be met by the salt industry and handed on to the consumer.

The Magnitude of the Problem

The iodine deficiency disorders (IDD) can be seen as an 'iceberg' (Fig.1.8) of effects in a community or population. In a severely iodine deficient area, cretinism with a prevalence of 1-10% is only the visible portion of an iceberg which includes an invisible but very substantial volume of effects due to lesser degrees of brain damage and cerebral hypothyroidism.

Quantitative estimates of the extent of lesser degrees of brain damage which effect learning at school are available from various studies in Indonesia, Ecuador and China. Ratios of three times the prevalence of the fully developed clinical picture of cretinism have been estimated from observations in both Indonesia and Europe. In China the ratio is considered to be higher (five times or more) in relation to a wider range of defects relating to mental and psychomotor status. This means that in a community with a prevalence of 1-10% of cretinism there will be 5-30% suffering from lesser degrees of brain damage (Fig. 1.8). (Hetzel 1989)

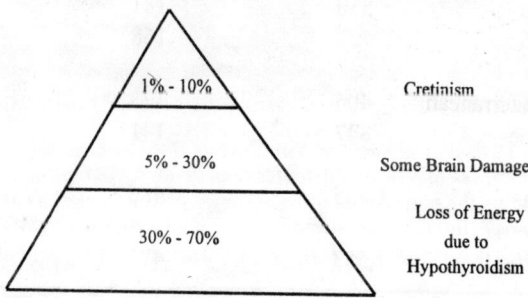

Fig. 1.8 The IDD iceberg showing the very large invisible 'hidden' component of Iodine Deficiency Disorders (IDD) associated with the small 'visible' components of cretinism.

Beyond this is the prevalence of cerebral hypothyroidism. Only rough estimates are available, suggesting that up to 70% in a severely iodine deficient area may be suffering from lethargy indicating some degree of cerebral hypothyroidism. Correction of this effect at the regional and village level by the use of iodized salt or iodized oil produces the dramatic 'coming to life' which has been noted in endemics in various parts of the world.

The 1993 estimated population at risk of iodine deficiency and population with goitre in the world by WHO & UNICEF regions is given in Table 1.6. The map of the world shown in Fig. 1.9 indicates all the iodine deficient areas as known by 1960. Since 1920, the effects of this iodine deficiency have been eliminated in many industrialized countries in North America, Northern Europe, Australia and New Zealand by the addition of iodine to the diet. The great challenge is to eliminate IDD from all countries by the year 2000 just as it has already been eliminated in most industrialized countries.

Table 1.6 *Estimate of population at risk of iodine deficiency and goitre in the world by WHO and UNICEF regions.*

WHO Regions

WHO Region	Population (millions)	Population at risk (millions)	Population with Goitre (millions)
Africa	550	181	86
Americas	727	168	63
Eastern Mediterranean	406	173	93
Europe	847	141	97
Southeast Asia	1,355	486	176
Western Pacific	1,553	423	141
Total	5,438	1,572	655

UNICEF Regions

UNICEF Region	Population (millions)	Population at risk (millions)	Population with Goitre (millions)
East & Southern Africa	261	90	51
Central & Western Africa	271	88	34
Middle East & North Africa	338	143	71
East Asia & the Pacific	1,724	557	212
South Asia	1,183	410	149
Americas & the Caribbean	444	168	63
Developed/ Industrialized	1,217	116	76
Total	5,438	1,572	655

Source: WHO, Global Prevalence of Iodine Deficiency Disorders, published jointly by WHO, UNICEF and ICCIDD, 1993.

Conclusion

In this review of the iodine deficiency disorders, their nature and magnitude, we realize what a challenge this global scourge represents. The costs in human, social and economic terms are overwhelming. We think of the personal tragedies of a family like the Chinese mother with her three cretin sons shown in Fig. 1.4, and this can be magnified by many millions when we realize that 20 million have been born with some degree of brain damage that can be so readily prevented by the correction of the iodine deficiency before pregnancy. The social and economic costs of such tragedies are incalculable.

In addition, there is, in developed countries and the more affluent minorities of developing countries, the economic cost of goitre and its investigation and treatment. This is an unnecessary burden on the public and private purse. The costs of large scale hypothyroidism, particularly cerebral hypothyroidism, cannot readily be calculated but must be enormous.

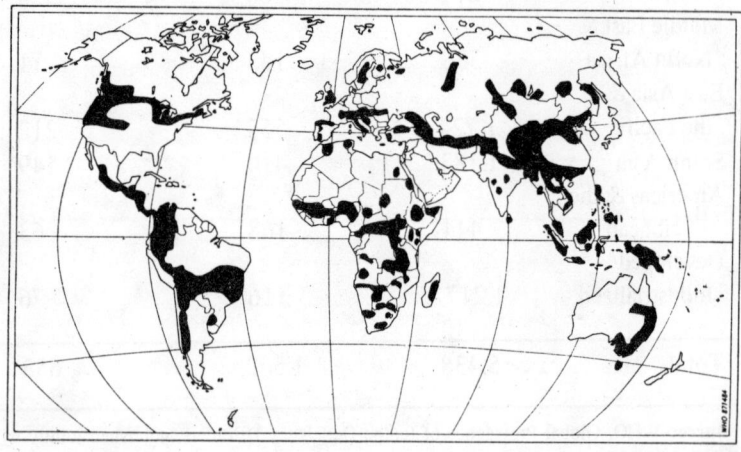

Fig. 1.9 The extensive land areas throughout the world that are iodine deficient. Successful elimination of IDD has been achieved in many industrialized countries by the addition of iodine to the diet in the form of iodized salt. The present challenge is to eliminate IDD in all countries of the world by the year 2000 (From World Health Organization with permission).

Yet we have easily available, adequate and proven methods to prevent the iodine deficiency disorders as shown by experience in a number of developed countries. Medical technology with iodized salt and iodized oil has been proved effective for mass application. So we have a great opportunity to eliminate this ancient scourge of mankind.

In the following chapters, the way in which this is gradually being achieved has been discussed.

In the second chapter we review the overall strategy that has been developed for the international public health programme.

In the third chapter we describe a partnership of organizations that has now come together to achieve the great goal of the global elimination of IDD. Most notable is the recent commitment by Kiwanis International in its first World Service Project to the elimination of IDD by the year 2000.

A detailed discussion of the various special components of a national IDD elimination programme follows - measurement (Chapter 4), iodized salt technology (Chapter 5), other alternatives to iodized salt technology in the form of iodized oil, iodized water and other modalities (Chapter 6) cost benefits (Chapter 7) from knowledge to policy to practice (chapter 8) and communication (Chapter 9). Then follows a more detailed discussion of planning and management for the countries in the 3 major regions of the world (Chapter 10).

After a review of the contribution by the major international agencies, WHO and UNICEF (Chapter 11), and by Kiwanis International (Chapter 12), we embark upon a regional review of the country programmes throughout the world (Chapter 13 to 19). Chapter 20 describes the monitoring and verification of progress towards the elimination of IDD by the year 2000 and beyond.

Chapter 21 reproduces the World Health Organization statement on safety of iodized salt and ICCIDD statement on safety of iodized oil.

The last section deals with the new alliances in the elimination of Iodine Deficiency Disorders. Chapter 22 describes IDD in the Livestock population and Chapter 23 is a report on the Future Search conference held in April, 1995 at Dhaka Bangladesh ; Partnership to End Hidden Hunger: Sustaining the Elimination of Iodine Deficiency Disorders.

This book reports great progress towards the goal. We from the ICCIDD together with WHO and UNICEF invite all men and women of good will to join in this great task which is such a special opportunity for our generation.

References

Boyages, S.C., J.K., Collins, G.F., Maberly and J.J., Jupp, 1989. 'Iodine deficiency impairs intellectual and neuromotor development in apparently normal persons'. In *Medical Journal of Australia* 150: 676-82.

Bautista, A., P.A., Barker, J.T., Dunn, M., Sanchez and D.L., Kaiser, 1982. 'The effects of oral iodized oil on intelligence, thyroid status, and somatic growth in school age children from an area of endemic goitre'. *American Journal Clinical Nutrition* 35: 127-34.

Delange, F., P., Valeix, R., Lagasse, J.P., Ermans, C., Thilly and A.M., Ermans, 1981. 'Comparison of the epidemiological and clinical aspects of endemic cretinism in Central Africa and in the Himalayas'. In Hetzel, B.S. and R.M., Smith eds. *Recent approaches to the problems of mental deficiency* pp. 243-64. Amsterdam: Elsevier.

Delange, F. et al., 1986. 'Regional variations of iodine nutrition and thyroid function during the neonatal period in Europe'. *Biology of the Neonate* 49:322-30.

Fierro-Benitez, R., R., Cazar, J.B., Stanbury, P., Rodriguez, F., Garces, F., Fierro-Renoy and E., Estrella, 1986. 'Long-term effect of correction of iodine deficiency on psychomotor and intellectual development'. In Dunn J.T., E. Pretell and C., Daza eds. *Towards the eradication of endemic goitre, cretinism, and iodine deficiency* pp. 182-200 Wasington: Pan American Health Organization.

Hetzel, B.S., 1983. 'Iodine deficiency disorders (IDD) and their eradication'. *Lancet* 2: 1126-29.

Hetzel, B.S., 1989. *The Story of Iodine Deficiency: an international challenge in nutrition.* Oxford/Delhi: Oxford University Press.

Hetzel, B.S., 1994. 'Historical Development of the Concepts of Brain Thyroid Relationship'. In Stanbury J., ed. *Iodine Deficiency and Brain Damage*. Philadelphia: Franklin Institute, (in press).

Kochupillai, N., and C.S., Pandav, 1987. 'Neonatal chemical hypothyroidism in iodine deficient environments'. In Hetzel B.S., J.T., Dunn and J.B., Stanbury eds. *The prevention and control of iodine deficiency disorders* pp. 85-93 Amsterdam: Elsevier.

Levin, H.M., E, Pollitt, R., Galloway and J., McGuire, 1991. 'Population health and Nutrition Division HSPR-19' Washington: World Bank.

Pfannenstiel, 1985. 'Direct and indirect costs caused by continuous iodine deficiency'. In Hall, R. and J., Kobberling eds. *Thyroid disorders associated with iodine deficiency and excess.* p. 447 New York: Raven.

Pharoah, P.O.D., I.H., Buttfield and B.S. Hetzel, 1971. 'Neurological damage to the foetus resulting from severe iodine deficiency during pregnancy'. *Lancet* 1:308-310.

Stanbury, J.B., 1994. In ed. *Iodine Deficiency and Brain Damage.* Philadelphia: Proceedings of a Symposium held at the Franklin Institute. 4-5 May 1993.

World Health Organization, 1990. Report to 43rd World Health Assembly. Geneva.

WHO/UNICEF/ICCIDD, November 1992. 'Indicators for assessing Iodine Deficiency Disorders and their control through salt iodization'. *Report of a Joint Consultant.* 3-5. WHO, Geneva. Document WHO/NUT/94.6.

2

Recent Progress in the Elimination of Iodine Deficiency Disorders

B.S. Hetzel

The goal of elimination of IDD as a public health problem by the year 2000 was accepted by the United Nations System in 1990 when two major decisions were taken.

The first major decision was the Resolution of the 43rd World Health Assembly (WHA) in Geneva (May 1990) calling for the elimination of IDD as a public health problem by the year 2000. The WHA is the annual meeting of 180 national government health authorities which decides the policy of the World Health Organization (WHO).

The second major decision was made by the World Summit for Children which met at the United Nations in New York (30 September 1990) and approved a Plan of Action for the future health and education of children throughout the world. This included the virtual elimination of IDD by the year 2000.

This Plan of Action was signed by 71 Heads of State who attended the World Summit. They were followed by 88 high level government representatives who also signed the Plan of Action making a total of 159 countries committed to the Plan.

This action by the World Summit for Children provides unprecedented support at the Heads of State level for progress towards the improvements in the field of child nutrition in all countries of the world. None of these goals will be easily reached, but there is considerable confidence and expectation that the elimination of IDD can be achieved by the year 2000 or possibly before this in many countries.

This confidence is there because the elimination of IDD has already been achieved by a number of developed countries and there has been rapid progress recently in many developing countries. The USA and Canada have eliminated IDD. Norway, Sweden, Finland, the United Kingdom, Australia and New Zealand have achieved this goal.

In this chapter we will consider the way an international programme for the elimination of IDD has developed. We begin with brief reviews of the successful national programmes in Switzerland and the USA where IDD has been eliminated.

By 1983 it was clear that there was an enormous gap between these countries and most countries in the developing world. To bridge this gap, a group of concerned professionals was formed in 1986. This group comprises the International Council for Control of Iodine Deficiency Disorders (ICCIDD) which is an International-Non Government Organization (NGO) - which has worked closely with WHO and UNICEF and thus led the crusade against IDD throughout the world.

This has been done through support for national programmes by the ICCIDD, WHO and UNICEF at global, regional and national levels. In this chapter we describe these developments and report the remarkable progress that has been made since 1986.

In the light of this progress and the strong political support that has now been provided, there is great confidence that the goal of elimination of IDD as a public health problem by the year 2000 might be achieved.

The story of the successful programme in Switzerland indicates the great benefits obtained from the elimination of IDD.

Elimination of IDD achieved in Switzerland

Over the centuries many travellers in Switzerland have reported on the high prevalence of goitre and cretinism (Burgi et al 1990). At the end of the eighteenth century, a survey was carried out by the order of Napoleon because of the large number of recruits who were found to be unfit for the French army. This initial survey revealed 4,000 cretins among 70,000 inhabitants in the canton of Valais. An example of a cretin subject is shown in Fig.2.1. This survey was followed by many others in the first half of the nineteenth century.

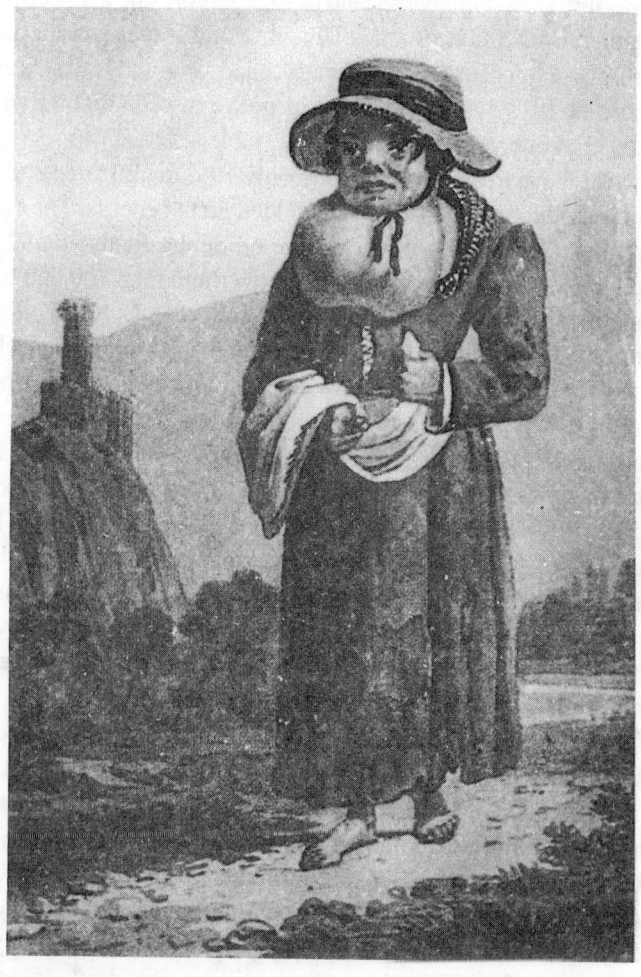

Fig. 2.1 Goitrous cretin woman from Martigny, Valais, Switzerland. Aquarelle painted by Almeraz in 1820. This young woman exhibits a very large goitre, squint, clenched fists suggesting a spastic state, with unkempt clothing indicating mental deficiency (From Merke 1984 with permission).

During the years 1886 to 1891, 8-11% of 19-year-old men were found to be unfit for military service owing to the symptoms causing large goitres–smaller goitres were not accepted as a reason for exemption.

After a series of surveys and studies carried out after 1891, iodized salt was introduced in Switzerland in 1922 largely due to the efforts of two general practitioners - Drs Hunziker and Bayard and a district surgeon Dr. Eggenberger. Dr. Hunziker had originally advocated the measure in 1915 when regression of goitre in school children was noticed after one year on sodium iodide tablets. There was regression in 75% of those treated compared to only 19% in untreated children.

The introduction of iodized salt yielded great benefits. The burden of cretinism had been a heavy charge on public funds–in 1923 the canton of Berne with a population of little more than 700,000 had to hospitalize 700 cretins incapable of looking after themselves. Following the introduction of iodized salt, deaf and dumb institutions were closed or used for other purposes. Between 1925 and 1947 the number of exemptions for military service dropped from 31 to less than 1 per thousand. No new cretins have been identified in births since 1950. Goitre has disappeared rapidly in the newborn, infants and school children. In some cantons, which allowed iodized salt only in 1952, incidences of goitre took much longer to disappear which clearly indicated that iodized salt had positive effects. Subsequent surveys revealed that isolated instances of deafness, mental deficiency and short stature, each without the other features of cretinism, also decreased. Adverse effects were minimal.

The original level of iodine introduced in 1922 was 3.7 mg iodine per kg. This was doubled twice in 1962 and 1980 to the present level of 15 mg per kg. In 1988, 92% of retail salt, and 76% of all salt for human consumption including the processed food industry was iodized, even though its use continues to be voluntary. Urine excretion of iodine (which is the best measure of dietary iodine intake), was earlier low - 18 to 64 µg/gm of creatinine per day, but is now normal (150 µg/gm of creatinine per day). It can be concluded that iodization of salt has been a highly cost effective measure and that Switzerland offers a very successful example to other countries especially in Europe.

Elimination of IDD in the USA

In the USA the introduction of iodized salt in 1924 followed the large scale pioneering experiments of Marine and Kimball (1922) carried out over the period 1916-20 on school girls in Akron, Ohio. It was based on the earlier experimental work of Marine who first said in 1915: 'Endemic goitre is the easiest known disease to prevent–it may be excluded from the list of human diseases as soon as society is determined to make the effort'.

Mass prophylaxis of goitre with iodized salt was first introduced on a community scale in Michigan in the USA in 1924. There was a fall in the average goitre rate from 38.6% to 9% by 1929 following the use of table salt containing 1 part in 50,000 of potassium iodide (20 mg/kg). By 1951 the goitre rate had dropped to only 1.4%. It was also reported that in 7 large hospitals in Michigan, thyroid surgery accounted for only 1% of all operations in 1950 as compared to 3.2% in 1939. No toxic symptoms of iodine prophylaxis were observed.

Since 1951, goitre has largely disappeared in the USA. A more recent factor has been the increase in iodine intake due to the addition of iodate to bread as an improver and the use of iodophors as a disinfectant by the dairy industry. This latter measure has also been extensively used in Northern Europe, the United Kingdom, Australia and New Zealand and has also been a contributory factor to the elimination of iodine deficiency in all these countries. But such changes have not occurred in Southern Europe and in developing countries (Hetzel 1989).

The success in the elimination of IDD in a number of industrialized countries led to efforts to control the problem in developing countries but until recently only slow progress has been made.

The Bridging of the Gap - International Action

There were a number of calls for the elimination of goitre by international organizations beginning with the World Food Council in 1974, followed by the General Assembly of the United Nations (1978) and the International Nutrition Congress (Rio de Janeiro 1978). After 1980 these were followed by the Regional WHO Committee for South-East Asia (1981, 1982), the Asia and Oceania Thyroid Congress (Tokyo 1982) and the Pan American Health Organization (1983) with similar recommendations (Hetzel 1989).

It is however disappointing to record that comparatively little happened over the decade 1974-1983 in response to these various resolutions. This clearly reflected the lack of urgency in regard to the problem in the midst of competing pressures from other more urgent health problems in developing countries, including particularly infectious diseases (smallpox, measles, tetanus, polio and the diarrhoeal diseases).

At that time it was difficult to get beyond the term 'goitre' in discussing the problem of iodine deficiency. By 1982, I realized that there was a big communication problem and that a new concept beyond that of goitre and cretinism was needed which would better reflect the increase in knowledge that had occurred over the preceding 25 years particularly in relation to brain development. After much pondering, including a stimulating visit to China and with the sympathetic encouragement of colleagues, I proposed the term 'Iodine Deficiency Disorders' (IDD) to denote all the effects of iodine deficiency on a population which could be totally prevented by the correction of deficiency (Hetzel 1983).

The announcement by the WHO of the global eradication of smallpox in 1980 also encouraged me to raise the possibility of the eradication of iodine deficiency disorders (Hetzel 1983).

The reasons why the eradication or the elimination of IDD was considered to be worthy of serious attention by governments and the major international agencies were the following:

(1) The **problem was of sufficient quantitative significance** to justify a major allocation of resources. This was justified by the well documented effect on brain development particularly during foetal life and early infancy and the evidence of serious effects on the population as described in the first chapter of this book.

(2) There were **effective preventive measures suitable for mass application** (iodized salt and iodized oil). This had been shown by the

use of iodized salt in developed countries and by many studies on the effect of iodized oil.

(3) There was an **available system for the delivery of technology** – through the salt industry, or the primary health care system, for iodized oil. This had been demonstrated in many countries. (see further Chapter 6)

(4) There were **practical methods for monitoring and surveillance** of the programme so that it could be effective. This was clearly demonstrable by checks of salt iodine and measurements of urinary iodine excretion.

These were the major components needed to justify an international nutrition programme.

These considerations led me to propose the objective of the eradication of IDD at the Fourth Asian Congress of Nutrition (Bangkok 1983) when serious attention was given to the problem as worthy of priority in international nutrition. In 1984 this led to my being invited by the Standing Committee on Nutrition (SCN) of the UN Agencies, through the Australian government, to prepare a state-of-the-art review of IDD and the possibility of successful prevention and control on a global basis. I duly submitted this report to the SCN office at FAO in Rome in February 1985.

In my report, I noted the great delay in the application of existing knowledge on IDD and its prevention, to the detriment of the many millions in developing countries who were suffering irreversible damage to brain development. To help bridge this gap, I proposed that an expert consultative group of scientists and other public health professionals be established to assist in the development of IDD control programmes at the national level (Hetzel 1985).

The decision to establish such a group, the International Council for Control of Iodine Deficiency Disorders (ICCIDD), was made in Delhi in March 1985 when I put the proposal to a group of ten consultants and advisers who were attending a WHO/UNICEF inter-country workshop on the control of IDD in South-East Asia (Lancet 1985).

The decision was made effective by the support of UNICEF which provided an initial grant of US$ 150,000 for the first two years and the

Australian government through its agency the Australian International Development Assistance Bureau (AIDAB), which made an initial grant of 42,000 Australian dollars for the support of a global secretariat in Adelaide. This AIDAB support was increased to 100,000 Australian dollars per year for 2 years (1987-89) and subsequently to 150,000 Australian dollars per year which has continued since. The UNICEF support has continued uninterrupted since 1985, while in 1991 the Canadian International Development Agency (CIDA) came forward with a grant of 500,000 Canadian dollars over the following three years, and in 1992 the Swedish Government made a grant of 200,000 Swedish kroners for two years. The World Health Organization has provided major support particularly for the series of joint meetings (WHO, UNICEF, ICCIDD) that have been held since 1985.

The International Council for Control of Iodine Deficiency Disorders (ICCIDD)

The ICCIDD consists of a multi-disciplinary global expert network of 350 scientists, public health administrators, technologists, communicators, economists and other experts, who are committed to assisting national governments and international agencies in the development of national programmes for the elimination of IDD as a public health problem. Over 200 are from developing countries. The ICCIDD logo is shown in Fig. 2.2.

From the outset, the ICCIDD has worked closely with the World Health Organization and UNICEF. At the inauguration, notable messages of support were received from both the Director General of WHO and the Executive Director of UNICEF. The ICCIDD has been recognized as the expert group by the UN system. Since 1987, it has reported annually to the Sub-committee on Nutrition (SCN) of the UN system (Administrative Co-ordinating Committee) (Lancet 1986).

In 1987 a special IDD Working Group (IWG) was established by the SCN with the following functions: (1) Monitoring the prevalence and severity of IDD in countries throughout the world; (2) Facilitating the launching of programmes for the control of IDD; (3) Help to mobilize international resources to support such programmes; (4) Monitoring the progress of national IDD control programmes.

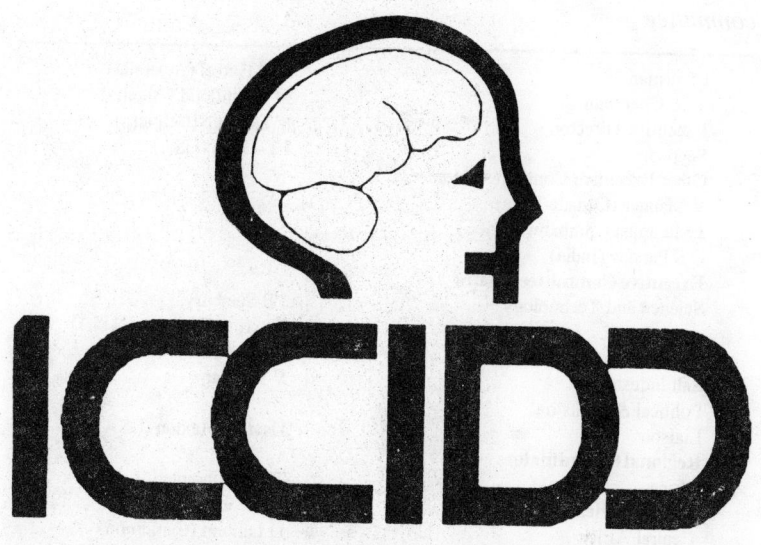

Fig. 2.2 The Logo of the International Council for Control of Iodine Deficiency Disorders. This shows the human brain within the skull which emphasizes the importance of the brain in the effects of iodine deficiency.

Since 1987 this group has met each year at the time of the SCN and full reports have been made to it by the ICCIDD.

The IWG has become a major channel of communication on IDD and national control programmes. The latest meeting (1993) in Geneva was attended by 34 representatives both from multilateral agencies including WHO, UNICEF, World Bank, World Food Programme, World Food Council, Food and Agriculture Organization and bilateral agencies (countries providing support for nutrition programmes Australia, Belgium, Canada, Sweden, Holland, Denmark, Italy, Switzerland).

The ICCIDD itself has a Governing Board of 39 members (Table 2.1) with more than half from developing countries and the international agencies. The Board meets annually, usually in conjunction with a regional meeting or a special workshop. The list of activities of ICCIDD are shown in Table 2.2.

Table 2.1 *Office bearers and board members of the ICCIDD executive committee*

Chairman	B S Hetzel (Australia)
Vice Chairman	M Benmiloud (Algeria)
Executive Director	F Delange (Belgium)
Secretary	J T Dunn (USA)
Other Executive Committee Members	
V Mannar (Canada/India)	
J Mutamba (Zimbabwe)	
C S Pandav (India)	
Executive Committee Chairs	
Science and Technology	J B Stanbury, Emeritus Chairman (USA)
Communication	J Ling (USA)
Salt Industry	V Mannar
Political & Industrial Liaison	David P Haxton (USA)
Regional Co-ordinators	
Africa	To be appointed
Western Africa	To be appointed
Central Africa	D Lantum (Cameroon)
East/South Africa	J Mutamba (Zimbabwe)
Americas	E Pretell (Peru)
South Asia & Pacific	C S Pandav (India)
China & Eastern Asia	Chen Zu pei (China)
Europe	F Delange (Belgium)
Eastern Europe & Central Asia	G Gerasimov (CIS)
Members of the Board	
M Asuquo (Nigeria)	G Maberly (PAMM/USA)
K V Bailey (WHO/Australia)	G Medeiros Neto (Brazil)
W J Blechman (USA)	R Mohan (India)
R Carriere (UNICEF)	M Ntambue-Kibambe (Zaire)
N Chawla (India)	S Ouais (Syria)
H Delisle (Canada)	A Pinchera (Italy)
R DeLong (USA)	C Pittman (USA)
R Djokomoeljanto (Indonesia)	M Rivadeneira (Ecuador)
O L Ekpechi (Nigeria)	K Siandwasi (Zambia)
M Girard (Canada)	C Thilly (Belgium)
F Kavishe (Kenya)	Van der Haar (USA)
B Kodyat (Indonesia)	H Viswanathan (India)

Table 2.2 *ICCIDD-global activities*

---

1. Advocacy of the Goal of Elimination of IDD
2. Expert Consultative Group for UN System
3. Global Multidisciplinary Network
4. Training of Professionals
5. Publications
6. Global Monitoring of Progress Towards the Goal
7. Applied Research and Development
8. Liaison with UN and Bilateral Agencies
9. General Co-ordination and Administration

The first meeting took place in Kathmandu, Nepal, in March 1986, when a review of all aspects of public health programmes was carried out. This led to the subsequent publication of a book (The Prevention and Control of Iodine Deficiency Disorders, BS Hetzel, JT Dunn and JB Stanbury (Eds.), Elsevier, Amsterdam 1987).

An Executive Committee was elected which included a Chairman, Vice Chairman, Executive Director and Secretary (Fig.2.3).

The Executive Director's position is full-time, the others being part time. The ICCIDD has Regional Co-ordinators for Africa, Americas, Asia (Southern & Pacific), China & Eastern Asia, Europe, Eastern Europe and Central Asia. In Africa three sub-regional Coordinators are responsible for countries in the West, for Central and South-Eastern areas. Each Regional or sub-Regional Co-ordinator is a member of the Board who makes an annual report on IDD activities in the region and also takes appropriate initiatives including consultancies to individual countries.

The ICCIDD has more than 350 members drawn from 70 countries with many different disciplines. Membership is free and open to qualified professionals interested in the elimination of IDD. Additionally, over 3,000 persons receive the quarterly IDD Newsletter.

At the global level the ICCIDD has been successful in greatly increasing the awareness of IDD as an international health problem of major importance. It is now recognized that iodine deficiency is the single most important cause of mental abnormality in the world today.

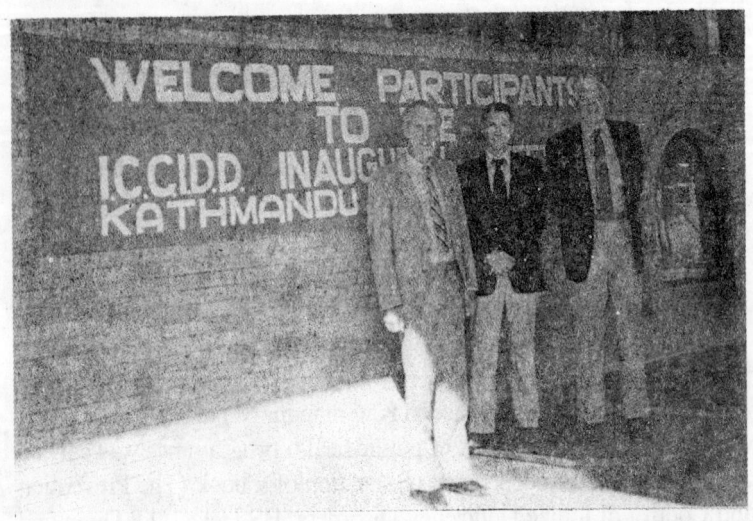

Fig.2.3 This shows the three office bearers of the ICCIDD at the Inaugural Meeting in Kathmandu, Nepal 23-27 March 1986. They are (from the right), Dr John Stanbury, Chairman; Dr John Dunn, Secretary; and Dr Basil Hetzel, Executive Director.

This was the major reason for the recognition of the problem by the World Health Assembly in 1986, and again in 1990, and by the World Summit for Children (1990), already mentioned at the beginning of this chapter.

The ICCIDD has held a series of Regional Meetings with WHO and UNICEF designed to foster the development of National Control Programmes. These are listed in Table 2.3.

Apart from this important role, the ICCIDD has collaborated closely with WHO and UNICEF in short-term training programmes for country programme managers in technical procedures such as ultrasonography, the measurement of thyroid size, laboratory methods for the measurement of urinary iodine excretion and blood TSH. Multi-disciplinary training for a longer term (up to 6 months) is carried out by the Programme Against Micronutrient Malnutrition (PAMM) jointly organized by the Centre for Disease Control (CDC) and the School of Public Health, Emory University in Atlanta, USA.

Table 2.3 *Major ICCIDD/UNICEF/WH0 meetings from 1985*

1985	Birth of ICCIDD	Delhi, India
1986	Inauguration	Kathmandu, Nepal
1987	Africa	Yaounde, Cameroon
1988	Scientific Meeting on Iodine and the Brain	Washington, USA
1989	Asia	Delhi, India
	China	Tianjin, China
1990	Africa	Dar-es-Salaam Tanzania
1991	10 ITC	* The Hague, The Netherlands
	Former USSR	Tashkent, Uzbekhistan
1992	Europe	Brussels, Belgium
1993	Middle East	Alexandria, Egypt
1994	Latin America	Quito, Ecuador
1995	Asia	Dhaka, Bangladesh

* Transferred from Islamabad, Pakistan, due to the Gulf War and associated with the 10th International Thyroid Congress (ITC)

The ICCIDD has also participated fully in various expert meetings concerned with different aspects of control programmes such as the precise criteria for elimination and the relation of IDD control to the global immunization programme.

Operational research has been another important activity including the determination of the optimal dosage level (duration and effectiveness) for the iodized oil when given by mouth and a simplified method for the determination of urinary iodine. These and other such studies have provided important guides for future public health practice.

Finally, publications have been very important to the creation of an informed group of professionals throughout the world. These include the IDD Newsletter published quarterly since 1985 (edited by J T Dunn), the book published from the inaugural meeting in Kathmandu (1987), The Story of Iodine Deficiency by BS Hetzel (1989) and The Practical Guide to Iodine Deficiency Disorders Control Programmes Eds. J T Dunn and F Van der Haar (1990).

The latter two books have been translated into French and Spanish. Translations of the Story of Iodine Deficiency are now completed in Arabic, Chinese, Japanese and Russian. Hindi translation of the book is under publication.

Further practical manuals on salt iodization and the measurement of urinary iodine levels have also been published.

All these activities at the global level are ultimately designed to be of help at the country level along with effective national programmes.

We will now focus our attention on the issue of an effective national IDD control programme. This is the special challenge that has to be met to achieve the goal of elimination.

National IDD Control Programmes

Since 1983 there has been a much better understanding of national IDD control programmes and this has led to a new momentum and effectiveness in their implementation.

The national programme is now seen as a social process with a number of components. Notable among these components is political will which has been obviously lacking in the past. Another feature is the need for communication and education of the community about the problem of IDD. This is all the more important because as soon as possible, developing countries should take on the total responsibility for funding as well as the administration of these programmes.

These various components can be shown in the form of a wheel (Fig. 2.4). The wheel must be kept turning to be effective. A number of steps are required to achieve success:

(1) **Assessment** of the IDD problem with estimates of the population at risk, the prevalence of goitre and cretinism, evidence of iodine deficiency from the measurement of urinary iodine excretion and measurements of the thyroid related hormone (TSH). These

measurements require suitable laboratories. Effects on livestock can also be noted. In addition, the nature and operation of the salt industry must be assessed to enable plans for salt iodization to proceed.

(2) **Communication** of the problem to the public and the politicians in terms they can understand – the effects on the growth and development of children, including the prevalence of the handicapped (cretins), reduced school performance, and reduced productivity and quality of life in adults. The effects on livestock can also be highlighted.

(3) **The development of a plan** including the salt industry, the educational system, and the media as well as public health professionals. Consumers should be represented. This requires an intersectoral commission with a chairman wielding sufficient political authority to implement the plan once it has been approved by the government.

(4) **Political decision** which includes an allocation of the necessary funds from the government sources within the country supplemented by external funds from bilateral and/or multi-lateral sources. As already mentioned, recent estimates indicate that the cost of iodized salt is upto 7 US cents per person per year (less than the cost of a cup of tea in many countries) and for iodized oil, 20 US cents per person per year. These costs are indeed modest compared to the benefits and they can be readily absorbed by the salt industry.

(5) **Implementation** including organization of the supply of iodized salt, iodized oil (if necessary), appropriate training and education programmes. An emergency phase using iodized oil may be required for a region with cretinism and severe iodine deficiency for the immediate prevention of cretinism and lesser degrees of brain damage.

(6) **Monitoring and evaluation** of the programme. This requires process indicators such as the delivery of iodized salt, checking its iodine content in the factory, on arrival at the destination and in the home. It includes determining iodine in the population by the measurement of iodine in the urine and the assessment of thyroid hormone output by the measurement of thyroid related hormones (TSH).

Outcome measurements include evidence of the reduction of goitre prevalence by palpation or by using ultrasonography for more accurate

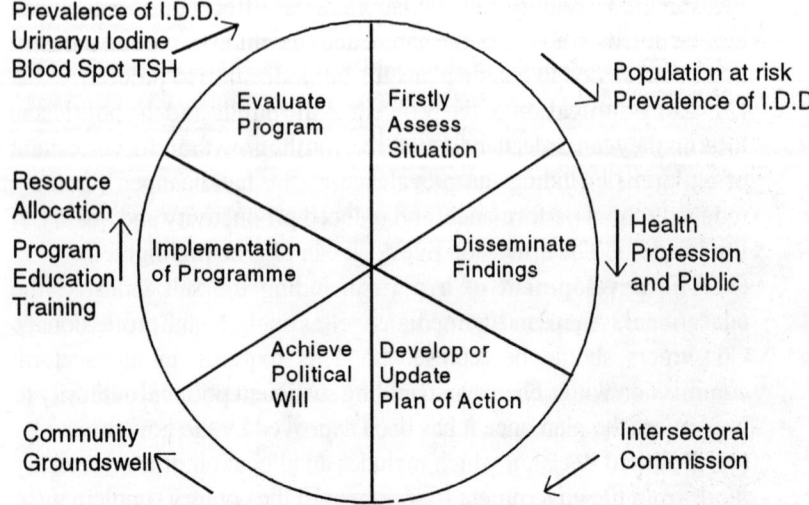

Fig. 2.4 The 'wheel' represents the continuous 'feed back' process involved in the national IDD control (elimination) programme. All 'actors' in the programme need to understand the whole social process.

assessment; the reduction of cretinism, including deafness and improved school performance. All these methods are being used to evaluate the programmes in a number of countries.

The final responsibility rests on national governments and the role of the international agencies is to work with national governments to assist them with appropriate advice, funding and training. But from the beginning the concerned country will have to incur expenditure from its own, often very scarce, resources.

This means that IDD control must compete with other health problems for priority. The recognition of the significance of IDD in social and economic terms is critical to IDD control receiving such priority attention. The economic benefits to both human and livestock populations were summarized in Chapter 1 and discussed in detail in Chapter 7. The costs of interventions with iodized salt (5 US cents/head/year, India 1989) and iodized oil (20 US cents/head/year, Indonesia 1986) must be regarded as modest in relation to the incalculable benefits with regard to the prevention of mental deficiency on such a large scale in severely iodine deficient populations.

These considerations are very important in rallying political support for IDD control. The remarkable cost benefit from the prevention of IDD has recently been noted in the 1992 World Bank Report on Health and Development.

Various aspects of National Programmes are fully described in Part II of the book.

Regional Support

An important factor in the new momentum of national IDD control programmes has been the support provided by Regional IDD working groups.

These groups were initiated by the ICCIDD. They began with the creation of the IDD Task Force for Africa at a Regional ICCIDD/ WHO/UNICEF meeting held in Yaounde in the Cameroon in March 1987, followed by Regional groups in SE Asia (1989), in the Middle East (1989), and national working groups in Indonesia and China (1989). More recently a group has been established in Latin America (1991) with particular reference to the Andean group of countries (Colombia, Venezuela, Ecuador, Peru, Bolivia).

These groups bring together regional representatives from WHO and UNICEF, together with the ICCIDD Regional Co-ordinator. They also include representatives from interested bilateral agencies* and non-government organizations. However, most important of all, they include representatives from the countries who share their experiences (Fig. 2.5).

These groups take responsibility for the promotion of national programmes, co-ordination, technical advice, monitoring progress, and providing assistance in raising funds for national programmes.

---

* Bilateral agencies refer to developed countries which provide aid directly to developing countries independent of international agencies such as WHO and UNICEF.

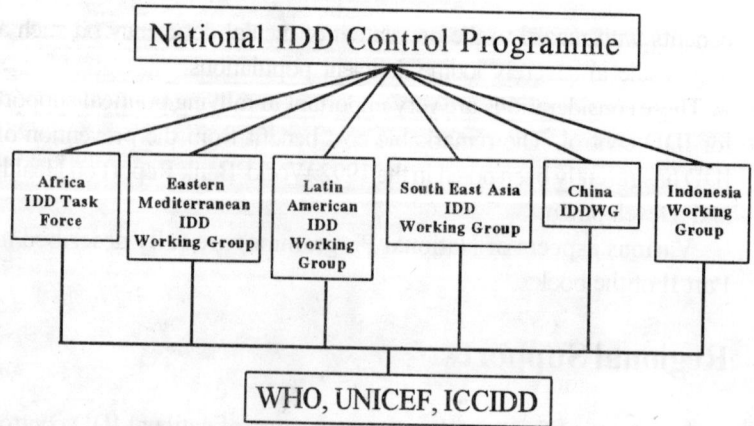

Regional Working Groups
Generally: include Countries, WHO, UNICEF, ICCIDD
Occasionally: Bilaterals, NGOs

Fig. 2.5 Network of regional IDD working groups (RIWG) providing support for national elimination programmes.

Experience over the past six years had indicated the great benefits provided by these regional working groups. This is particularly true of Africa (Chapter 10). Detailed descriptions are available in the later chapters of this book devoted to particular countries.

IDD and the United Nations System

The sequence of events leading to recognition of IDD as a major priority within the health targets of the UN System is listed in Table 2.4. This recognition has been the major achievement of the ICCIDD since it was founded in 1986 to bridge the gap between available knowledge regarding the elimination of IDD and its application in national IDD elimination programmes.

As we have noted the first step was the proposal of the concept of iodine deficiency disorders to denote all the effects of iodine deficiency on growth and development at the population level that could be eliminated by the prevention of iodine deficiency (Hetzel 1983).

Table 2.4 *ICCIDD and the United Nations system*

1983	IDD : Iodine Deficiency Disorders Concept
1986	ICCIDD : International Council for Control of IDD, Formal Inauguration, Kathmandu
1990	ICCIDD Global Action Plan for The Elimination of IDD By The Year 2000, United National Nutrition Subcommittee, Paris
1990	World Summit for Children United Nations, New York 71 Heads of State, Total of 159 Governments Plan of Action Adopted Included Elimination of IDD
1991	Ending Hidden Hunger Policy Conference on Micronutrient Malnutrition, Montreal 55 Countries
1992	45th World Health Assembly, Geneva National Strategies for Overcoming Micronutrient Malnutrition

The recognition of the great gap between available knowledge for the elimination of IDD and its application in developing countries led to the creation of the ICCIDD in 1985 with the formal inauguration in Kathmandu, Nepal in 1986.

From its inception the ICCIDD had worked closely with the WHO and UNICEF as described in the last section. An inter-agency Global Action Plan for the elimination of IDD as a public health problem by the year 2000 was put forward by the ICCIDD and endorsed by the UN Subcommittee on Nutrition (made up of all the UN agencies and the bilaterals) in February 1990. In May 1990 the 43rd World Health Assembly passed a Resolution accepting the goal of elimination of IDD as a public health problem by the year 2000. The Resolution included commendation of the work done by the ICCIDD.

The Executive Board of UNICEF also accepted the goal of 'virtual elimination of IDD by the year 2000'.

As already noted the World Summit for Children meeting at the United Nations, New York, included the elimination of IDD in the Plan of Action for the future health and education of children throughout the world. This Plan was signed by 71 Heads of State and 88 nominated representatives of other governments. This represents an unprecedented commitment by governments to the future health and well being of all children the world over.

Following the World Summit, a Policy Conference on Micronutrient Malnutrition 'Ending Hidden Hunger' was held in Montreal (10-12 October 1991) with full participation by the Board of the ICCIDD.

The meeting was hosted by the Canadian Government and was attended by representatives from 60 countries nominated by Heads of State on the invitation of the Director-General of WHO and the Executive Director of UNICEF. There was a total attendance in excess of 300. Six members of the Board of the ICCIDD presented papers.

The meeting provided greatly increased visibility for IDD and the ICCIDD. The ICCIDD was seen as having provided an effective model through its global multi-disciplinary network of scientists, health professionals and technologists, its global and regional structure and its record of facilitating national IDD national programmes.

There is already evidence that the Conference has made a major impact on a number of countries.

In May 1992, the 45th World Health Assembly adopted a Resolution on 'National Strategies for Overcoming Micronutrient Malnutrition' which commended the models developed by the ICCIDD at country and regional levels as being highly advanced and therefore particularly suitable for developing stronger support for programmes for overcoming Vitamin A deficiency and anaemia.

The goal of elimination was also included in the Plan of Action adopted by the International Conference on Nutrition (Rome 1992).

Progress Towards Elimination

Let us now take stock of the progress achieved since the creation of the ICCIDD in 1986. Much of this progress has been attributed to the ICCIDD working closely with WHO and UNICEF in all parts of the world.

Fig. 2.6 shows the Map drawn up in 1991 following the 1990 Resolution at the World Health Assembly calling for elimination of IDD by the year 2000.

It indicates four categories of IDD control at country level: countries which have already achieved elimination, countries where IDD is probably improving with control programmes (South America, Southern Africa, Asia), countries without national control programmes - (Africa and Europe) where IDD persists, and countries where data is not available as in the case of the former USSR.

The map indicates steady progress but there is still a long way to go before elimination can be achieved.

Since the World Summit for Children at the United Nations in 1990, UNICEF, WHO and ICCIDD have agreed on a series of targets to be met over the next 10 years in order to achieve the objective of the elimination of IDD as a public health problem by the year 2000.

For 1995, it has been agreed that the realization of the objective requires that all countries should have National Intersectoral Commissions operating national programmes with universal access to iodized salt, based on the measurement of the iodine content of salt. Measurement of the iodine content in salt requires only a simple chemical procedure (with a mobile kit) which is being made readily available through schools and other organizations for household use. More extensive observations are being made at retail and factory level.

Criteria for tracking progress towards the World Health Assembly/World Summit goal have now been agreed upon following extensive consultation between ICCIDD, UNICEF and WHO.

In Table 2.5 the country status of IDD and salt iodization programmes is shown as reported (WHO, 1994).

Table 2.5 *Progress with universal salt iodization**

Countries with IDD	118
Countries with no IDD	51
Countries with no data	14
Total	183
Countries with salt iodization programme	82

* WHO Report to SCN meeting, New York (1994).

This will be determined initially by measurements showing adequate salt iodine, and normal urinary iodine excretion as a measure of the actual consumption of iodine. This will be followed in due course by a demonstration of normal thyroid size (preferably by ultrasonography to provide an objective indicator) and normal levels of thyroid related hormones (TSH) (See further Glossary and Chapter 4).

What then is the present state of progress towards the elimination of IDD in the world today?

Europe. Elimination has been achieved in many, but not in all countries. Germany, Italy, Spain, Poland, Romania, and the CIS (former USSR), and others still have to make their control programme fully effective for the whole of their iodine deficient population.

Latin America. The objective of the establishment of National IDD control commissions, with IDD control units, has been achieved in nearly all countries. Significant challenges remain in Peru and Central America. Great progress has recently been made by Ecuador and Bolivia.

SE Asia. National programmes are now operating in most countries. India, Indonesia, Nepal, Myanmar, Thailand and Bangladesh have made good progress but still have some distance to go to cover their whole population.

Africa. There is still a long way to go with significant problems in no less than 45 countries including 6 in Northern Africa. The spectacular progress made since the establishment of the IDD Task Force for Africa encourages confidence that the 1995 objective may be achieved. With

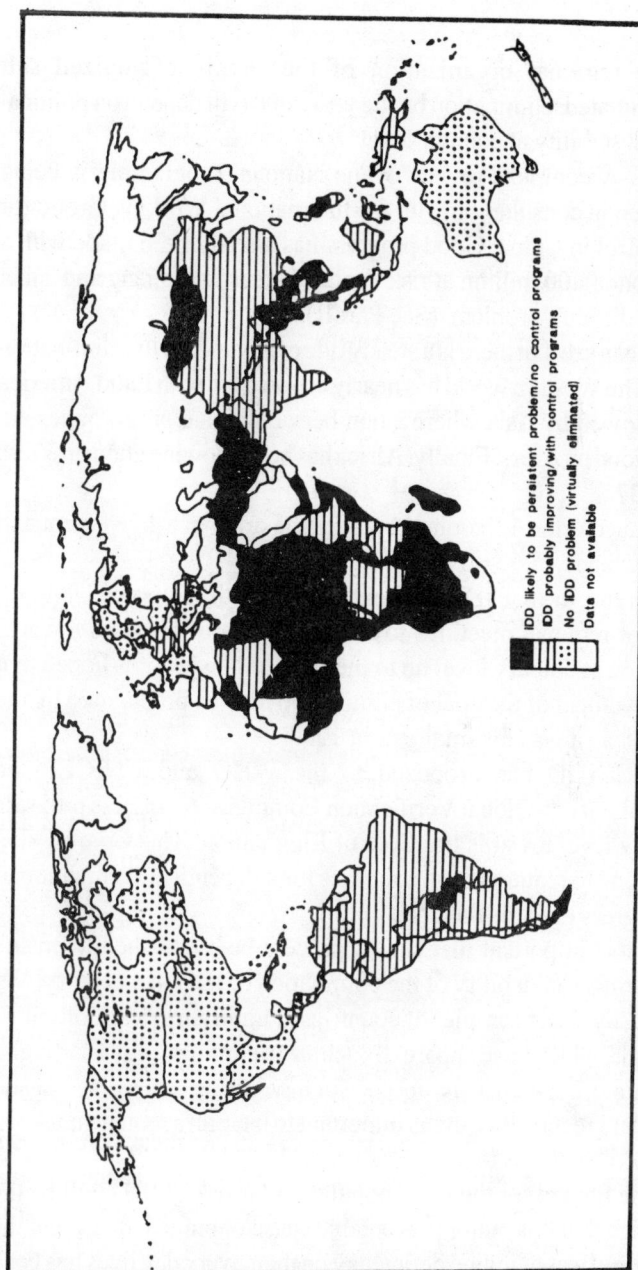

Fig. 2.6 The map shows the active progress of national IDD elimination programmes throughout the world. Countries are grouped into 4 categories. (see text) (From WHO (1990) with permission).

effective regional organization of the supply of iodized salt already initiated, elimination by the year 2000 will depend on political and social stability at country level.

China. A complete review of the National Programme is being undertaken in consultation with the International Working Group for IDD Control in China. Good progress has already been made with a population of 400 million at risk. Isolated areas in Sinjiang and Tibet remain a difficult problem. (See Part II).

So we can see that there is a steady tide of advance in the elimination of IDD. The Western world has nearly achieved it, with Latin America next, followed by Asia where a number of national programmes are making good progress. Finally, Africa has been showing good progress since 1987.

Continued effort is required both for the original achievement and its maintenance.

To this end, the ICCIDD has now planned with WHO and UNICEF a series of regional meetings to review reports of progress towards elimination at country level up to the year 2000 when it is hoped that the achievement of the goal of elimination may be proclaimed by the WHO just as it was for smallpox in 1980!

The ICCIDD has proposed to the WHO and UNICEF the establishment of a Global Verification Commission to assess progress at country level towards the Goal of Elimination. This Commission will respond to requests from countries for independent verification of their progress towards the goal.

It is most important that such a process be established to ensure longer term sustainability of the elimination of IDD in a country. We have already seen examples of countries in Latin America, Colombia, Guatemala, which have apparently achieved elimination at a particular point in time, but then in the absence of monitoring, control is lost and the problem recurs. It is just as important to have an adequate intake of dietary iodine as it is to have clean water!

But the reward for the large populations at risk of IDD will be the knowledge that this major preventable cause of brain damage and the deadening effect of iodine deficiency on their every day lives has been removed. It will be a great triumph in the field of public health, comparable to the eradication of smallpox and the progressive elimination of infectious diseases through the Expanded Programme of Immunization.

References

Burgi, H., A., Supersaxo and B., Selz, 1990. 'Iodine deficiency diseases in Switzerland one hundred years after Theodor Kocher's survey: A historical review with some new goitre prevalence data'. *Acta Endocrinologica.* 123: 577-90.

Dunn, J.T. and C., Van der Haar, 1990. *A Practical Guide to the Correction of Iodine Deficiency. ICCIDD Technical Manual.* Netherlands.

Hetzel, B.S. 1983. 'Iodine Deficiency Disorders (IDD) and their eradication'. *Lancet* 2: 1126-29.

Hetzel, B.S. 1985. 'The Iodine Manifesto'. *IDD Newsletter* 1:1-2.

Hetzel, B.S. 1989. *The Story of Iodine Deficiency: An international challenge in nutrition.* Oxford/Delhi: Oxford University Press.

Hetzel, B.S., J.T., Dunn and J.B., Stanbury, Eds. 1987. *The Prevention and Control of Iodine Deficiency Disorders.* Amsterdam: Elsevier.

Lancet 1985. World Health 2: 846.

Lancet (1986). 'Inaugural meeting of International Council for Control of Iodine Deficiency Disorders' 1: 1164.

Marine, D. and O.P., Kimball, 1922. 'The prevention of simple goitre in man'. *American Journal of Medical Science* 163-634.

Merke, F. 1984. *The history and iconography of endemic goitre and cretinism.* Lancaster MTP Press. (originally published by Hans Huber, Berne, in 1971).

World Health Organization 1990. *Report to 43rd World Health Assembly.* Geneva.

World Health Organization 1992. *Report to 45th World Health Assembly.* Geneva.

World Summit for Children 1990. New York United Nations.

3

The Conquest of Iodine Deficiency through a Global Partnership of People, Governments, International Agencies, The Salt Industry, Kiwanis International and Micronutrient Initiative

B.S. Hetzel

There has been a remarkable increase in the momentum of IDD control programmes over the past ten years. In spite of the immense magnitude of the threat to human potential posed by iodine deficiency, great progress has been made through a global partnership which has now come into being between people, governments, agencies and the expert multi-disciplinary network of the ICCIDD. Most recently, the salt industry has joined the partnership through a link established with the ICCIDD, while in 1993, Kiwanis International along with UNICEF adopted the virtual elimination of IDD as their World Service Project for the next five years.

In this chapter we describe this global partnership in detail with reference to the opportunity for greater co-ordination and more effective action that will facilitate the achievement of the great goal of elimination.

The partnership includes the following:
(1) People in countries where IDD is a public health problem.
(2) Governments of countries where IDD is a public health problem.

(3) The international agencies particularly WHO and UNICEF, which are specifically committed to assisting countries achieve the goal of elimination of IDD by the year 2000. In addition to WHO, UNICEF, other United Nations Agencies–the World Bank, UNDP, WFP and FAO are now playing a significant role.

(4) The International Council for Control of Iodine Deficiency Disorders (ICCIDD) which has come to occupy a central expert role in the establishment of effective national programmes and in the monitoring of progress towards the goal of elimination of IDD at the country level in association with WHO and UNICEF.

(5) The bilateral agencies of developed countries which have included national programmes for IDD control in their development programmes. These include Australia, Belgium, Canada, Germany, Sweden, Holland, Italy and the USA.

(6) Kiwanis International – an international world service club which has adopted the elimination of IDD as its international project for the next five years in collaboration with UNICEF and the ICCIDD.

(7) The salt industry which has now formed a working relationship with the ICCIDD.

(8) Micronutreint Initiative – its mission is to facilitate the achievement of virtual eliminiation of IDD by supporting effective and sustainable programme actions.

People in Countries where IDD is a Public Health Problem

The leaders in this partnership are clearly the people themselves who have the problem. (Fig. 3.1) It is a tragic fact that the people of many countries in the developing world are not fully aware of the problem that they have. The deadening effects of brain hypothyroidism combined with the geographic isolation of so many iodine deficient communities means that the problem is just not known to the people most affected. However, it is also true of Europe where the serious risk of widespread iodine deficiency on brain development in foetal life and early infancy is not generally understood.

This indicates that arousing community awareness is the major step required in country programmes. This applies to the local community and to the wider regional and international community. Different methods are required at each level.

The tragic situation shown in the photograph (Chapter 1) of the Chinese mother with four sons, three of them cretins, is reproduced over and over again throughout the large populations at risk all over the world.

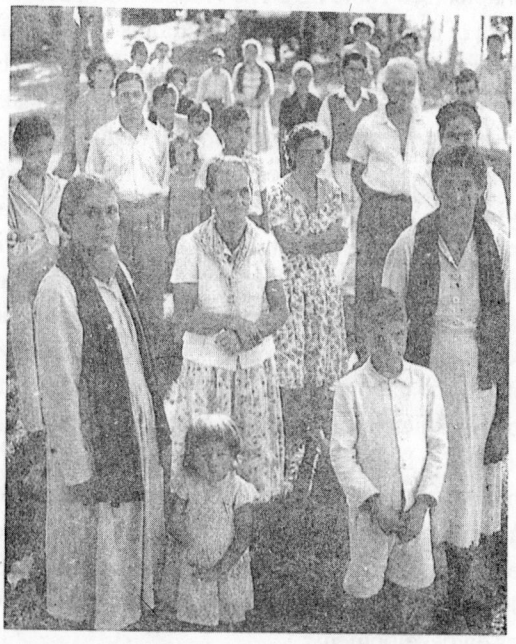

Fig. 3.1 As seen in this Bolivian community, IDD can affect people of all age groups.

The message that such situations can be totally prevented needs to be broadcast using every media resource. Now that transistor radios are so widely distributed there are new opportunities for effective media campaigns. Such campaigns are of course already operating in developing countries for the sale of aerated soft drinks, cigarettes, beer and other widely used products of Western civilization and are very effective.

There should be no hesitation in spelling out the personal and social dimension of the tragedies consequent on mental deficiency as the major effect of iodine deficiency on human development.

The impact of iodine deficiency on a village community and the benefits of its correction are vividly illustrated in the story of Jixian village in north-east China (Heilongjiang province), already referred to in the first chapter (see Table 1.3). The village known as the 'village of idiots' because of the high prevalence of cretinism was regarded with contempt by surrounding villages. The school children were backward, productivity was very low, and the young women from surrounding villages refused to marry young men from Jixian.

All this changed within a few years after the introduction of iodized salt in 1978. Cretins were no longer born, productivity increased, there was a drive for improving the run-down facilities of the village, the school performance of children improved and young women from surrounding villages began to marry young men from Jixian. These changes occurred at a time of new initiatives for economic development at the provincial and national level. But without the elimination of the effects of iodine deficiency, the people of Jixian would not have been able to benefit fully from these initiatives.

Such experience at the local community level has been noted in other countries such as India, Indonesia and Bangladesh. Indeed the correction of iodine deficiency may make village communities more restless and less compliant! This provides a great opportunity for education programmes on development.

There are significant community groups which could provide leadership in arousing awareness about IDD. The problem is above all one affecting women and children. The IDD problem should be taken up by the well organized women's movements in many countries. Women have previously provided outstanding leadership in connection with other health problems.

Another resource would be groups of disabled persons. An example is the Chinese Disabled Persons Federation of which the Chairman is

Mr Deng Pu-fang, son of Mr Deng Xiaoping, the famous Chinese leader. The International League against Mental Handicap is composed of national groups in both developed and developing countries. These groups often include people in leadership positions.

A well informed community can apply significant political pressure for effective IDD control programmes at the regional and national level. This has already been noted in considering the model of a national programme. The perception of IDD at the community level as affecting productivity, the quality of life, and the performance of children at school can be very persuasive with politicians especially when accompanied by data on the economic costs of not having an IDD control programme.

An educated community will also create a demand for iodized salt and the salt industry will respond to this demand as has occurred in developed countries.

As we have seen in earlier chapters, the achievement of iodine deficiency elimination is often not sustained due to political instability affecting the public health sector. There may be ineffective and inefficient monitoring and many other problems may occur. The only insurance in the long term is the awareness of the community at risk of the proven means by which this risk can be removed. This question of sustainability is considered again later in this chapter when the creation of a Global Verification Commission is discussed.

An adequate dietary intake of iodine is just as important for the maintenance of health and well being as many other public health measures such as clean water, clean food and public hygiene.

In concluding this discussion, let us remind ourselves of the new importance of 'People's Power' in causing social and political change in our world today. The collapse of the communist regimes in eastern Europe and the former USSR, the collapse of the Marcos dictatorship in the Philippines and the very recent developments in Italy all indicate the 'power of the people'. The influence of the international media has undoubtedly been very important in all these developments. At best, they indicate a new awareness of human values as the highest priority.

We can confidently expect new momentum in the drive for improved public health including the elimination of IDD as a result of this new climate of 'people power'.

Governments of Countries with Significant IDD Affecting the People

The responsibility for a decision regarding the introduction and maintenance of an effective national IDD elimination programme rests ultimately with the elected government of the country. Governments are sovereign and it is to governments that the case has to be made. Governments, in their decision-making are influenced by community perceptions as well as the advice of professionals, together with economic considerations.

One reason for the neglect of the IDD problem has been the fact that it is often found in the more remote parts of a country where people have little political influence. Another reason has been the lack of perception of the importance of the IDD problem in human, social and economic terms. This limited perception has now been revised as evidence mounts of the personal, social and economic cost of IDD to the people of the country affected. This cost has been spelt out in detail in the earlier chapters of this book–it is very high for developed countries as well as developing countries as the data already cited from Germany indicates. By contrast, the cost of IDD control programmes is indeed modest. The cost of not having a programme is very great compared to the cost of the programme. Governments need to be aware of these major advantages of the prevention of IDD.

The decision of a government to have a national IDD control programme involves the setting up of a multisectoral IDD control commission. This involves health, education, industry, planning, finance, commerce and media sectors. The key figure is the chairman of the Commission who should be at the ministerial level if possible, with the political authority and support of the Cabinet. Similar considerations apply to other health problems as the WHO has been pointing out for some years. Health problems require a multisectoral approach–it is not just 'public health policy' but a 'healthy public policy'–and such policy belongs to the mainstream of government.

Of course, pressures for expenditure come from areas other than health–these include defence needs–for instance armaments of various types which consume far too much of the health budgets of many developing countries.

In developing countries, according to the UNDP, some 20% of Central Government expenditure is devoted to defence. In the mid 1980's military spending in developing countries exceeded the expenditure on health and education combined. At a time of national budget cuts, the US$ 200 billion the developing world spends annually on the military has largely been protected. Arms are often a major source of external debt–military debt accounts for more than a third of the total debt in several large developing countries.

These are the realities that need to be borne in mind in relation to future health and education expenditure by developing countries. There is an urgent need for a more human approach to national budgets in many developing countries. But the same applies to developed countries as well.

It has been estimated by UNICEF that all child malnutrition could be ended by an additional expenditure of US$ 25 billion which would remove widespread illiteracy and preventable disease. Such a big figure has to be compared with other big items in the costs of development. It is slightly greater than the expenditure proposed for the new Hong Kong airport. It is about the same as the agreed support package to be provided by the group of seven (G7) for Russia alone. It is less than what Europeans spend on wine and less than what Americans spend on beer each year!

The control of IDD is in fact rather cheap in comparison to many other problems. The extra cost of salt iodization is low–normally in the range of 2-7 US cents per kilogram which is less than 5% of the retail price of salt in most countries (see further Chapter 5). This means that the cost of salt iodization can sooner or later be transferred to a large extent to the salt industry and the consumer.

A major step forward in securing a higher priority for expenditure on children's health and education was the World Summit for

Children held at the United Nations on 30 September 1990. This was attended by 71 Heads of State together with senior representatives of 88 other governments. This meeting was convened by a group of six Heads of State under the chairmanship of the President of Mali and the Prime Minister of Canada.

At the World Summit, the 71 Heads of State followed by the other governments, signed a Declaration and approved a new programme for the improved health and education of children throughout the world. This list of goals included the virtual elimination of IDD by the year 2000.

This is an unprecedented commitment by Heads of State to give priority to the needs of children.

The World Summit for Children in 1990 was followed by a further commitment by 60 Heads of State who nominated delegations to the Policy Conference on Micronutrient Malnutrition held in Montreal, Canada (October 1991). The recent International Conference on Nutrition (Rome, December 1992) was attended by government delegations from 160 countries.

At the level of Ministers of Health of more than 160 governments, the World Health Assembly in 1990 also adopted the goal of elimination of IDD as a public health problem by the year 2000. This has provided future endorsement of the World Summit Goals.

This new level of political commitment at the national level has made the achievement of the goal of elimination of IDD much more of a possibility than before. Examples are set by Indonesia, the Philippines and China.

In Indonesia, President Suharto announced a trebling of the expenditure on IDD control in January 1992.

In the Philippines, president Fidel V Ramos, (see/refer to Fig. 5.8) speaking at a National Advocacy Meeting on 'Ending Hidden Hunger' in June 1993, noted recent progress in ensuring that no baby is born physically or mentally handicapped because of iodine deficiency and called on his government to fully support IDD elimination.

In China, a National Advocacy Meeting on the elimination of IDD was held in the Great Hall of the People with the sponsorship of Premier Li Peng (21-24 September 1993).

All Provincial Governors with their staff attended the meeting in addition to representatives of the international agencies including WHO, UNICEF, UNDP, the World Bank and ICCIDD. The meeting was chaired by Madame Peng Pei Yung–one of the five members of the States Council. The Vice Premier, Mr Zhu rong Ji, made a commitment on behalf of the Chinese government which was followed by speeches of support from the international agency representatives including UNDP and the World Bank. Mr Zhu subsequently, at a special meeting of the Provincial Governors, assured them that the Central government would provide the necessary funds to secure an effective elimination programme. It is clear that the Chinese government has recognized the major hazard of the effects of iodine deficiency on early brain development in the light of its one child family policy.

At a regional level, this commitment to the elimination of IDD has also been made by the South Asian Association for Regional Co-operation (SAARC) including Bangladesh, Bhutan, India, Maldives, Nepal, Pakistan and Sri Lanka. It has also been made by the Organization for African Unity (OAU) in Cairo (1993) and the Organization of American States in Latin America (Bogota 1992).

The ICCIDD, together with WHO and UNICEF, is providing advice and help to national governments with the necessary expertise required for effective national IDD control programmes. As described in the previous chapter, regional IDD working groups are now functioning throughout the world attended by national government representatives for a regular review of their programmes.

The United Nations Agencies

The World Health Organization (WHO)

The WHO was founded in 1948 to be the specialized United Nations agency concerned with health in all its aspects for all peoples. In the WHO charter, health is defined as a 'complete state of physical, mental and social well-being and not merely the absence of disease or infirmity'. From this is derived the WHO's imperative of prevention.

The WHO is an inter-governmental organization which derives its authority from the World Health Assembly made up of government representatives meeting annually in Geneva where they receive reports on the state of health of the world's peoples. The WHA decides policy for the organization.

The WHO provides the necessary global network of expertise on all major public health problems. This expertise is provided both by its specialized staff as well as a large number of consultants called in for varying periods to provide advice on special problems. The WHO has given much attention to the problem of iodine deficiency since its foundation.

Resolutions passed at the World Health Assembly are binding on governments to implement them. In the case of IDD there was a WHA Resolution in 1986 sponsored by the Australian government pointing to the feasibility of the prevention and control of IDD. In 1990, another WHA Resolution accepting the goal of elimination of IDD as a public health problem by the year 2000 was passed and this was further reinforced in 1992 when a resolution adopting national programmes for combating micronutrient malnutrition (including IDD, Vitamin A and Iron deficiency) was also passed.

A major function of WHO is now the global monitoring of progress in IDD elimination at country level. A comprehensive system for doing this has now been drawn up and is in the process of being tested in 35 countries. This question is further discussed in part IV.

New developments in computer and information technology greatly expedite this monitoring process so that up-to-date data can be rapidly processed and incorporated with earlier data to give a clear picture of the progress towards the goal. (See further Chapter 11).

In May 1993 the ICCIDD proposed to WHO and UNICEF the establishment of a Global Verification Commission. This will provide the final necessary framework for the co-operation and commitment of national governments to the goal of elimination of IDD and to the sustainability of that goal.

The precedent for such a Global Verification Commission is the WHO Global Commission on the eradication of smallpox. This Commission and its Regional Expert Committees carried out the verification and certification of the goal of eradication of smallpox throughout the period 1965-1980. The historic and epoch making announcement of the achievement of the goal of eradication was made at the World Health Assembly in 1980.

It is the hope of all of us concerned with the elimination of IDD that such an announcement will be possible by the world Health Assembly when it meets in the year 2000. This will require the verification of over 100 countries with IDD public health poblems as having achieved elimination.

In contrast to smallpox, which has finally been eradicated (there are no more infected humans who could transmit the disease), we know that IDD could easily recur if there was a relaxation of the monitoring of salt iodization due to any one of a variety of factors. Hence there is the need for continued vigilance through the maintenance of the Global Verification Commission which will be able to ensure the sustainability of IDD elimination.

UNICEF

UNICEF has a special mandate to improve the welfare of children and women. It has therefore a broader mandate than WHO which is primarily concerned with health.

The basic operation of UNICEF is at country level by contrast with WHO, where the basic operations are at the regional level. In each of the countries UNICEF has a country representative who has the authority to negotiate with the government on the country programme for which there is a financial allocation approved by the Executive Board which meets annually in New York.

As mentioned earlier in this book, it was the Executive Director of UNICEF, Mr Henry Labouisse, who in 1978, declared to the International Union of Nutritional Sciences meeting in Rio de Janeiro that 'Iodine deficiency is so easy to prevent that it is a crime to let a single child be born mentally handicapped for that reason.'

Before and since that time UNICEF has given high priority to the IDD problem. Emphasis has been laid on salt iodization and communications aspects.

The combination of UNICEF and WHO has been of great importance to the recent achievement of the goal of child immunization. The achievement of world coverage of 80% of children was announced at the UN Headquarters in 1991. This great triumph has been estimated to have saved the lives of 3 million children. UNICEF at country level and WHO at the regional level have provided very successful complementary inputs which are being reproduced with the IDD control programme. The Director General of WHO and the Executive Director of UNICEF jointly convened the Policy Conference on Micronutrient Malnutrition at Montreal, in September 1991.

Since the policy meeting at Montreal in 1991, UNICEF has been allocating increased funds to IDD country programmes along with increased allocation for the other major micronutrient deficiencies (Vitamin A and Iron). Strong leadership by the Executive Director, Mr J P Grant, has led to the adoption of the goal of universal access to iodized salt by a number of countries by 1995.

This mid-decade goal has led to the greatly accelerated activity at country level which has already been discussed in Chapter 2.

Other UN Agencies

There are three other major UN agencies which have included the correction of iodine deficiency in their programmes:

The World Food Programme (WFP)

The World Food Programme(WFP) provides food aid on a massive scale which is valued at more than US$ 1 billion per year. This food goes to refugees, displaced persons, assisted projects, food assisted development projects and emergency operations.

The need for supplementation of food--particularly with iodized salt–is now well recognized. For example, the WFP has been supplying 137 tonnes of iodized salt over five years to the road workers of Bhutan and another 14 tonnes to the boarding schools for both primary and post-primary students. A similar programme operates for mothers and school children in Bolivia.

The need for concurrent nutrition education programmes is also being recognized.

The United Nations Development Programme (UNDP)

This agency is concerned with overall economic development which has been defined as a process of enlarging people's choices. Opportunities to earn a greater income is one choice, but in addition, there are important choices for education, health, environment and political and economic freedom. All are significant for human development.

From the 1990 Human Development Report it is clear that there has been substantial progress in developing countries over the last 30 years. This includes an overall increase in life expectancy by 16 years, an increase in adult literacy by 40%, and per capita nutrition levels by over 20%. These improvements took nearly a century to achieve in industrialized countries.

The challenge for the next decade is not only to improve survival, but also to improve the personal and social development of the children who have survived. This includes the elimination of iodine deficiency as the most common preventable cause of mental defect. The UNDP has now accepted this message and is proceeding to act on it by including IDD control in its country programmes. This has occurred notably in China.

The International Bank for Reconstruction and Development (IBRD)

The **World Bank** has now included IDD control programmes in its country programmes. This is the most significant development. The Bank's basic mission is to reduce poverty and accelerate growth, clearly the elimination of IDD is an essential pre-requisite for this to occur. The bank is also now providing core support for the ICCIDD.

The International Council for Control of Iodine Deficiency Disorders

This international non-government organization (NGO) has provided a global multi-disciplinary network of expertise since 1986. As we have seen, the ICCIDD has worked closely with WHO and UNICEF since its inception. The ICCIDD has played a key role through advocacy which has led to the acceptance by the UN system of the international importance of the IDD problem and the feasibility of its elimination.

The ICCIDD is recognized by the UN system as the expert body on all aspects of iodine deficiency and the prevention and control of iodine deficiency disorders. In 1990 the ICCIDD put forward the inter-agency plan which was endorsed by the UN Subcommittee on Nutrition and has since guided activities at the global, regional and national level.

The ICCIDD by virtue of its expertise occupies a central role in the partnership that has now come into being to achieve the goal of elimination.

As we have already noted, the ICCIDD has now proposed the formation of a Global Commission to WHO and UNICEF for the assessment and verification of progress towards the goal at country level. A resolution to this effect has now been transmitted to the Director-General of WHO and the Executive Director of UNICEF for their formal approval, following favourable informal exchanges on the subject held earlier.

The ICCIDD has now as an International-NGO negotiated an official relationship with the WHO in place of the informal relationship already existing since the initial recognition by the Director-General of WHO at the inauguration of the ICCIDD in Kathmandu, Nepal in 1986.

The structure and functioning of the ICCIDD has been described in Chapter 2. In relation to its role in the global partnership, there is a close liaison with UNICEF country offices so that its expertise can be available with minimum delay to country programmes. The same applies to WHO Regional and country offices, and bilateral agencies where the Regional IDD Working Groups provide the appropriate strategic focus.

An important development is that expert ICCIDD Regional co-ordinators have expressed their willingness to work half time in the regional and country offices of the WHO and UNICEF.

Governments of various countries have shown willingness to render help in making the national programmes more effective.

The ICCIDD proposes to carry out a series of regional reviews of progress at country level towards the goal of elimination in collaboration with WHO and UNICEF. Particular attention will be given to the mid decade goal of 95% salt iodization by December 1995.

The first region selected is Latin America. The Director of PAHO has indicated his approval, and criteria for the assessment of progress are being finalized following the WHO/UNICEF/ICCIDD/ Consultation on IDD Prevalence and Programme Indicators meeting in Geneva (3,4 November 1992).

The result of this review was reported to a joint PAHO/WHO/ UNICEF/ICCIDD Regional meeting on the elimination of IDD in Latin America to be held in Quito, Ecuador (9 - 11 April 1994).

The ICCIDD proposes to carry out similar reviews of progress towards the goal with reports to regional meetings (held jointly with WHO and UNICEF) in the years leading up to 2000.

The Bilateral Agencies

As already noted in Chapter 2, the relevant bilateral agencies comprise those international development programmes of specific countries which include nutrition and particularly national IDD control programmes in their portfolio of aid projects.

The relevant countries that are currently contributing support for IDD control are Australia, Belgium, Canada, Holland, Italy, Sweden, and the USA.

Australia, through its Australian Agency for International Development (AusAID) has contributed to the support of the ICCIDD since its inception in 1985. In 1992 the agency carried out a review of the ICCIDD with the help of an external consultant. The agency received a very favourable report, and the support has been increased.

In addition, Australia has had a notable bilateral programme with the People's Republic of China for the development of technical expertise to assist in the massive national IDD control programme in that country. A sum of 2.6 million Australian dollars was provided over a period of five years (1986-1991) which resulted in the establishment of four monitoring centres (Tianjin, Harbin, Giuyang and Xining) for IDD status and the state of control programmes at provincial level—over 40 professionals were trained in various aspects of the national programme (Management, data processing and laboratory technology) at the Westmead Medical centre in Sydney. This programme has made a very significant contribution to China's herculean task of IDD control.

More recently Australia has provided support for IDD control in Vietnam and is about to undertake further assistance with national programme development in that country.

Belgium, through the Belgian Co-operation Programme, has provided major support through UNICEF for the control programmes of the five sub-Andean countries (Venezuela, Colombia, Ecuador, Peru and Bolivia). These programmes are progressing well with a sub-regional co-ordinator. Earlier Belgium has supported several national programmes in Africa including Zaire and Burundi.

Canada, through the Canadian International Development Agency (CIDA), has also provided major support for the ICCIDD since 1991. In addition, Canada was the sponsor of the Micronutrient Policy Meeting in Montreal 'Ending Hidden Hunger' (1991). CIDA has also supported individual country level efforts–Salt Iodization Workshops in Botswana and Senegal in 1992, in Central America in 1993 and the National Control Programme in Bangladesh. Finally, support is being provided for the development of a global strategy on salt iodization.

The Netherlands, through its international co-operative programme, is supporting national control programmes in Tanzania, Zimbabwe and Malawi. In addition, Holland has supported the publication of a series of practical manuals on various aspects of IDD control. General guides on urinary iodine methodology and salt iodization have now appeared, to be followed by others. These guides are being translated into French and Spanish.

Italy, has provided major support for the earlier joint WHO/UNICEF Nutrition Support Programme which in its later stages provided support for IDD control programmes in Latin America and Africa.

Sweden, through the Swedish International Development Agency (SIDA), is providing core support for the ICCIDD as well as supporting the national programmes in Tanzania and Zimbabwe.

USA, through the US Agency for International Development (USAID), had until very recently not provided any support for IDD control, although it has provided strong support for the investigation of Vitamin A deficiency. However, the US Senate and the US congress passed a Foreign Aid Bill in late 1992 which provided for an annual allocation of US$ 25 million for micronutrient malnutrition including Vitamin A, Iodine and Iron. Of this amount, up to US$ 13 million could be available for national IDD control programmes.

Following this notable step, USAID has advertised (June 1993) a major project – 'Opportunities for Micronutrient Nutrition Initiatives' (OMNI) which provides for the expenditure of up to US$50 million over a five year period. Other special projects which are also being negotiated with the ICCIDD are concerned with a global strategy, global monitoring and scientific meetings and research. Support is also being provided for the Programme Against Micronutrient Malnutrition (PAMM) in Atlanta.

It will be clear from this brief listing of support by the bilateral agencies that an increased volume of resources has become available from bilateral agencies. This support is most encouraging and will fully utilize the available resources of professional manpower for the great task ahead.

The Salt Industry

The formation of a working relationship between the ICCIDD and the international salt industry dates from a meeting held at the 7th International Symposium on Salt, held in Kyoto (6-9 April 1992). The Symposium brought together about 600 delegates from the salt industry and related activities all over the world.

A special symposium was held on the iodine deficiency disorders for the information of all the delegates.

An informal special meeting then took place which was attended by 16 representatives of the international salt industry who were particularly concerned about the production of iodized salt for human consumption.

The representatives present agreed to remain in communication with the ICCIDD on all the technical aspects of salt iodization.

A roster of consultants was established for technical advice to the ICCIDD and to agencies.

It was pointed out that the demand for iodized salt was increasing and so there was a need to increase production.

A subsequent resolution by the International Board of the ICCIDD in 1993 has recommended the iodization of all salt for human consumption which is exported to countries with an IDD problem. Letters with this recommendation have been sent to the senior executives of major international salt companies.

It is clear that the salt industry has an important role to play in achieving effective salt iodization. ICCIDD/UNICEF/WHO/CIDA workshops in Africa for the salt industry held in Botswana (April 1992) and in Senegal (October 1992) have led to an increased demand for the production of iodized salt.

Kiwanis International

Kiwanis International, dating from 1916, consists of all chartered local Kiwanis Clubs made up of Kiwanis members. The official motto is 'We Build'. A short description of its activities is given in Chapter 11.

Kiwanis International, after careful consideration, has adopted the elimination of IDD by the year 2000 in collaboration with UNICEF and the ICCIDD as the objective of the first Kiwanis International World Service Project. A campaign plan has been adopted with a fund-raising target of in excess of US$ 50 million over the next five years. An extensive education and promotion programme has now begun following the announcement at the World Kiwanis International Convention (Nice, June 1993). (Fig. 3.2)

The World Service Project will be carried out in partnership with UNICEF. A Campaign Cabinet has been appointed with the Executive Director of the ICCIDD as Adviser. Most of the funds will go towards country programme support via UNICEF.

Kiwanis groups have already made visits to observe IDD control programmes in Bolivia, the Philippines and Ghana.

The project is seen as the first step in the Kiwanis commitment to 'Young children: Priority one' which focusses on long term gains in children's physical and mental health.

This decision by Kiwanis International is of far reaching significance. It provides not only a major funding source, but will lead to an international community fully educated on the elimination of IDD. Apart from the U.S.A, which has 8,000 clubs, strong clubs in Japan, Korea, Taiwan and many other countries, provide an international input of the greatest importance. The ICCIDD is already mobilizing its full support for the education programme throughout the world through its global multi-disciplinary network.

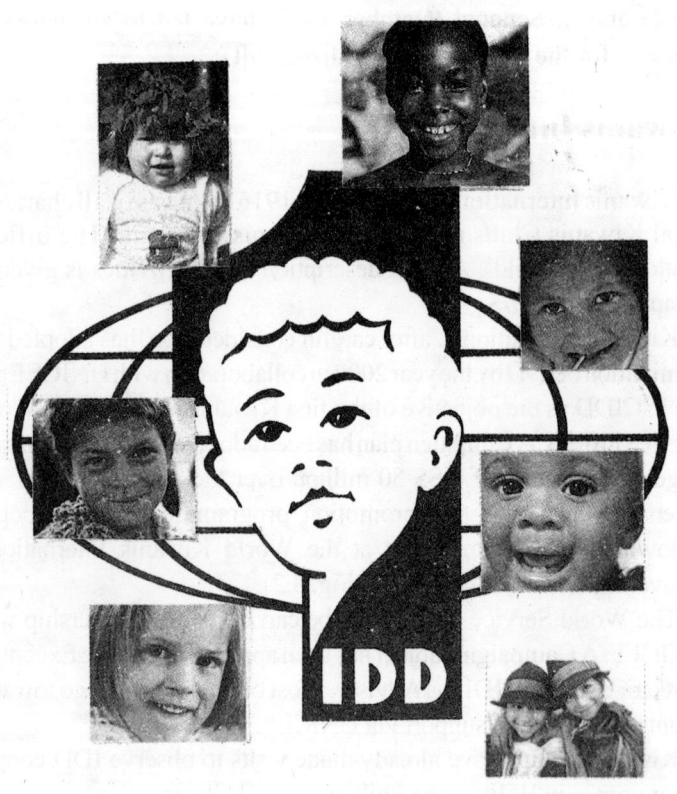

Fig. 3.2 Iodine: The Kiwani Solution. A campaign to virtually eliminate Iodine Deficiency Disorders by the Year 2000.

Micronutrient Initiative

Micronutrient Initiative (MI) was established in 1992 as an international secretariat by its principal sponsors: Canadian International Development Agency (CIDA), International Development research Centre (IDRC), United Nations Children's Fund (UNICEF), United Nations Development Programme (UNDP) and the World Bank. The MI is housed within the IDRC in Canada. The mission of the MI is to

facilitate the achievement of the following goals related to the elimination of micronutrient malnutrition by supporting effective and sustainable programmatic actions:
* virtual elimination of iodine deficiency disorders
* virtual elimination of vitamin A deficiency and its consequences, including blindness
* reduction of iron deficiency anemia in women by one-third of the 1990 levels.

The MI programme framework for 1995-1998 provides for support in five areas considered critical to national and global efforts in eliminating micronutrient malnutrition (MM).

Advocacy and Alliance Building

Information presentation to policy makers and donors to generate committment and increased funding; promotion of MM elimination at key internaitnal meetings; motivaiton and involvement of the food industry; formation of partnerships between government, consumers, industry, expert groups and international agencies at national and international level.

Development and Application of Technologies

Development of appropriate technology for medium and small-scale food producers and field testing; technology transfer and licensing issues; development of quality assurance and control systems; monitoring of intervention of effectiveness; promotion of micronutrient fortification of food aid.

Regional and National Initiatives

Assistance in developing/refining country proposals; support for responsive and proactive information systems at the country level; increasing access to information by MM field staff; brokerage of technical assistance and funding.

Capacity Building

Consultnat identification and orientation; preparation of a roster of consultants in different areas of expertise; development of training skills and facilities at the regional and country level curriculum development.

Resolution of key operational issues
Operations research topics of global relevance; activities that will help in the timely resolution of issues critical to policy and/or programme formulation.

Conclusion

What a unique partnership we now have for this great enterprise! It includes the people and governments of affected countries, the international and bilateral agencies, the Kiwanis Club members and the international salt industry. The ICCIDD has been privileged to be able to co-operate and help facilitate this remarkable development.

PART II

National Programmes for the Elimination of Iodine Deficiency Disorders

4

Measurement of Iodine Deficiency Disorders

J.B. Stanbury and A. Pinchera

Measurement of the extent of iodine deficiency disorders (IDD) in population indicates the extent and severity of the problem. It also indicates progress in the elimination of IDD. Measurement of IDD, therefore, provides key information in deciding whether a programme is required for IDD elimination. Once having initiated such a programme, measurement is required to demonstrate its effectiveness.

Identification of an individual with an iodine deficiency disorder can be made only in an epidemiological context as part of a community problem. It is not possible, with one exception, to attribute a disorder in an individual patient to iodine deficiency unless that subject is a member of a community in which other similar disorders are found. The exception is the typical cretin with neurological damage in whom the findings are those that are typical and unique to endemic neurological cretinism (see Chapter 1). In such an instance it might be possible to make a positive diagnosis outside the context of an endemia.

An endemic of IDD may be suspected when there are anecdotal accounts from particular regions of the presence of goitre or of retarded individuals who seem to show the features of endemic cretinism. The absence of such testimony or rumours is useful, but is no guarantee that IDD does or does not exist, because IDD of significant degree may escape casual detection. Whenever there is a suspicion of IDD, it is necessary and important that direct and objective information on IDD status be assembled. IDD is so pervasive and often so subtle, and also so important to community health that detection cannot be left an uncertainty: its presence or absence must be ascertained by measurement.

Measuring the presence of IDD

Several methods are employed in quantifying the extent and severity of IDD. These are listed in Table 4.1 and described in the following paragraphs.

Table 4.1 *Methods employed in the epidemiological measurement of the iodine deficiency disorders*

* Thyroid size by palpation of the thyroid

* Thyroid size by ultrasonography

* Urinary excretion of iodine

* Thyroglobulin concentration in the blood

* Thyrotropin (TSH) concentration in the blood

* Thyroid hormones (thyroxine and triiodothyronine) concentration in blood

* Radioiodine uptake

* Prevalence of cretinism

Sampling

The investigator intent on detecting or measuring IDD must identify the target population group. This may be a country or a region, or it may be a smaller population unit. A sample size must be selected so that numbers will be representative and statistically valid. The sample size will depend on the error in the measuring instrument and on the variability of the parameter within different sub-regions and not in others. This information is essential in order to have a perception of the extent and severity of the problem and for devising strategies for prevention. A common method for assessing IDD prevalence is the "probability proportionate to size" (PPS) cluster method.

Precise guidelines for assessing IDD prevalence are discussed in detail in the report of a joint ICCIDD/UNICEF/WHO consultation on Indicators for assessing Iodine Deficiency Disorders and their control through salt iodization. (Document WHO/NUT/94.6)

Endemic goitre: Palpation of the thyroid

Palpation of the thyroid for size has been the standard technique for measuring endemic goitre. School children, because of their accessibility and large numbers, have generally been selected and their thyroid sizes measured by experienced surveyors.

Goitre size has been estimated according to preset criteria which are described in Table 4.2. Strict adherence to this classification has enabled a limited degree of comparability among surveys in different regions. As indicated in Table 4.2 larger goitres may not need palpation for a diagnosis, provided that conditions such as rolls of fat in the neck region mimicking thyroid enlargement are excluded. Thus, a classification as a 'thyroid invisible at a distance' is unacceptable unless accompanied by careful palpation.

There are several advantages to palpation as a method of measurement. It is a technique that requires no instrumentation, can reach large numbers in a short period of time, is not invasive and makes relatively limited demands on the skills of the surveyor.

Nevertheless, palpation has some outstanding disadvantages. There is high level of inter-observer variation especially in low grade goitres i.e. grade 0 and grade 1. This has been demonstrated by studies of experienced examiners where misclassification can be as high as 40%.

Table 4.2 *Simplified classification of goitre*

Grade 0 :	No palpable or visible goitre
Grade 1 :	A mass in the neck that is consistent with an enlarged thyroid that is palpable but not visible when the neck is in the normal position. It moves upward in the neck as the subject swallows. Nodular alteration(s) can occur even when the thyroid is not enlarged
Grade 2 :	A swelling in the neck that is visible when the neck is in a normal position and is consistent with an enlarged thyroid when the neck is palpated

Source: From the report of a Joint WHO/UNICEF/ICCIDD Consultation on 'Indicators for Assessing Iodine Deficiency Disorders and their Control through salt iodization' Geneva, November 1992. Document WHO/NUT/94.6.

An effort to lend objectivity and quantitation to palpation has been made (Gaitan and Dunn 1992). The palpated thyroid is outlined with a felt pen on paper applied to the neck, and then the area of the outlined gland is measured. This technique is an advanced one, but in one large trial was not found to offer any major advantage.

Why has palpation not proved to be entirely satisfactory?

Fundamentally, the thyroid is not easy to feel, and it is not easy to translate a felt gland into weight or comparative size. Such difficulty is more pronounced in men as opposed to women because of the greater development of neck muscles hindering palpation in males. There is observers' fatigue, especially when dealing with large numbers of subjects with normal or only slightly enlarged glands. Finally, as noted above, inter-observer discordance has proved the inadequacy of palpation.

Goitre represents the integration of events extending overtime—it is a historical relic that does not necessarily indicate the present state of iodine nutrition. A recent survey in rural Ecuador demonstrated that goitre had vanished among the youth of a community who had received iodine prophylactically, but was present in many older persons whose goitres were established before the iodine programme was begun. Those goitres were relics of the iodine metabolism of two or more decades earlier.

Palpation is most useful as an initial signal that IDD may be present and as an indicator that more refined assessment is needed. If palpation suggests that IDD is a problem, then one of the methods of measurement in the following paragraphs are employed.

Recently palpation has been carried out in Tanzania by school teachers as an initial screening procedure before an expert survey is made. More experience is required for an evaluation of this sort.

Thyroid size by Ultrasonography

Objectivity can be introduced into goitre surveys by ultrasonographic measurements as used in other medical investigations, for example in antenatal care. This technique is being used with increasing frequency. It gives a quantitative measure of thyroid volume that is largely free of observer bias (Fig. 4.1). The procedure is not invasive, and can be used to measure several hundred subjects in a day. Its accuracy diminishes when the gland is quite large, but in such instances precise volume is not important for epidemiological purposes. The technique can be easily learnt within a few days. The use of ultrasonography by providing an objective measurement of thyroid volume, may in some cases show that concern for IDD is unwarranted, and accordingly an expensive programme of prevention could be avoided (Gutekunst 1990).

The disadvantages of ultrasonography are a requirement for training, the cost of the instrument (a satisfactory portable machine can be purchased for about fifteen thousand US dollars) and the problem of transport from centre to survey site. Ultrasonography is rapidly replacing palpation, and has thrown doubt on the validity of many older surveys.

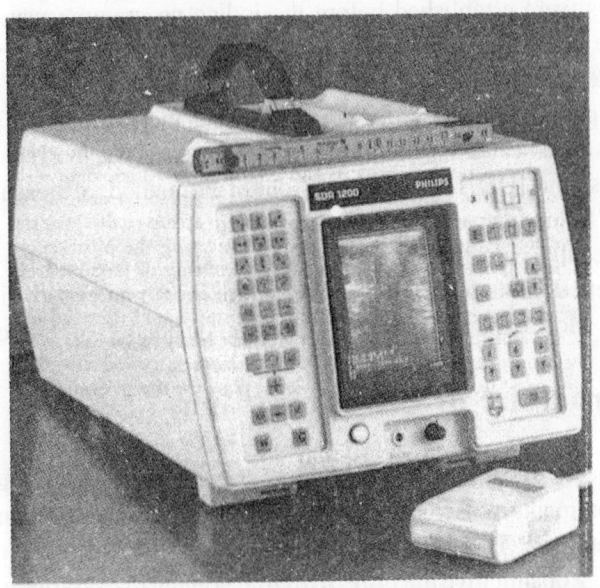

Fig. 4.1 Closeup view of the small portable ultrasonography instrument.

Urinary excretion of iodine

For nearly half a century the benchmark method for determining the state of iodine nutrition has been the measurement of the excretion of iodine in the urine. Approximately 90% of ingested iodine is excreted in the urine. While it is not generally possible to obtain twenty-four hour samples of urine, measurements of concentration in a casual sample from 40-50 subjects is an excellent surrogate. Keying iodine excretion to creatinine excretion has not proved to be helpful because of variations in creatinine excretion with nutritional status so that this ratio is no longer used.

The advantages of assessment by this method are that the method is entirely objective, it is non-invasive, and it provides information on the one factor that can be addressed directly, i.e., iodine supply to the individual. The excretion of iodine indicates the recent but not precisely the immediate intake of iodine. Samples need not be processed immediately: they can be held until they are returned to the laboratory, or they can be shipped to a distant processing point.

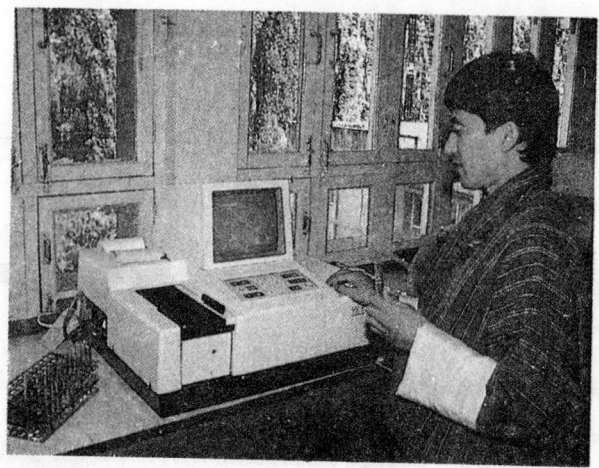

Fig. 4.2 Estimation of urinary iodine concentration in a laboratory in Bhutan. (With permission from "Iodine Deficiency Disorders - The Bhutan Story" ; Directorate of Health Services, Ministry of Social Sciences, Royal Government of Bhutan, 1992).

The problem with iodine excretion is that it requires a laboratory geared to providing accurate determinations, and it incurs some expense. Recent developments have much simplified measurements of iodine in the urine, making it easier and within the limitations of a modest budget. Nevertheless, a skilled technician specially trained in this technique is required, as is laboratory space set apart exclusively for this purpose. Similarly, it is also necessary that in order to maintain continuing quality control, checking with a central laboratory is done.

Table 4.3 *Epidemiological criteria for assessing the severity of IDD based on median urinary iodine levels*

Median value ($\mu g/l$)	Severity of IDD
< 20	Severe IDD
20 - 49	Moderate IDD
50 - 99	Mild IDD
≥ 100	No deficiency

Source: As for table 4.2

There is, of course, the initial expense of equipping the laboratory.* The estimation of urinary iodine concentration in the laboratory in Bhutan is given in Fig. 4.2.

The results of a survey must be interpreted. In general, if the median concentration is below 100 µg/l there is a strong suspicion of IDD in the region surveyed. If the value is below 50µg/l there is almost surely IDD, and if it is below 20 µg/l, the problem is a serious one demanding immediate attention (Table 4.3). Alternatively one can employ a set of criteria wherein the fraction of subjects below a given level specifies the immediacy and seriousness of the problem.

Measurements of thyroglobulin concentration

The thyroid gland leaks thyroglobulin into the blood at a rate roughly dependent on its size. Recent studies have indicated that measurement

---

* John Dunn and colleagues have prepared for general distribution, a manual on the determination of iodine in urine. This is available free of charge from ICCIDD; with the latest techniques up to 200 samples can be processed in a day.

in serum can grossly mirror the size of the thyroid in regions where IDD is found. Increased concentrations of serum thyroglobulin have been found in goitrous subjects, and especially in those with larger goitres. This reflects to some extent the degree of chronic thyroid stimulation by TSH and is also related to the development of autonomous thyroid function.

The advantages of a thyroglobulin assay are its objectivity and reliability. The method has the disadvantages that it requires invasion (a blood sample), and that the measurement, being a radio-immunoassay, necessitates special laboratory expertise, special equipment, and a supply of the radio-labeled antigen. It appears to be a promising and potentially useful indicator of IDD, but has as yet not been thoroughly validated for epidemiological assessment (Fenzi et al 1985).

Measurements of thyroid stimulating hormone (TSH)

The thyroid stimulating hormone (TSH) is secreted by the pituitary and controls the thyroid gland function. Newly introduced ultrasensitive methods for measuring the concentration of thyrotropic hormone in the blood permit accurate assays within and below the normal range, and a fine discrimination in the zone between normal and slightly elevated values. Since thyroid enlargement in IDD is presumed to depend on a response in TSH to a deficiency of iodine, hypothetically serum TSH concentration should reflect iodine deficiency, and perhaps would do so more accurately and immediately than goitre size itself. TSH concentration might be an immediate indicator of hormone production, which in turn should reflect iodine nutrition.

Several factors blur this simplistic view. Because the thyroid has an enormous capacity to store iodine and buffer the hormone secretion rate, serum TSH values may not reflect recent dietary iodine supply, or deficits incurred more remotely in time. Indeed, in most endemias, measurements of serum TSH concentrations of subjects with endemic goitre, or of those living in endemic goitre areas, have been well within normal limits.

An alternative use of TSH as a signal of IDD is in the newborn. This procedure is now widely used in developed countries to screen for the occurrence of congenital hypothyroidism. This condition is associated with a defect in the production of thyroid hormones due to the absence of the thyroid, a small or misplaced thyroid, or a defect in the biochemical machinery in the thyroid for the production of thyroid hormones.

The importance of an adequate level of the thyroid hormone for normal rapid brain development in the foetus and early infancy has already been pointed out (Chapter 1) in relation to iodine deficiency.

If there is adequate iodine intake, congenital hypothyroidism occurs at a rate of about 1 in 4,000 births (0.025%). As already pointed out in Chapter 1, if iodine intake is inadequate then the rate may increase to 1% or even up to 10% of births, which indicates a massive threat to brain development. This measurement then can be used as a population indicator of IDD quite apart from its use as a screening measure for individuals.

On the other hand, if there is a very low rate of detection of neonatal hypothyroidism, then this can be cited as evidence that the elimination of IDD has been achieved. These data are readily available in many developed countries where universal screening of newborns is well established. Other developed countries still have to establish universal coverage while in most developing countries such a procedure has not yet been established.

There are several problems with this approach. First, this method requires sophisticated laboratory backup and an organized programme of sample collection. Also, if one initiates an investigation by screening newborns, then the data will inevitably be too slow in arriving for recognizing a possibly dangerous presence of IDD. Further, this would probably be a method that might appear less severe, but is nonetheless important, because most of the results would be insufficiently high to raise the suspicion of neonatal hypothyroidism. Finally, any programme that involves blood samples carries the risk of unclean needles and the implied risk of hepatitis or the acquired immunity deficiency syndrome (AIDS). The card used for collecting blood spots for serum thyroid stimulating hormone estimation is shown in Fig. 4.3.

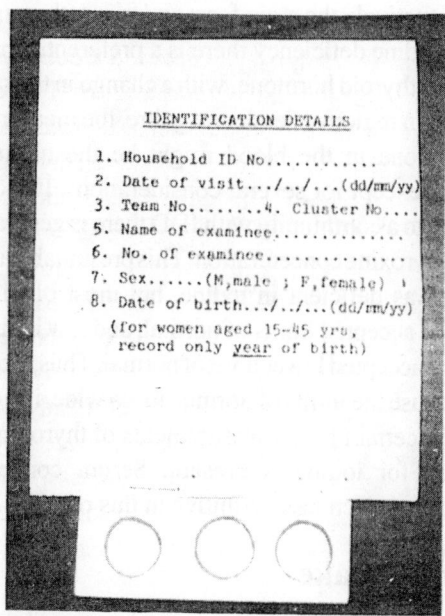

Fig. 4.3 The card used for collecting blood spots for estimation of Serum TSH levels. (With permission from "Iodine Deficiency Disorders - The Bhutan Story"; Directorate of Health Services, Ministry of Social Sciences, Royal Government of Bhutan, 1992).

In spite of these reservations, once established, neonatal screening for congenital hypothyroidism provides useful information particularly in developed countries. A mild iodine deficiency in a given area may be disclosed by the finding of a median neonatal serum TSH within normal limits, but relatively high when compared with an iodine sufficient control area. Moreover, a shift to the left, i.e., to lower values, of neonatal TSH screening data after the instituting of iodine prophylaxis should provide an indicator of the adequacy of the preventive programme.

Measurements of Thyroid Hormones

The objective of the thyroid system is to supply to the body an appropriate amount of the thyroid hormone, of which thyroxine represents quantitatively the main form and triiodothyronine the most active form. In iodine deficiency there is a preferential production of the less iodinated thyroid hormone, with a change in the ratio between serum T_3 and T_4. In regions of endemic goitre, the measurement of the amount of hormone in the blood might be the ultimate tool for measuring IDD, except for several considerations. If iodine is given prophylactically to a community with IDD there is generally a net rise in mean serum thyroxine concentration. This presumably indicates that the population was deficient in iodine, but most often this change occurs within the accepted limits of normal, and few individuals have values below the accepted lower limit of normal. Thus, from the results of a survey, because the limits of normal are so wide, it would be quite impossible to be certain from measurements of thyroxine alone, that IDD or a need for iodine is present. Serum concentrations of triiodothyronine are even less definitive in this regard.

Radioiodine Uptake

Early studies on the pathophysiology of endemic goitre used radioiodine uptake to demonstrate the ambient lack of dietary iodine as reflected in the avidity of the deprived thyroid for radioiodine. An elevated radioiodine uptake shows that at the moment of testing, the thyroid lacks iodine. It may take days or weeks of daily supplements of iodine to restore the uptake to a level consistent with normal gland function.

The radioiodine uptake test would remain a first-line tool for measuring the need for iodine if it were not for certain disadvantages. Such disadvantages are: its use requires rather expensive and cumbersome apparatus, trained observers, and a supply of the radioisotope. The test also entails a small radiation exposure to both subject and investigator.

Prevalence of Cretinism

The frequency with which cretins occur in a targeted area, has been proposed as a measure of the presence and severity of IDD. This might serve admirably if the rate is sufficiently high and statistically reliable numbers can be obtained in reasonable time, and if the observers are sufficiently skilled in recognizing cretins apart from others with physical findings that superficially resemble those of cretinism. The clinical findings of cretinism are variable. The spastic paralysis which tends to spare the distal ends of the extremities and other subtle and unique features of the endemic cretin may not be easily identified without experience and careful instruction.

If endemic cretins constitute one percent of the population then there has clearly been an IDD problem, but this is no guarantee that the population is still at risk. Dietary habits may have changed. It is always necessary to search for evidence of an existing or recent state of iodine deficiency.

Ancillary Signals of the Presence of IDD

There are several epidemiological findings that are consistent with IDD, and indeed are part of the IDD spectrum, but their identification and measurement cannot be employed for identifying or measuring the presence or severity of an endemia. High pre-or peri-or post-natal death rates are caused by iodine deficiency. If one of these is observed and other causes are not immediately apparent, one should consider iodine deficiency and screen for it by one of the techniques described above. Similarly, endemic deaf mutism should require screening for iodine deficiency. Poor intellectual performance in school children in a community should stimulate a consideration that it is part of an IDD endemia. None of these three findings could be translated into a method for field testing for the presence of IDD: they are too crude and too often attributable to other causes, but when they are present they should suggest iodine deficiency as a possible factor.

Measurement of the Severity of an IDD Endemia

When an endemia of IDD has been identified it is necessary to know its severity in order that the urgency of intervention with a prophylaxis programme can be judged. If the endemia is severe then there is great urgency to prevent the further devastating occurrence of cretins or neurologically damaged individuals in the community. This might call for an urgent and immediate programme with iodized oil, because this can begin almost immediately, and further mental and physical retardation can be stopped at once. Generally programmes of prevention with iodized salt take months or longer to implement because of the need to obtain the concurrence of governments and of the salt industry, to obtain the financing and the equipment for iodizing the salt, to develop a distribution and marketing system, and to promote the use of iodized salt by the general public.

Guidelines for classifying endemias appear in Table 4.4. Should there be any question concerning where a given endemic fits, then the decision regarding prophylaxis should incline to greater concern and appropriate action, rather than the reverse.

Measuring Progress towards Elimination

It is not sufficient to identify an endemia of IDD: once a preventive programme has been instituted it is essential that its progress and continuation be carefully monitored. Too many national and regional programmes have begun with much enthusiasm and have achieved some success, only to fail for lack of continued surveillance. To prevent mental defect, elimination of IDD must be carried out.

Salt Iodine

The adequacy of a prophylactic programme should be continuously checked. This can be done by monitoring the distribution of iodized salt to the population at risk and the actual iodine content of table salt at the consumption level. A technique which has been highly successful in Ecuador depends on the country-wide continuous monitoring of the iodine content of table salt. In this way, a continuing flow of salt of good quality with respect to iodine content is ensured at the dealer as well as the household level. A laboratory in the capital city receives samples

Table 4.4 *Summary of IDD prevalence indicators and criteria for a public health problem*

Indicator	Target population	Severity of public health problem (prevalence)		
		Mild	Moderate	Severe
Goitre Grade > 0	SAC[a]	5.0-19.9%	20.0-29.9%	≥ 30%
Thyroid volume > 97th percentile by ultrasound[b]	SAC	5.0-19.9%	20.0-29.9%	≥ 30%
Median urinary iodine level (µg/l)	SAC	50-90	20-49	< 20
TSH > 5 µU/l whole blood	neonates	3.0-19.9%	20.0-39.9%	≥ 40%
Median Tg (ng/ml serum)[c]	C/A[d]	10.0-19.9	20.0-39.9	≥40

[a] SAC = school aged children

[b] Normal thyroid volume size values will be available from WHO and ICCIDD in 1995

[c] Different assays may have different normal ranges.

[d] C/A = children and adults

Source: From the report of a Joint WHO/UNICEF/ICCIDD Consultation on 'Indicators for Assessing Iodine Deficiency Disorders and there Control through Salt Iodization' Geneva, November 1992. Document WHO/NUT/94.6.

of salt at frequent intervals from stations situated around the country. Any breakdown in the flow of iodine to the consumers is quickly identified. The weakness of this method is that only commercial salt is monitored. Occasionally other sources of salt may be introduced, especially if there is a significant price differential between the iodized and the uniodized salt. This happens especially where there are sources of salt from cottage industries. Monitoring of salt iodine at household level provides a final check—recent programmes have included monitoring of household samples brought to school by school children with mobile kits (See Chapter 7).

The mid-decade goal for the elimination of IDD calls for universal access to iodized salt by the end of 1995. The acceptance of this goal by WHO, UNICEF, the ICCIDD and by national governments has produced a great acceleration of effort to involve the salt industry in a partnership as already described in Chapter 3.

Other methods for checking the effectiveness of a preventive programme include the periodic assessment of iodine intake by measuring urinary iodine excretion and evaluation of the clinical and hormonal response. This in turn may be performed by epidemiological surveys of goitre prevalence or by monitoring blood TSH in newborns wherever neonatal samples are available.

Summary

The traditional method for measuring an endemic of iodine deficiency disorders is to assess goitre prevalence by palpating the thyroid gland of a representative sample of the population, usually of school children. This technique lacks precision, and is being replaced by other methods, including ultrasonography, measurements of the urinary excretion of iodine, and assays of thyroid related hormones in the blood. Measurement of the urine excretion of iodine is perhaps the most useful and reliable method.

The severity of an endemic is assessed by the results of surveys, especially those using the excretion of iodine. This is important in indicating the urgency with which prophylaxis should be introduced.

If there is an IDD problem sufficient to require prophylaxis either with iodization of the salt or by administration of iodized oil, then it is necessary that the course of the endemic and the supply and distribution be monitored on a continuing basis. This can be done by monitoring the iodine content of table salt and by measuring urinary excretion of iodine or be supplemented by one of the other methods for measuring hormonal response. In this way the necessary criteria for the elimination of IDD can be demonstrated.

References

Delange, F. 1989. 'Iodine nutrition and congenital hypothyroidism'. In : Delange, F., D.A., Fisher and D. Glenoer eds. *Research in Congenital Hypothyroidism.* New York: Plenum Press. p.173.

Dunn, J.T., H.E., Crutchfield, R., Gutekunst, A., Dunn, P., Bourdoux, E., Gaitan, M., Karmarkar, O., Pinda, Pino, R., Suwanik, 1993. *Methods for measuring iodine in urine.* ICCIDD.

Fenzi, G.F., C., Ceccarelli, E., Macchia, et al. 1985. 'Reciprocal changes of serum thyroglobulin and TSH in residents of a moderate endemic goitre area'. *Clin. Endocrinol.* 23: 115.

Fenzi, G.F., L.F., Giusti, F., Aghini-Lombardi, L., Bartalena, et al. 1990. 'Neuropsychological assessment in school children from an area of moderate iodine deficiency'. *J. Endocrinol. Invest.* 13: 427.

Gaitan, E. and J.T., Dunn 1992. *Epidemiology of iodine deficiency. Trends End. Metab.* 3: 170.

Gutekunst, R. 1990. 'The value and application of ultrasonography in goitre survey'. *IDD Newsletter.* 6: 4.

Stanbury, J.B. Ed. 1993. *Iodine Deficiency and Brain Damage.* Philadelphia: Proceedings of a Symposium held at the Franklin Institute, 4,5 May 1993 (in press).

WHO/UNICEF/ICCIDD November, 1992. 'Indicators for Assessing Iodine Deficiency Disorders and their Control through Salt Iodization'. *Report of a Joint Consultation.* 3-5. WHO, Geneva. Document WHO/NUT/94.6.

5

The Iodization of Salt for the Elimination of Iodine Deficiency Disorders

M.G. Venkatesh Mannar

Introduction

Iodine is an essential dietary nutrient that helps the body to manufacture thyroxine the hormone that regulates normal growth and development. The quantity of iodine required by an individual is minute 150-200 micrograms per day which amounts to a pinhead a month or a teaspoonful for a lifetime! And yet iodine deficiency is one of the major health problems faced by the developing world with more than one billion people at risk.

Lack of iodine in the diet causes a spectrum of disorders that include goitre, stunted physical growth, mental retardation, lassitude, impaired hearing, speech and movement. Women exposed to iodine deficiency suffer more miscarriages, stillbirths and decreased fertility. Insufficient iodine supply to the foetus can result in reduced birth weight and reduced resistance endangering the very survival of the child. Apart from these health consequences, iodine deficiency can also produce socio-economic retardation. Communities whose members are mentally slow, less vigorous and more difficult to educate, are low in productivity. Livestock need iodine too. Iodine deficiency could cause reduced milk and meat yields from animals and lower wool production from sheep. All this can be prevented. Today it is possible to eliminate IDD by ensuring a steady and continuous supply of iodine to the entire population. These simple techniques and procedures have been effectively used in some countries to eliminate IDD as a public health problem. Yet iodine deficiency is a major health problem in many other countries.

The challenge today is to determine how the available knowledge can be applied towards establishing systems which can deliver iodine to the entire population on a continuous and self-sustaining basis. If iodized salt containing the required concentration of iodine is widely available and consumed in a community, there will, in a year's time, be no further birth of cretins or children with subnormal mental and physical development which can be attributed to iodine deficiency. Goitres in primary school children and young adults will begin to shrink and even disappear altogether. Children will be more active and perform better at school. Further enlargement of the thyroid in adults will be prevented. Recognising this unique opportunity, the World Summit for Children called for the virtual elimination of iodine deficiency by the year 2000. As a prerequisite to achieving this goal, there has been international commitment to ensure universal iodization of all salt for human and animal consumption by 1995.

Rationale for Food Fortification

Unlike nutrients like iron, calcium or the vitamins, iodine does not occur naturally in specific foods; rather, it is present in the soil and is imbided through foods grown on that soil. Iodine is irregularly distributed over the earth's crust resulting in acute deficiencies in areas like mountainous regions and flooded riverines. The problem is aggravated by accelerated deforestation and soil erosion. This deficiency cannot be corrected. The food grown in iodine deficient regions can never provide enough iodine to the population and livestock living there. There are indeed rare examples of foods rich in iodine such as certain types of sea weed and sea fish; but these are not accessible to everyone. Thus iodine deficiency results from geological rather than social and economic conditions. It cannot be eliminated by changing dietary habits or by eating specific kinds of foods. Rather the correction has to be achieved by supplying iodine from an external source. This can be done in two ways; by periodic supplementation of iodine-deficient populations with iodized oil (capsules or by injections) or by fortifying a commonly eaten food with iodine. While both strategies are effective, oil supplementation is a short term strategy to be used in hyperendemic areas where supplies of iodized salt may not always reach on time. In all other situations, the iodization of salt is the long term and sustainable solution which will ensure that iodine reaches the entire population and is ingested on a regular basis. Fortification of foods has been extremely successful in eliminating a number of micronutrient deficiencies in the developed world.

Why Iodize Salt ?

In the rural areas of many developing countries, where iodine deficiency is most severe, the populations are largely dependent on subsistence foods. Their diet is typically based on one or two cereals, tubers or pulses as the staple food. If the household has any livestock, it may also consume some dairy products. It is this dietary and economic context that must be considered while choosing a vehicle for iodine to reach such populations.

Over the past 60 years, in the effort to introduce iodine regularly into the daily diet, several foods have been considered as possible vehicles. These include salt, bread, sweets, milk, sugar and water. Among these, salt has become the most commonly accepted owing to a variety of reasons:

* It is one of the few commodities that comes closest to being universally consumed by almost all sections of a community irrespective of economic level. It is consumed at approximately the same level throughout the year in a given region by all normal adults. Thus, a micronutrient like iodine introduced through salt will be administered to each individual at a uniform dosage throughout the year.

* In comparison to other food commodities whose production is widely dispersed, the production of salt is limited to few production centres. In many remote areas of the world, salt is one of the few commodities that comes from outside the area, thereby lending itself to processing on an economical scale and under controlled conditions. By adding a fixed dosage of a micronutrient like iodine to salt at centralized locations, a majority of the population all over a region or country will ingest the nutrient in physiological amounts continuously with no additional effort.

* The mixing of an iodine compound with salt is a simple operation and produces no adverse chemical reactions. The equipment required is not complicated, and is easy to operate and maintain.

* The addition of iodine to salt (usually as potassium or sodium iodide/iodate) does not impart any colour, taste or odour to the salt. In fact iodized salt is indistinguishable from uniodized salt.

* The cost of iodization is low: normally in the range 2-7 US cents per kilogram which is less than 5% of the retail price of salt in most countries. (Table 5.1)

Table 5.1 *Average cost of salt iodization*

Component	Range (US$/Ton)	Average (US$/Ton)
Iodine Compound	0.50-1.5	1.0
Processing	2.35-5.5	4.0
Packing material	0.00-4.0	—
Overheads	0.60-1.5	1.0
Amortization	0.50-2.5	1.5
Total	3.95-15.0	7.5
Cost of iodization	0.4-1.5 US cents/kg or 2-8 cents per person per year	
Retail price of salt	US$ 0.25 - US$ 1.00/kg	
Cost of iodization as a percentage of retail price	2-32%	

Since iodine is required in very minute quantities (150-200 micrograms), the dosage of iodine in salt is extremely small. Salt consumption could be anywhere in the range of 5-20 grams a day within a given region or country. Normally the iodine concentration in salt is fixed in the range of 30-100 micrograms of iodine in one gram of salt. This dosage is determined after taking into account anticipated iodine losses during transport and storage. Iodized salt needs to be packed in waterproof bags or containers and labeled, indicating the name and address of the producer and the date of manufacture to enable monitoring.

In certain parts of the world, there are populations that do not consume salt from a regular production source. They collect rock salt or saline twigs (that are locally available and are boiled to extract the salt). Sometimes brines are boiled to produce small quantities of salt sufficient for the household. It is difficult to make salt available to such populations but improved marketing and availability of commodities for these populations should encourage them to purchase salt.

Once the iodization of salt is quantitatively established as a permanent measure in a country, it eliminates iodine deficiency disorders and continues to provide each individual his daily iodine needs and prevents recurrence. The introduction of iodine through salt has been successful in eliminating the problem of iodine deficiency in a number of countries for over 60 years.

Historical Background

The idea of using salt as a vehicle for the addition of iodine to the diet began in Switzerland in the 1920's and was soon followed by the USA (Michigan) where there was a major problem with goitre. The mixing of iodine as iodide with salt was easily added to the automated procedure at the final stage of processing before it was packed. The concept gained ground and many salt companies in the USA, Canada, Australia and certain European countries began iodizing their salt. This practice continues even today. In many countries like the USA, distribution remains voluntary.

When the concept of salt iodization was transferred to developing countries, it was believed that the problem could be solved with the same ease. Therefore, by the late fifties, salt iodization programmes had been initiated in several Central and South American countries. While some countries in that sub-continent showed remarkable progress in combating the problem, bottle necks persisted in others. In certain countries in Central America, the problem was successfully eliminated but subsequently recurred when government commitment to the programme and monitoring slackened. By the early 1990's, countries with logistic constraints such as Ecuador and Bolivia systematically identified and overcame these problems.

In Asia, although action was initiated in the 1950's and 1960's, progress was minimal until the late seventies. Subsequently, with increasing awareness of IDD and its consequences, several governments reappraised their programmes. This led to a systematic identification of the bottlenecks and the streamlining of iodization programmes in several countries. Since the early eighties, China has implemented a successful programme targeted at the endemic areas covering about 300 million people and recently took a decision to expand the programme to cover the entire country. India adopted a policy of universal iodization of all salt in the country in 1984. Currently, over 500 million people living in the endemic regions of India receive iodized salt. Indonesia faces constraints in its salt iodization programme as it has a large number of scattered small salt producers in its islands and has had to supplement this with a large iodized oil injection programme. Several other countries like Bangladesh, Philippines and Thailand are in the process of establishing iodization facilities at all of their salt processing units. Bhutan's salt iodization programme has successfully overcome an extremely severe IDD problem in the entire country.

In Africa, general awareness has been quite recent–less than seven years. Salt iodization programmes have been initiated in Ethiopia, Kenya, Tanzania and Cameroon. Several other countries including Nigeria, Zaire, Zambia, Ghana, Zimbabwe and Malawi are planning control programmes. In sub-Saharan Africa, several countries do not produce their own salt and rely partly or wholly on imports. This has prompted the development of a regional strategy to ensure that salt is iodized at the production sources in South Africa, Namibia, Mozambique, Eritrea, Sudan, Ghana and Senegal. Countries in different regions of the continent are also co-operating to establish common standards for salt purity, iodine level, packaging and labelling.

The Iodization Process

The production of common salt (or sodium chloride) is one of the most ancient and widely distributed industries of the world. Salt is produced by mining solid rock deposits or by the evaporation (by the sun's heat or by using artificial means) of sea water, lakes or underground brines. The salt produced is ground to a powder or refined before being packed and offered for sale. Sometimes the salt is compressed into blocks to facilitate transportation and marketing. The purity of salt varies over a wide range depending upon the source, method of manufacture and refining techniques adopted. In developed countries and an increasing number of developing countries, salt is refined in modern automated plants. In less developed countries, salt production is essentially a cottage scale operation adopted by hundreds or thousands of producers along sea coasts or saline lake shores.

The process of iodization consists of mixing salt with a determined quantity of a compound of iodine usually potassium iodate or iodide (Fig. 5.2). The iodine compound could be mixed in a dry form or in solution form. In hot, humid environments where salt quality and packaging are less than ideal, potassium iodate is the preferred iodine compound. The equipment required consists of relatively simple measuring devices, feeders and mixers. While iodization can be easily done in an automated refinery, it would call for the significant upgradation and reorganization of small cottage units (Fig 5.3).

In most countries, the salt producing units are concentrated around a few areas. Often the iodine deficient areas are widespread and are at a considerable distance from the salt production centres. Salt moves from production to consumption centres by different modes of transport. Distribution patterns are complex and erratic; under these circumstances it is difficult to regulate a dual market comprising iodized and non-iodized salt or a target programme aimed at the iodization of salt earmarked for the endemic areas. The workable solution in most cases

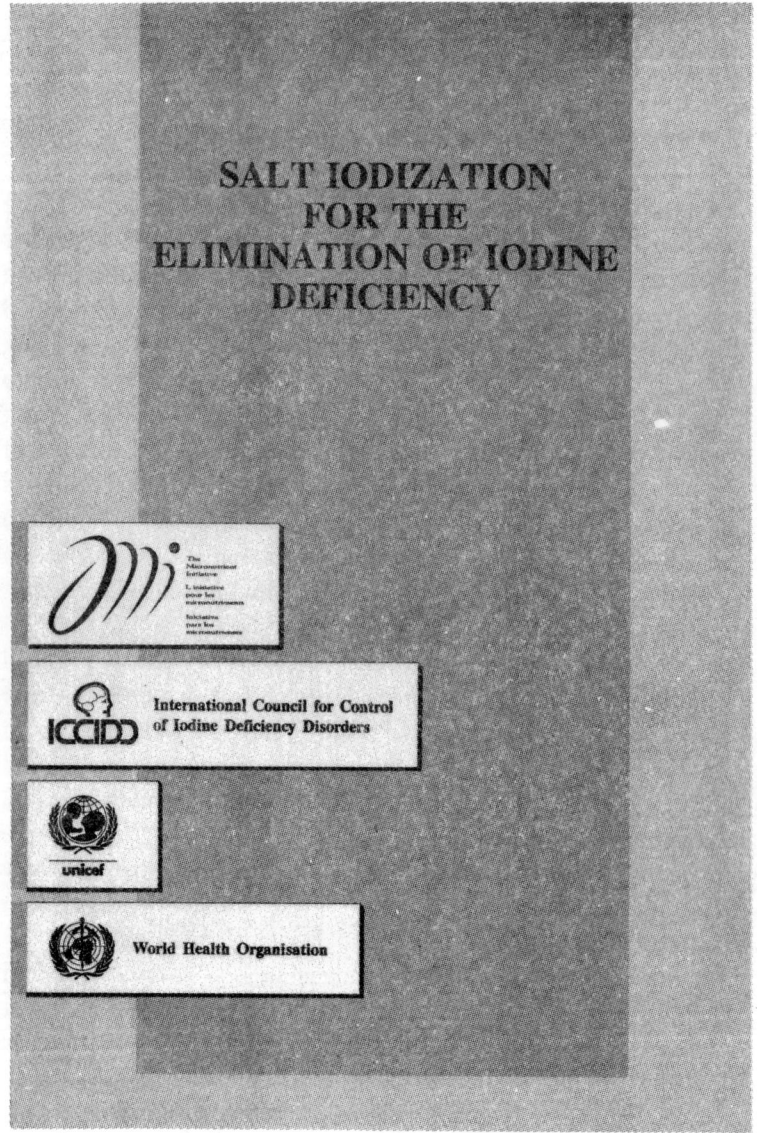

Fig. 5.1 Salt iodization for the elimination of iodine deficiency - A joint publication by ICCIDD/MI/UNICEF/WHO, 1995 which decribes in detail salt production and iodization, quality control, monitoring and marketing.

is the universal iodization of all the salt produced. The iodization should also include salt for livestock consumption.

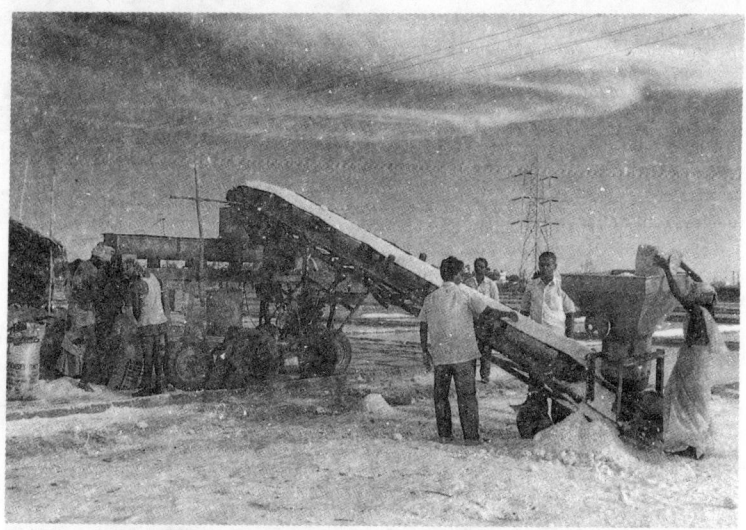

Fig. 5.2 A spray-mix iodization unit operating in Tuticorin, India.

By and large, the consensus is in favour of locating the plant at the production point or refining point just prior to packing the salt. Under proper iodization and packing conditions, iodized salt has been found to retain at least 75% of the iodine after nine months of storage. (Fig. 5.4) Once the iodization at source is accomplished at the prescribed level and the salt is packaged properly, losses during transit and storage will not be significant.

Salt Production and Distribution

Key considerations include:
* Salt producers are often a heterogeneous group consisting of private companies, co-operatives and individuals who may be operating outside any legal or administrative framework.

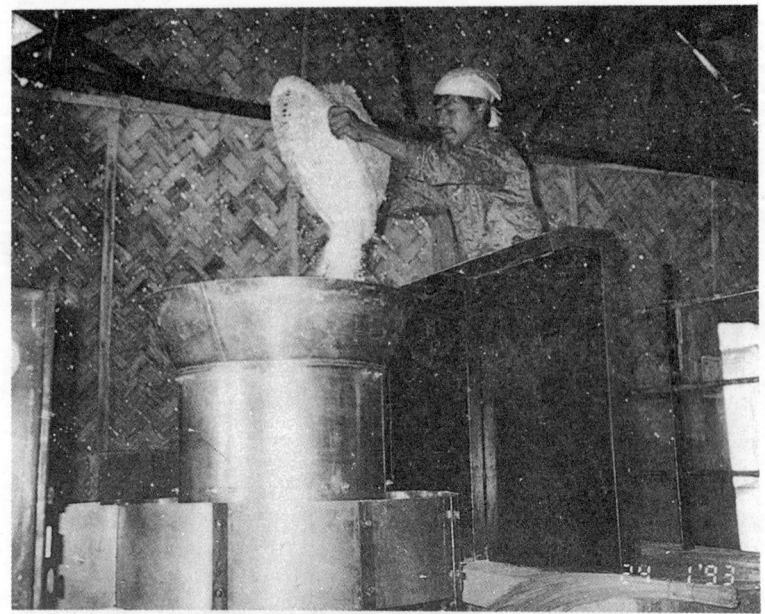

Fig. 5.3 Worker feeds an iodization plant in a salt refinery near Dhaka in Bangladesh.

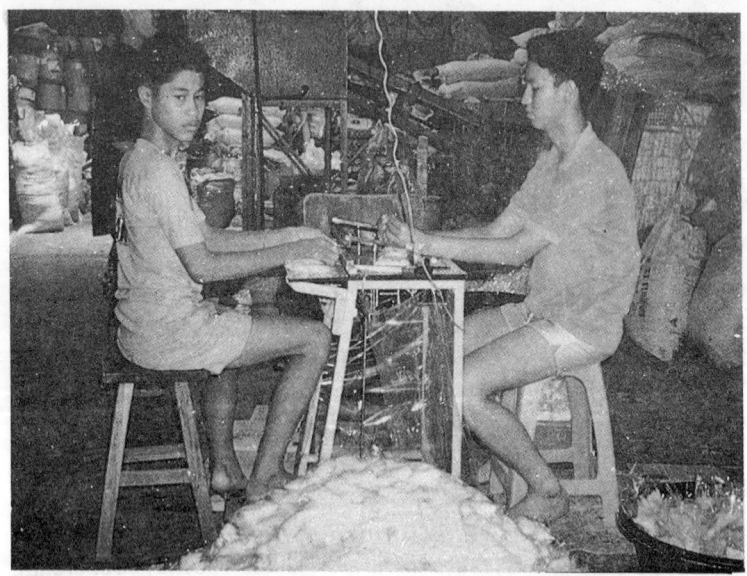

Fig. 5.4 Operation of an iodized salt packing line near Bangkong in Thailand.

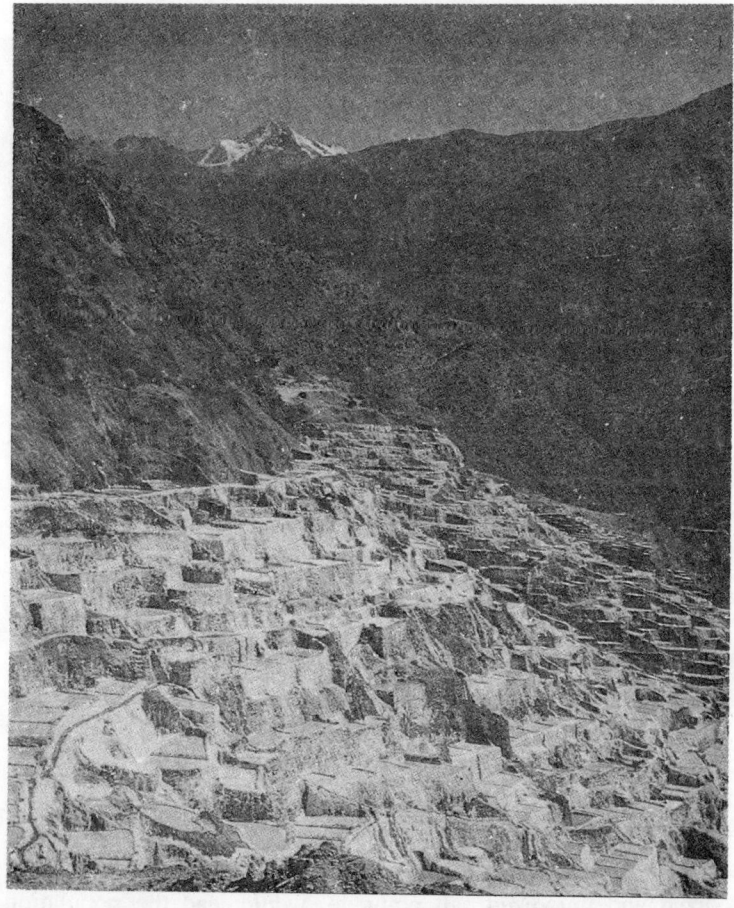

Fig. 5.5 Several thousand workers operate small salt ponds on the mountain in Maras, Peru.

* Multiple small salt producers and erratic distribution patterns make management of the programme difficult. (Fig.5.5)
* Primitive methods of production leads to poor salt quality, for example, with large crystals and impurities which affect iodine retention in salt. Visible impurities prompt householders to wash salt before cooking resulting in the loss of virtually all iodine.
* Inadequate packaging, for example in jute rather than high-density polyethylene, which aggravates iodine losses during transport, handling and storage.

The approach to these issues would be on the following lines:

i) Small farms should be brought under a system of registration by which they should periodically report to the appropriate local government authority on their area of operation and production and despatch figures (destination-wise) for monitoring of the distribution system.

ii) Wherever possible the small manufacturers should be organized into co-operatives for producing and marketing their salt. Where they are dispersed, the iodization and marketing of the iodized salt alone could be done on a co-operative basis. Long term financial support for equipment and supply of iodate may be required.

iii) Technical assistance should be made available to plan for and help upgrade the technology of production and processing of salt in such a way that its iodization would be easy.

Support Measures

Every successful salt iodization programme depends upon a number of support measures to enhance its effectiveness:

(i) **Advocacy and communication:** At the outset, there is the problem of inadequate awareness at several levels regarding the magnitude of the problem and its alleviation through salt iodization: at the policy making level, among medical professionals, the salt sector and the general public. Lack of awareness in a dual market, where both iodized and uniodized salt compete, would lead the population (especially the rural poor) to choose the uniodized salt even if it is only marginally cheaper. This can be overcome by assessing current knowledge, attitudes and practices towards IDD as well as salt purchase and consumption. Based on these perceptions, a comprehensive communications programme can be developed to address the different target groups. The object is to create a demand 'pull' for iodized salt to which the salt industry and trade will have to respond.

(ii) **Economic and Marketing incentives:** During the initial stages of the development of a programme, there will inevitably exist a dual market in which cheaper uniodized salt will compete with the more expensive iodized salt. (Fig. 5.6) Since the creation of consumer demand for the fortified product can be done only over a period of time, several countries have offered a package of assistance and incentives to producers during this crucial interim period.

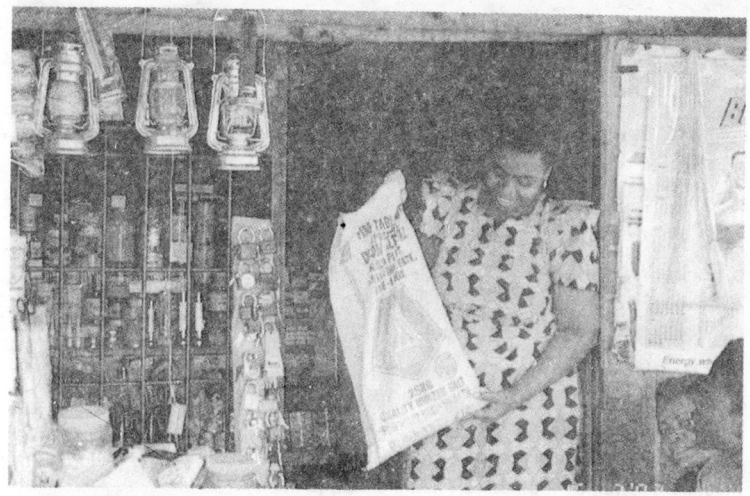

Fig. 5.6 Grocery store owner near Jos in Nigeria displays her stock of iodized salt.

(iii) **Legislation:** Programmes need to be supported with legislation mandating the universal iodization of all forms of salt (both for human and livestock consumption) and outlining enforcement procedures and penalties for noncompliance with specified salt quality, packing, labelling and iodine levels.

(iv) **Monitoring:** The success of the programme depends upon ensuring the specified iodine content in the salt at the consumer level. Towards this end, iodine levels in salt need to be monitored periodically from production to consumption (Fig. 5.7). Areas in which iodized salt is consumed less should be targeted for intensive education.

(v) **Administration and Co-ordination:** There should be adequate administrative, technical, financial and marketing support for the production and marketing of iodized salt, and also advocacy and monitoring. Usually a national advisory committee draws up a master plan and periodically reviews implementation.

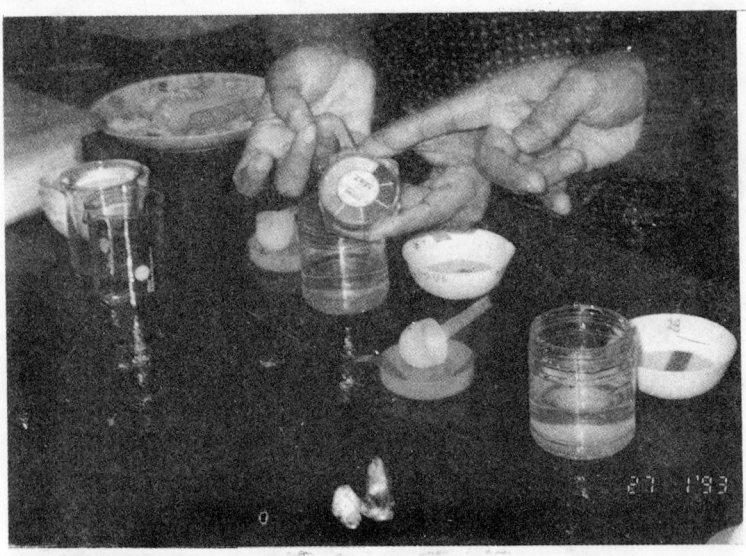

Fig. 5.7 Testing of iodized salt using a simple kit.

A specially appointed multisectoral IDD Commission is required to supervise the programme as described in other chapters in this book.

Characteristics of Effective Salt Iodization Programmes

While salt iodization is technically a straightforward process, its sustained large scale implementation calls for changes within political, administrative, technical and socio-cultural spheres.

Although in some countries, this process has run smoothly, others have been struggling for many years to establish effective salt iodization programmes. Information available on the experiences of various countries indicates that certain key issues have a bearing on the success of national programmes:

i. Policy support: Several health and nutrition programmes compete for priority action by policy makers. Raising the level of awareness about the problem and the effectiveness of its control within a short period through salt iodization has been an important factor in generating political will to support serious control and monitoring efforts. Awareness has been created by assessing and making available epidemiological information regarding IDD prevalence and the meaning of the data to high level politicians and bureaucrats. Initial promotion of the programme by convening a National Advocacy meeting and/or issue of a statement by the Head of State has been extremely effective in Philippines (Fig. 5.8) and China. Resolutions by regional groups like South Asian Association for Regional Co-operation (SAARC), Association of South East Asian Nations (ASEAN) and the Organization for African Unity (OAU) in Africa, calling for universal salt iodization, have also been effective in initiating action.

ii. Involvement of multiple sectors in the planning and administration of salt iodization programmes: While the responsibility for initiating, co-ordinating and monitoring an IDD elimination programme rests primarily with the health sector, its planning and implementation calls for the active involvement of other sectors like industry, trade, planning, transport, legislators, communicators and educators, in order to implement and integrate iodization into the salt production and distribution system. In countries like India, Sri Lanka, Bangladesh and Nepal, the industry sector is assigned the role of planning and implementing the iodization programme with the health sector providing financial and impact monitoring support.

iii. Strong advocacy with the salt manufacturing and trading community: Since the salt sector is a key player in the project, its motivation and involvement is an essential prerequisite. In several countries, the salt industry needs communications support and orientation, as well as technical, marketing and financial support. The commitment of one refiner in Cameroon who processes almost the entire requirements of that country and three or four neighbouring countries as well has led to effective iodization of all salt in that region. Strong support for salt iodization is a hallmark of Bolivia's small salt manufacturers. Organized into co-operatives, they receive ongoing technical support and educational workshops that foster commitment to the goal of IDD elimination. Similarly, Ecuador has placed emphasis on establishing good relationships with producers, explaining the goals of fortification and instituting annual information and motivation meetings. The Bangladesh Small Industries Corporation which oversees salt iodization in that country is in constant touch with salt crushers to understand their problems and needs. In India, workshops are held specifically for salt producers and traders to understand their problems. The Salt Commissioner in the Ministry of Industry has several officers who deal exclusively with the iodization programme. In China, a major UNDP/UNICEF assisted project has recently been launched to upgrade the salt industry to facilitate effective iodization.

iv. **Well conceived IEC campaigns incorporating a social marketing approach to educate consumers, generate demand for and to encourage the use of iodized salt:** In both Ecuador and Bolivia, rural consumers in particular had to be convinced of the importance of iodine to their health, since they had to expend scarce resources to pay the increased cost of iodized salt. A long-standing cultural acceptance of goitre as a normal condition in Bolivia and an absence of knowledge about the less obvious manifestations of IDD had to be addressed in educational strategies. Using a social marketing approach enhances the IEC component, by focusing messages on the perceptions and attitudes of consumers. In each case, the content of the educational messages are restricted to a few basic ideas. The actual communication of these messages occurs in a variety of ways—media, radio, television, traditional drama forms and one-on-one counselling. The use of multiplier educators—teachers, village health volunteers and local political leaders trained by IDD control programme staff, proved to be highly effective in Bolivia and Ecuador. IEC campaigns have greatly assisted programmes in Tanzania and Bangladesh.

v. Economic and marketing incentives: In almost all countries potassium iodate is provided free of cost to producers at least for the first 3 - 5 years. Thereafter the subsidy is phased out. In addition, Brazil has donated iodization equipment and provides technical assistance in production and quality control to producers. Bolivia guarantees the sale

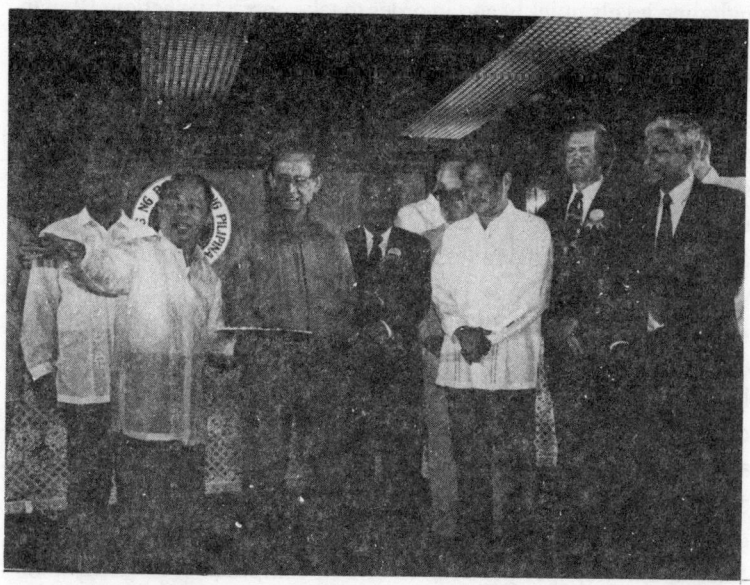

Fig. 5.8 Advocacy plays a big role in salt iodization programmes. President Ramos inaugurating the programme in the Philippines.

wagons for iodized salt movement and promotes marketing by progressively banning the entry of uniodized salt into the endemic of iodized salt once it is produced. India offers priority allotment of rail wagons for iodized salt movement and promotes marketing by progressively banning the entry of uniodized salt into the endemic States. Bhutan and Ethiopia provide even the packing material free of charge. Compared with most consumer products, salt fortification subsidies are small but play a crucial role during initial promotion. Their withdrawal has to be in a phased manner. In some countries like Indonesia and India, sudden withdrawal of the iodate subsidy led to problems.

vi. Monitoring of iodine levels in salt: Frequent testing of iodine levels at iodization plants and periodically at intermediate points in the distribution network, retail outlets and the household level has been characteristic of countries with successful programmes. Ecuador and Brazil sampled salt on a weekly basis at production plants during the early phases of the Fortification programme in order to detect variability in iodine levels quickly and in order to take corrective action. Bhutan has developed a systematic monitoring and reporting system for iodine levels at the production level, at important distribution (retail) points and at consumer level. The reports are reviewed centrally every month and correctives initiated where required. The involvement of other sectors like NGO's, voluntary organizations, and schools in the salt monitoring, using the low cost field test kits is another useful exercise and helps increase awareness and community participation.

vii. Legislation and enforcement: By legislation, Bolivia and Brazil have fairly successfully precluded the use of cheaper, unfortified animal salt by rural populations (while at the same time providing the benefits of iodine to livestock in iodine deficient regions). Enforcement of the regulation has proved critical to ensuring the quality of iodized salt, especially in countries such as Bolivia, where there are multiple small producers. When identified by inspectors, uniodized salt is confiscated or destroyed. In Ecuador, legal sanctions in the form of fines and newspaper publication of non-compliant brand names are used for purposes of quality control. For many years in Kenya, uniodized salt was allowed in the market as long as it was labeled as 'lacking a necessary nutrient'. This legal loophole was plugged in 1988.

viii. Financial and technical assistance by external donors: This has been critical to the success of initial and often ongoing efforts for salt iodization in many countries. In almost all developing countries, international financing has been responsible for the establishment of IDD elimination programmes under which salt iodization is implemented. External technical consultations and international training of national technical staff involved in all phases of the fortification contributed to the development of iodization activities. External financial support for the import of iodization equipment, quality control accessories and iodine for an initial period has also been a key input. International agencies have also played an important co-ordinating role between the different sectors.

ix. Programme monitoring: Systems should be functional from the outset of the iodization programme with rapid analysis and dissemination of data to keep the managers informed of the decisions regarding mid-programme changes and corrective actions at production sites. Ecuador and Bhutan analyse their cumulative salt sampling data at regular intervals and communicate results to the involved industry representatives and health personnel.

x. Programme leadership: In Bolivia and Ecuador, the role that individual leadership played in the progress of salt fortification programmes deserves note. Perseverance during early years of governmental inaction despite the knowledge of goitre prevalence, and willingness to participate at the local level programme activities characterizes the administration of both the country programmes.

xi. Regional co-operation: An innovative regional strategy has been initiated for countries in sub-Saharan Africa to ensure that all salt produced for human and animal consumption is iodized at source. Salt producing and importing countries from 9 southern and central African countries met in April 1992 to work out a regional strategy to ensure that all salt produced for human and animal consumption is iodized at a uniform concentration. A similar meeting for the west and central African countries was held in October 1992. Similar meetings are planned for other regions like central America and south-east Asia.

Salt Industry Participation in IDD Elimination

Over the past decade there has been a world wide movement by consumer groups to raise the industry's conscience to participate in tackling social and environmental problems. The industry has responded to this call by including these considerations as part of its corporate philosophy. Viewed from this angle, IDD elimination presents an opportunity for the salt industry to derive economic and social benefits for itself while simultaneously providing a social benefit to the community by fortifying the salt it produces and sells.

Salt iodization programmes are a unique example wherein an industry and trade which have so far been working in a largely commercial environment are required to participate and play a leading role in a health intervention endeavour. In order to have an effective and sustained salt iodization programme, it is vital for the Health Ministry and the salt industry to work in close collaboration, explicitly understanding and recognizing each other's view points, concerns and interests.

Conclusion

Iodine deficiency disorders are still a major public health problem in many countries of the world, in spite of the fact that the technology available for its prevention makes this problem the most amenable of the nutritional deficiencies to quick and effective control.

The goal of universal iodization of all human and animal salt in the world by the end of 1995 is a lofty target. However, it can be achieved with strong political commitment and industry motivation supported by effective and continuous monitoring and regulation. We are on the threshold of eliminating the scourge of iodine deficiency disorders from the earth and should institute sustainable systems supported with essential technical and financial inputs to ensure that it will never recur in future.

6

The Use of Iodized Oil and other Alternatives for the elimination of Iodine Deficiency Disorders

J.T. Dunn

The objective of any iodization programme is to correct iodine deficiency as quickly, effectively and economically as possible. In concept, both the problem and its solution are straightforward—people are iodine deficient and therefore need to receive more iodine. As pointed out in the preceding chapter, salt is a nearly ideal vehicle for iodization. Its advantages include a universal, constant human need for salt, the relative ease of controlling its access and delivery, and the availability of simple effective technology for iodization. Prompt implementation of salt iodization is easy in countries where there is controlled access to salt, high quality salt and packaging, and a receptive government, public, and producers. In other countries, implementation of salt iodization may be a tortuous process as at least several years may be required to overcome logistic, political and economic constraints. In such countries an aggressive drive for salt iodization should be pursued, but at the same time alternative measures for prompt and temporary correction of iodine deficiency are also needed. These major alternatives, in approximate order of importance, are iodized vegetable oil, iodized water, iodine drops or tablets, and fortification of other foods.

Iodized Oil

Iodized vegetable oils have long been used as contrast dyes in diagnostic X-ray procedures. One of the most widely used, Lipiodol, contains 480 mg of iodine, covalently bound to 1 ml of poppy seed oil. Its use for the correction of iodine deficiency resulted from the observation of its persistence in the body after a single injection in patients suffering from lung diseases. This led to the suggestion of its use by a chest physician in Papua New Guinea, Dr D Jamieson, to one of his patients Dr John Gunther, at that time Director of Public Health. It was seen as particularly appropriate for people living in isolated and severely iodine deficient mountain villages where salt distribution was difficult to achieve.

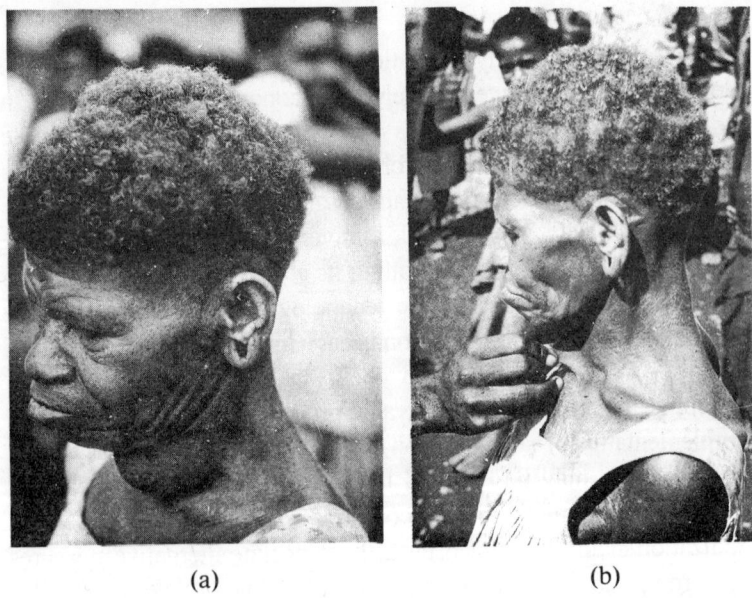

(a) (b)

Fig. 6.1 Subsidence of goitre in a New Guinea woman three months after the injection of iodized oil. This is accompanied by a feeling of well-being due to a rise in the level of the thyroid hormone in the blood. This makes the injections very popular (From Buttfield and Hetzel 1967 with permission).

Several field trials followed which indicated that a single injection of iodized oil would prevent goitre over a period of 3 years (McCullagh 1963) and provide adequate correction of severe iodine deficiency for over 4 years depending on the dosage used. Regression of goitre is often observed (Fig 6.1). Removal of hypothyroidism leads to greatly increased vitality (Fig 6.2. Buttfield and Hetzel 1967). The measure has now been widely used throughout the world in maternal and child health units (Fig 6.3).

Recent years have brought increasing attention to the oral administration of iodized oil. This route is logistically more attractive than the intramuscular one because it does not require skilled injectors, needles or syringes, and avoids transmission of diseases such as AIDS and hepatitis. However, the duration of the effect is shorter, because there is no intramuscular storage. In most instances the advantages of oral administration outweigh its drawbacks, except in geographic areas where the group targeted for iodized oil administration is very difficult to reach, and the longer duration of the effect of intramuscular oil is particularly valuable.

Several recent studies have examined the optimal dose and duration of effect for oral iodized oil. In one investigation in young adults, small doses containing 120 mg of iodine seemed satisfactory for coverage for a period of six months to a year. A collaborative study of school children in Algeria, India, and Peru showed that a dose of 480 mg of iodine is barely adequate for a year's coverage, and half that dose gave satisfactory coverage for six months. A new preparation, Oriodol, from Guerbet, the manufacturer of Lipiodol, appears equally effective for oral administration and is less expensive because the pharmacological requirements for oral use are less stringent.

As an example, Nepal has had an intramuscular iodized oil programme for more than 15 years. Each year specific districts are targeted for administration. Local residents familiar with the area and its customs are trained in injection techniques. They then move in two-person teams throughout the district, injecting as many people in the targeted area as possible, relying heavily on local civic and health authorities for assistance in making contact. Iodized oil administrations are usually

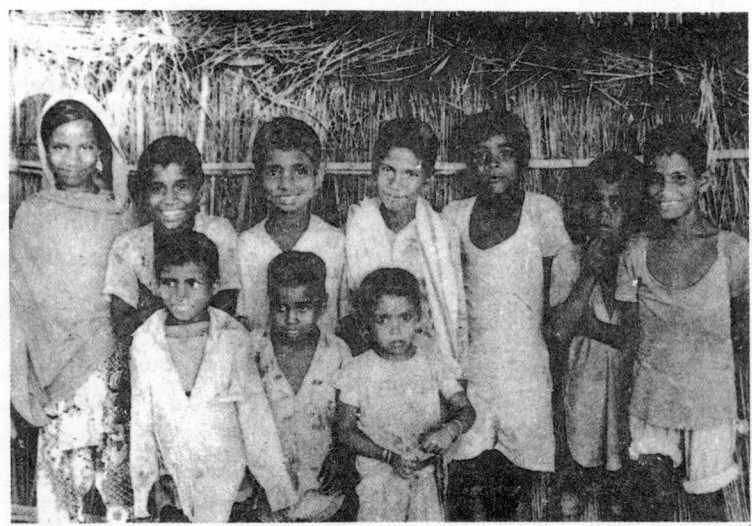

Fig. 6.2 A group of lively Indian children from Deoria, Utter Pradesh, India who had received iodized oil injections six months before this photograph was taken (From Hetzel 1989 with permission).

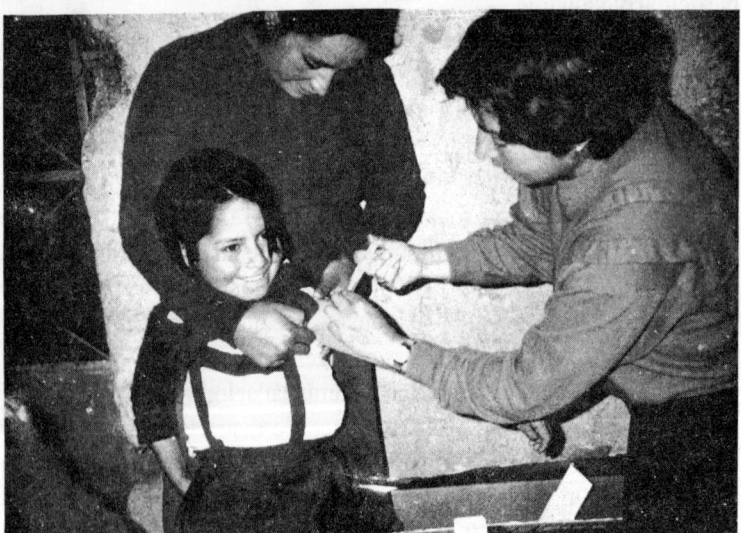

Fig. 6.3 Young girl in Bolivia receiving an injection of iodized oil in a maternal and child health clinic. Large quantities of iodized oil have been given in these clinics throughout the world (From Hetzel 1989 with permission).

repeated after four or five years. A programme begun in Zaire in the late 1970's involved three mobile teams that moved throughout the iodine-deficient area injecting as many subjects as possible. Injections can also be administered through the primary health care system rather than by specialized teams.

Campaigns with oral iodized oil have also been conducted either by specialized teams or through the primary health care system. A recent example is Bolivia, where 1.5 million doses of oral iodized oil were administered over a period of several months, targeting rural areas with significant iodine deficiency and that were unlikely to have access to iodized salt for several years. This rapid distribution was possible through the involvement of community members who were designated to link up with more centralized health authorities. In many other countries, oral iodized oil is distributed through the primary health care system, either as part of regular contacts for other health matters or in specialized campaigns.

Compared to iodized salt, iodized oil has several distinct disadvantages. First, oral administration requires direct contact with every targeted subject and this takes more effort and expense than mass prophylaxis through the salt distribution channels. Also, the oil is given only at infrequent intervals as compared to the constant daily ration which is received with iodized salt. Therefore, body stores of iodine will be quite high shortly after administration and then taper off to low levels later on. While bolus administration is unphysiologic, the human body can fortunately tolerate large amounts of iodine with few significant complications. The major advantage of iodized oil administration is that it can be implemented immediately, and does not involve the complexities of altering salt production and trade. Thus, the usual places for iodized oil are for areas of significant iodine deficiency where iodized salt is unlikely to be successfully implemented soon and correction is needed promptly. In many such areas the iodized oil programme will be necessary for at least several years, and for some remote areas it may be semi-permanent (Dunn 1987)

The strategy for administering iodized oil must be tailored to the particular situation of the individual country or region. Lipiodol currently costs about US$0.14 for a 200 mg iodine capsule or for a 200 mg solution; each syringe and needle for injection costs about US$0.30. Oriodol, in a dispenser, costs about US$0.04 for 200 mg. The most important goal is to prevent brain damage in the developing human. Therefore, the target groups in order of priority are women of childbearing age, neonates, young children, older children and adult men.

Frequently, it is not possible to exclude a group, such as village men, so that it is more practical to administer the iodized oil to everyone.

Iodized Water

Water, like salt, is a dietary necessity, and must be consumed daily. Therefore, water is another physiologically ideal vehicle for introducing iodine. Its big drawback as compared to salt is that sources of drinking water are ubiquitous and therefore, very difficult to control. Nevertheless, under favourable circumstances, water iodization is a reasonable method for the correction of iodine deficiency.

Several techniques are available. The simplest one adds drops from a concentrated iodine solution, usually in the form of potassium iodate or potassium iodide, to standing water in vessels used for drinking. This method has been introduced by Dr Romsai Suwanik of Bangkok. It is widely used in schools of northern Thailand and even in households. Such an approach costs only the price of the iodine solution itself, but it requires constant supervision at the local level to see that the correct amount of iodine is actually added (Dunn 1987).

Another method at the community level is the introduction of porous polymer vessels containing iodine into the water supply, either in hand pumps or into open well water. The design of these containers allows the potassium iodide solution within the vessel to be slowly released into the well water. This system can run free of trouble for about a year (Fisch et al 1993).

In still another approach, a portion of the water flowing through pipes is diverted through a canister packed with crystals of iodine, and then reintroduced into the mainstream. The amount of iodination can be controlled by the amount of water diverted through the canister. This system has been applied in Thailand, Malaysia, and Sicily, among others countries. It requires some maintenance and monitoring of iodine levels, but is easy to operate and very inexpensive, even though most tap water is not used for drinking (Squatrito et al 1986).

Iodine at a level of 500 µg/l has been used in community water supplies to reduce bacterial pollution. This iodine is available to the thyroid, and will certainly correct any iodine deficiency present, without any apparent problems from excessive iodine intake. In Sicily the iodine level in the water was set at 50 µg/l, somewhat below levels that are bactericidal. A mild medicinal taste was described when the iodine concentration was greater than 200 µg/l, but there were no complaints when it was below 120 µg/l. There has been continued interest in the possibility of using iodine to correct iodine deficiency and purify water at the same time. Many rural communities in developing countries share both the problems; so a joint solution would be attractive, and further investigation is needed. Only iodine in the chemical form is effective; potassium iodide and potassium iodate are not.

One of the first programmes of water iodization was implemented in Rochester, New York, 70 years ago. Bags of sodium iodide were simply thrown into a reservoir's inflow stream several times over two five-week periods each year. This approach was successful as shown by adequate iodine levels in the water consumed in the city and a decrease in goitre prevalence in school children.

Direct Iodine Supplements

The circumstances where iodized salt or other alternatives are not readily available, iodine supplements in the form of tablets or drops can successfully correct iodine deficiency. In Germany, for example, tablets containing from 100-500 mg of potassium iodide are available for daily consumption. In Sucre, Bolivia, local health authorities have mixed concentrated solutions of potassium iodide and distributed them to schools and households with instructions on proper daily administration. Such daily dosing with iodine is highly effective and relatively inexpensive. Its major drawback is that it requires the constant attention of responsible individuals to see that the iodine is actually ingested. This supervision is difficult to maintain in most public health programmes in developing countries.

Recent efforts have examined the longest interval feasible between administrations of iodine. As a historical example, the first organized attempt at prophylaxis in this century was made in Akron, Ohio, by Marine and Kimball. They gave school children 180 mg of sodium iodide over a ten-day period twice a year, and observed a marked decrease in goitre. A current trial using either potassium iodide or Lugol's iodine in school children in Bolivia and Zimbabwe is showing that administration of 8 mg of iodine every two weeks or 29 mg every month provides adequate iodine levels, and that 148 mg every three months is barely adequate. Thus, in some settings, such as schools, it would appear quite feasible to administer potassium iodide or Lugol's iodine every month, or perhaps every three months. Given the supervision of a responsible person, the administration itself is quite cheap. Lugol's solution contains about 6 mg of iodine per drop. It is widely available in rural pharmacies for use as a wound disinfectant and can be easily adapted for oral prophylaxis of iodine deficiency. This approach is worth remembering in circumstances where a responsible person, such as a medical missionary or nurse, is available and can oversee the programme with minimal financial resources. However, it will be difficult to apply to a large population because of the high demands on individual responsibility.

Other Alternatives

In principle, virtually any food can be used for fortification with iodine. Salt and water are especially suitable because they are a dietary necessity that everyone must consume. The problem with using other foodstuffs as vehicles is that their intake is not essential, and frequently they are not consumed by those most vulnerable to iodine deficiency – women, children, the poor and the isolated.

Therefore, it is not often that other foodstuffs deserve serious consideration as primary vehicles for correcting iodine deficiency. Occasionally, however, special circumstances in a particular community may justify their use.

One example is the iodization of brick tea in Tibet. This beverage is widely consumed by children and women as well as by men. The sources of production and distribution are easier to control than those for salt. Thus, for this population, brick tea provides a workable alternative. Its success depends on the accuracy of the assurance that women, children, and poor isolated families all drink enough brick tea to obtain adequate iodine.

Iodine has also been added to bread, sugar, and candy. Although it is effective, each of these foodstuffs risk maldistribution in the diets of a community, and therefore, wide variations in iodine intake may result.

Interest in fortifying food with iodine is increasing. This development is welcome when the iodized food is viewed as an addition rather than as an alternative to iodized salt. Usually this fortification will be in processed foods and beverages that are more likely to reach the urban affluent rather than the poor rural communities with iodine deficiency. However, such additional fortification can help in areas where the iodized salt programme is absent or not working well. Even if a fully effective salt iodization programme is in place, additional iodine from foods is unlikely to have adverse effects, because the safety level for iodine tolerance is very high.

Dietary diversification deserves a mention as a passive alternative or addition to iodized salt. This occurs when iodine is occasionally introduced into foods for commercial rather than health reasons. For example, iodate was widely used in the United States and elsewhere as a bread conditioner in the baking industry. Iodine finds its way into meat and dairy products through the use of iodine solutions in cleaning udders and from iodinated medicines used for treating cattle disease. Various grain grown in iodine-sufficient fields may provide supplementary iodine when ingested in iodine-deficient areas, as well as elsewhere. Advances in food preservation and transportation now make iodine-rich foods from the ocean more easily available in the inland areas that frequently harbour iodine deficiency. Many vitamin preparations add iodine specifically, and other medicines may have iodine as part of the chemical formulation.

A combination of these factors has eliminated iodine deficiency in many industrialized countries such as the United States. However, these sources depend on commercial rather than health trends, and it is unreliable to base an iodine deficiency correction programme solely on them.

In summary, salt is generally the best vehicle for iodine prophylaxis. When its effective implementation is delayed, the most useful alternatives are iodized oil, iodized water, iodine tablets, or Lugol's iodine. Oil, tablets, or solution involve the disadvantages of repeated administration, direct contact with each individual and target, and changing the amount of iodine availability between doses, but they can be administered promptly without waiting for the delays associated with restructuring the salt industry.

References

Buttfield, I.H. and B.S., Hetzel, 1967. 'Endemic Goitre in Eastern New Guinea with special reference to the use of iodized oil in prophylaxis and treatment' *Bull World Health Organization*. 36:243-62.

Dunn, J.T. 1987. 'Iodized oil in the treatment and prophylaxis of IDD'. In Hetzel, B.S., J.T., Dunn and J.B. Stanbury eds. *The prevention and control of iodine deficiency disorders*. pp.121.

Fisch, A., E., Pichard, T., Prazuck, et al. 1993. 'A new approach to combating iodine deficiency in developing countries: the controlled release of iodine in water by a silicone elastomer' *Amer. J Public Health*. 83:540-45.

McCullagh, S.F. 1963. 'The Huon Peninsula Endemic: I. The effectiveness of an intramuscular depot of iodized oil in the control of endemic goitre'. *Med J Australia*. 1:767-79.

Squatrito, S., R., Vigneri, F., Runello, A.M., Ermans, R.D., Polley, S.H., Ingbar, 1986. 'Prevention and treatment of endemic iodine-deficiency goitre by iodination of a municipal water supply'. *J Clin Endocrinol Metab*. 63:368-372.

7

The Economic Benefits of the Elimination of IDD

C.S. Pandav

Iodine Deficiency Disorders (IDD), one of the three important micronutrient deficiencies are a major health problem of the world. The wide spectrum of the disorders that IDD encompasses, both in man and animals results in its having a significant impact of the social and economic development of the population. For the control of IDD, certain inputs in terms of money, material and manpower are needed. A programme for the control of IDD is worthwhile only if the costs detailed in controlling it are lower than the benefits which accrue as a result. This chapter examines the costs and benefits of elimination of IDD.

Until recently the problem of iodine deficiency was being viewed as limited to goitre. As pointed out in Chapter 1, this view however no longer adequately reflects the current knowledge on the subject as we know that iodine deficiency causes a spectrum of disorders (Hetzel 1987). Its most important effects are on the growth and development of the foetus, the neonate and the child. These effects are manifested as endemic cretinism (characterized most commonly as mental deficiency), milder forms of mental and motor impairment, stillbirths and neonatal deaths. Goitre is important because it serves as a marker for the severity of iodine deficiency. In the wake of the information available and knowledge of the subject, the prevention and control of IDD justifies a much higher priority. Apart from minimizing human misery, the prevention of IDD would mean that more and better education can be imparted to children, greater productivity can be achieved, and a better quality of life would be possible for the millions living in the iodine deficient areas of the world.

As pointed out in Chapter 1, iodine deficiency is a major impedment to human development (Hetzel 1988). However the positive aspect of this disease is that it is easily preventable.

There is overwhelming evidence available to prove that IDD can be successfully prevented by iodine supplementation. All strategies for the prevention and control of iodine deficiency are ultimately based on some form of iodine supplementation. Iodized salt and iodized oil (by injection or orally) are suitable for the correction of iodine deficiency on a mass scale.

Priority target groups which are at high risk are women in the childbearing age group of 15 to 44 years and children in the age group of 0 to 14 years.

In some cases, IDD control programmes have been successfully integrated into the existing primary health care systems. In Nepal, for example, innovative approaches of recruiting local health personnel for iodized oil injection programmes have been adopted. In other countries such as India and Bhutan, the monitoring of iodine content in salt has been integrated with the primary health care system (Acharya 1991). The results of controlled trials with iodized salt in the Kangra valley in India by Sooch and Ramalingaswami et al (1965) and (1973) have demonstrated prevention and reduction in the prevalence of endemic goitre. A controlled trial with injections of iodized oil in Papua New Guinea has demonstrated the prevention of cretinism provided the injection was given before pregnancy (Pharoah et al 1971). Controlled trials of iodized oil in Zaire (Thilly et al 1980) have shown a reduction in perinatal and infant mortality and an improvement in birth weight. In a number of iodization programmes a reduction in stillbirths has also been reported (McMichael et al 1980).

Economic Evaluation

Considering the scarcity of resources, especially in the developing countries, there is a greater responsibility on society to strike the most favourable balance between the health benefits achieved and the cost incurred. Here, the concept of cost implies the sacrifice society must make by choosing one programme in preference to an alternative. The link between the scarcity of resources and sacrifices can be best described as 'opportunity cost', that is, when a resource is used for one purpose, the opportunity to use it for another purpose is lost. Economic analysis is important in the planning and execution of the IDD programme as it focuses on the cost efficient use of resources.

It places a monetary value on the results of the correction of iodine deficiency and allows a comparison with the benefits from the use of resources for other health programmes and other programmes for the benefit of society.

Economic evaluation in the health care sector consists of comparing two or more health care interventions in terms of their cost and consequences. There are two objectives in the economic evaluation: first; to introduce resources consideration into the analysis and to assess the opportunity cost of new procedures and programmes (preventive, diagnostic, therapeutic, rehabilitative) second; to develop a framework within which the costs of the new procedures or programmes can be compared to their benefits. These characteristics of the economic evaluation make a valuable contribution to rational decision making. The objective of economic evaluation is to identify the alternative that yields the greater benefit for the given cost.

Types of Economic Evaluations

There are three types of economic evaluation or analyses.
(i) cost-effectiveness analysis
(ii) cost-utility analysis
(iii) cost-benefit analysis

The process of identification, measurement and valuation of costs associated with each alternative are identical in all three methods. The difference is only in the way the consequences (outcome) of the alternative are measured and valued (Fig. 7.1). However, in any given economic evaluation, the consequences of different alternatives must be measured in the identical units.

Cost-effectiveness analysis provides for the choice of the most effective strategy at the least cost. Here the outcome is measured in natural units, i.e., life years gained, the number of cases of cretinism averted. The measure of efficiency is the cost per unit outcome obtained. This is also known as the cost- effectiveness ratio. The alternative with the smallest cost-effectiveness ratio is technically the most efficient one for the desired outcome.

In **Cost-utility analysis,** outcomes are expressed in such a manner that the qualitative as well as quantitative dimensions of the health outcome are considered. The outcome measures most often measured are: quality adjusted life years (QALY) or health years equivalent (HYEs). The measure of efficiency is the cost per QALY or the cost per HYE. The cost utility analysis can be viewed as a step beyond cost effectiveness analysis in which the objective is to measure outcome in such a manner that both life years gained and the quality or desirability of those life years are reflected.

Cost-benefit analysis is a useful tool to establish the priority of a particular health service action. In this both inputs and outputs are measured in monetary terms. Cost-benefit analysis is probably most useful for health programmes that have a major impact on economic development.

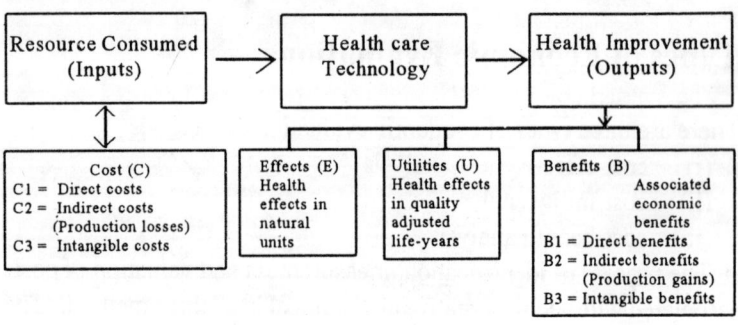

Fig. 7.1 Components of economic evaluation.

Source: Adapted with kind permission from Methods for the economic evalution of health care programmes edited by M F Drummond, G L Stoddart and G W Torrance.

In economic analysis the first step is to estimate the cost of the intervention that is being used for control or prevention. In order to control IDD, iodine supplementation either by an iodized salt programme or an iodized oil programme would be in operation ad infinitum and hence costs for these programmes will be incurred in perpetuity. The iodized salt programme has capital costs as well as annual operating costs. The capital costs are incurred at the beginning of the programme. The iodized oil programme has no capital costs and the operating costs are incurred only for the first year of the five year injection cycle.

Therefore, one of the main objectives in the economic evaluation of IDD control programmes is to calculate the costs of the salt programme and iodized oil programme for a 'given year'. This would constitute the equivalent annual cost. The next step is the identification, measurement and valuation of the consequences of the prevention programme that is being adopted. For this purpose the consequences related to preventing IDD can be classified as follows:

i) Those related to the changes in physical, social or emotional functioning, that is, health effects.

ii) Those related to the change in resource use, i.e., costs averted and productivity gains.

iii) Those related to the change in the quality of life of patients and their families.

The averted costs to the government health care system are in the form of reduced treatment costs associated with the prevention of IDD. The productivity gains are measured by the human capital approach. In this approach, the health care programmes are viewed as an investment in people. This investment enables the people to be more productive and to increase their material well-being. The increase in productivity associated with better health status, therefore, is one kind of benefit.

The full consequences of IDD, however, go far beyond the cost averted and lost work time and cannot be realized in these limited measures of the benefits of the IDD control programmes. These are the ones to which monetary value could be assigned and therefore are the only ones that explicitly enter the cost benefit analysis. However, there are benefits associated with health outcome itself. People prefer to be healthy. A comprehensive 'willingness to pay' methodology could potentially capture all these benefits associated with an improved health outcome.

Table 7.1 *Effects of iodine intervention and measurements of benefits**

HUMAN POPULATIONS	
Effects	Benefits
Reductions in: 1. Mental deficiency 2. Deaf-mutism 3. Spastic diplegia 4. Squint 5. Dwarfism 6. Motor deficiency	1. Value of higher work output in the household and labour market. 2. Reduced cost of medical and custodial care 3. Reduced educational costs from reduced absenteeism and grade repetition and higher academic achievement by studies.
LIVESTOCK POPULATIONS	
Effects	Benefits
Increase in: 1. Live births 2. Weight 3. Strength 4. Health (less deformity) 5. Wool coats in sheep	1. Value of higher output of meat and other animal products 2. Value of higher animal work output

* From Levin et al (1991).

None of the studies on the economic benefits of IDD elimination have considered the impact it has on livestock. Farm animals are equally at risk to the spectrum of iodine deficiency disorders at all stages of growth and development, from conception to adult physical performance in farm animals. Reproductive failure is the outstanding manifestation of iodine deficiency in farm animals. Foetal development may be arrested at any stage, leading to either death and resorption, abortion and stillbirth, or the birth of young ones that are weak, often associated with prolonged gestation and retention of foetal membranes. More kids are born to iodine-sufficient goats and they are twice as likely to survive as those born to iodine-deficient goats.

In addition to the reproductive disturbances described, infertility, both male and female, has been associated with goitre and shown to respond to iodine therapy in iodine deficient areas. The full effects of iodine supplementation are shown in Table 7.1. The consumption of iodized salt by the farm animals will add to the economic productivity of the population. Thus the cost-benefit ratio of iodine supplementation programmes will increase significantly, making a programme a worthwhile investment, not only for better human resource development, but also to add to the economic contribution from the farm animal sector.

Economic Evaluation of IDD in Different Countries

Information on economic evaluation of IDD in Germany, Ecuador and India with a case study from one of the states – Sikkim is briefly described in the following section.

Germany

Direct and Indirect costs caused by Iodine Deficiency

The study on direct and indirect costs caused by iodine deficiency by Pfannensteil (1985) examines only the cost of IDD and as such is only a descriptive one. There is no comparison of alternatives. Expenses incurred by different agencies for the diagnosis and treatment of endemic goitre have been taken as costs i.e. the view point is that of the health (insurance) agencies, both public and private.

In 1981 the total expenses incurred in the diagnosis of endemic goitre by social security companies, private insurance companies and the government was 510 million DM. Since 90% of the goitre in Germany is due to iodine deficiency, 459 million DM were attributed to the costs incurred for the diagnosis of endemic goitre.

The costs of the treatment of endemic goitre was estimated by totalling expenses on thyroid hormone replacement, hospital expenses for the treatment of goitre, and payments made by the employers or insurance companies to the patients who were unable to work as a result of surgery. In all 680,000 days were spent in the hospital by goitre patients amounting to 150 million DM. The payment by insurance companies to these patients as compensation was 45 million DM. A sum of 65 million DM were spent on the drugs (mainly hormones). Thus the total costs of the treatment of endemic goitre in Germany for the year 1981 was 260 million DM.

In short, a total expense of 710 million DM was incurred in 1981 in Germany for the complete management of endemic goitre. The importance of this descriptive study is that it identified the costs required for the treatment of endemic goitre in an iodine deficient environment.

Cost and benefits of goitre prevention

The annual costs for the diagnosis and treatment of goitre due to iodine deficiency for Germany (unified) for the year 1992 was 2 billion DM (Gutekunst 1990). As a part of the strategy under the national goitre control programme, early detection by paediatric standard examination, prenatal care and routine health checks would be carried out. The investigation to be done for early detection was ultrasonography and those detected as having endemic goitre would be put on iodide.

These measures would in total cost 122 million DM. These measures would reduce the problem of endemic goitre by 70%. Thus the costs averted would be 70% of 2 billion DM (1.4 billion DM). Thus by spending 122 million DM, 1.4 billion DM could be saved or a cost benefit balance of 1.3 billion DM would result per year.

Ecuador

Cost Benefit Study of Iodine Supplementation programmes for the prevention of Endemic Goitre and Cretinism.

The study on Cost Benefit of iodine supplementation programmes for the prevention of Endemic goitre and cretinism by Correa (1980) evaluated the relationship between endemic goitre, endemic cretinism, intelligence (measured by IQ) and the income of the population with and without an iodine supplementation programme. The costs of iodine supplementation programmes were taken from different published studies and as well as personal communication. The cost per person per year ranged from US$ 0.0025 to US$ 0.100 in these studies. For intramuscular iodized oil, the estimated cost was US$ 0.4338 per person per year.

Among the consequences, the study assumed benefits of the iodine supplementation programmes on higher earnings associated with reduction in mental deficiencies. From the data on goitre and cretinism, the IQ of the population was estimated.

Information available on the impact of iodine supplementation programmes in the form of iodized salt and iodized oil in Ecuador and Peru was used to estimate the impact of iodine supplementation on endemic cretinism and the average IQ. On the basis of this estimate, it was found that an iodine supplementation programme can effect an increase in the mean IQ of the goitrous population by 10.92 points. Subsequently the relationship between IQ and per capita income was estimated. These results were used to estimate the impact of changes in IQ generated by iodine supplementation on per capita income and these constituted the estimated economic benefit of iodine supplementation programmes.

Since the increased IQ of the children would produce economic benefits only after several years, in the computations it was assumed that such increase would begin to take place 15 years later. In agreement with the assumption about costs, it was assumed that the benefits of the programme would be received in perpetuity, after the initial delay of 15 years. According to this study, the benefits of reducing mild iodine deficiency among children, in terms of improvements in their lifetime earnings, considerably exceeded the costs of the interventions.

Hershman (1986) used the data from the above study in Ecuador to estimate the relationship between the incidence of cretinism and the overall IQ of the population. Using regression analysis, he calculated the change in the IQ of the population that would occur if the incidence of cretinism decreased. The impact of the change in the IQ on per capita income was calculated. It was estimated that a 20% reduction in cretinism would lead to a 4.7% increase in the per capita income.

This estimate was used to calculate the aggregate effects in the following example: A country has an annual per capita income of US$ 1,000 and has a population of one million with a prevalence of 5% cretinism. A 20% reduction in cretinism (that is to 4%), in the population would increase the annual per capita income to US$ 1,047. This translates into an increase of US$ 47 million in national income. This study examined only the consequences and is therefore an outcome description study.

India

India is the second most populous country in the world, with a population of 834 million (1991 census). IDD constitute a major public health problem for the country. India with its average national goitre prevalence of 7.3% is estimated to have 167 million at risk for IDD, 54 million with goitre, 2.2 million suffering from endemic cretinism, and 6.6 million with milder neurological deficits, making it one of the most important endemias in the world (WHO/SEARO 1985).

Out of 457 districts in the country, 239 (60%) districts have been surveyed for IDD. 197 districts are IDD-endemic areas. These districts cover all the states and union territories in India.

A National Goitre Control Programme (NGCP) was launched in 1962. The programme was limited to areas where the prevalence of goitre was high, namely in the sub-Himalayan areas. The measures were mainly baseline surveys, provision of iodized salt and re-surveys.

But restriction on the sale of uniodized salt in certain specific areas was found to be administratively difficult.

As the surveys done under the programme indicated that the problem was nation wide, the Universal Iodization Programme was implemented in 1986.

The main strategy adopted by NGCP for the control of IDD was by salt iodization programmes. Thus, if an economic analysis of IDD and its control is done, the cost would be the cost relating to salt iodization programmes. The benefits could be the prevention of the different consequences of IDD.

The cost of a salt iodization programme included the cost of:

- Land and buildings
- Iodization plants and equipment
- Potassium iodate
- Labour, supervision and administration
- Maintenance and electricity
- Monitoring
- Communication campaigns

Calculations were based on the following assumptions:
(1) The total requirement of iodized salt for the country (6 kg/person/year) is 5 million tons.
(2) Production capacity of salt per plant was 25 tons per day and the total number of working days in a year would be 160 days.

A discount rate of 10% per annum was assumed in the analysis.

Capital costs of land, building and equipment were converted into amortised capital cost. The total annual cost of the programme was Rs. 12,896 million at 1991 prices. The amortized cost of the programme was calculated, i.e., the equivalent annual cost discounted over the 60 year period. This cost did not include the cost of monitoring the programme and communication.

The benefits of IDD control included improved neurological, mental, auditory, and speech capabilities as well as skeletal growth. This results in higher work productivity, reduced costs due to reduced absenteeism and grade repetition and higher achievement by students. Consequences of iodine deficiency in a community are not only restricted to humans. Confining the economic analysis to humans would result in an under estimation of the benefits of IDD control programmes. The benefits of the control of iodine deficiency in livestock populations include an increase in the number of live births, higher birth weight, less deformities and thicker wool coats in sheep. A higher output of meat and other animal products and higher animal work output are other benefits.

For calculation of the IDD load in India, using an epidemiological model and assuming a life expectancy of 60 years and the crude birth rate at 33 per 1,000 population, 42,000 new cases of cretins and 126,000 stillbirths and abortions would occur every year if no control programme is launched (WHO/SEARO 1986).

Calculations of the costs of management of IDD were based on the assumption that:

(1) Only 10% of the affected people seek health care.

(2) Only people with visible goitres (Grade 2) seek treatment.

(3) Costs include physician costs and cost of the treatment.

(4) Endemic cretins visit a health facility only once in a lifetime and no treatment is available for them.

Using the above assumptions, the total cost of management of patients with IDD was Rs. 342 million.

Loss in productivity was based on the following assumptions.

Cretins have 55% less productivity compared to the normal unaffected adult. A person suffering from mild iodine deficiency will have 5% less productivity. Severely impaired cretins require full-time care. The minimum wage per person is Rs. 16 per day. The number of working days in a year is 183 and 90% of the population in the 15-59 years age group is engaged in productive work.

The total productivity loss averted is estimated to be Rs. 3906 million : Rs. 1699.2 million each for endemic cretins and those who look after severely affected cretins and Rs. 504 million for recoupment of productivity loss by averting mild IDD. The cost of the salt iodization programme is Rs. 1296 million and the benefit of the salt iodization programme in terms of improved productivity and money saved on the management of IDD is Rs. 4208 million (Rs.3906 million + Rs. 342 million). The cost benefit ratio is therefore 1:3. Thus, there seems to be ample justification for having a salt iodization programme in India.

Sikkim (India)

Sikkim is a small hilly state in India. The entire state lies in the severely iodine deficient zone in the eastern Himalayas. A detailed IDD prevalence survey with a household as the basic sampling unit, was carried out. The overall goitre prevalence observed in the survey was 54% and cretinism prevalence was 3.5%. (Sankar et al 1993)

An economic evaluation of the following three alternatives for the control of iodine deficiency disorders in Sikkim was made: (Pandav et al 1991)
1) no preventive programme (NPP);
2) iodized salt programme (ISP); and
3) iodized oil programme (IOP)

The primary outcome measure of the IDD control programme was the prevention of the irreversible IDDs. The secondary outcome measure was the prevention of endemic goitre. In order to compare goitre prevalence in the different alternatives, a new unit of measure, 'visible goitre person years' (VGPY) was introduced. Two methods of economic analysis were applied: cost-effectiveness analysis and cost-benefit analysis. The analyses were carried out from the view point of the community of Sikkim.

The total cost of the iodized salt programme for a 'given year' was Rs. 1,612,174 including the annual equivalent cost and annual operating cost required for the salt iodization; annual equivalent cost and operating cost for monitoring and the annual operating cost of a communication campaign. The major portion of the cost was accounted for by the salt iodization (64%) with monitoring (18%) and communication (18%) equally sharing the remaining cost.

The whole population of Sikkim is at risk of IDD. The 1991 census estimated the total population at 403,612. The per capita cost of iodised salt programme is Rs. 4 per person per year.

In the iodised oil programme an iodized oil injection is given every five years. Hence, all the costs are incurred in the beginning of that programme, that is occur at year "0". The total costs of different components of the iodized oil programme for Sikkim is Rs. 5,237,870. Based on the observation that iodized oil injection gives protection against IDD for five years, the annual equivalent cost for a "given year" of the Programme, using 10% disocunt rate for IOP is Rs. 1,256,114.

Iodized oil constituted 51%, salaries health worker 12%, syringes and needles 10%, interns' expenses 7%, communication 6% while travel costs accounted for 14% of the totla cost of iodized oil programme. The cost per beneficiary (people at high risk - children and women in reproductive age group) was Rs. 5.20 per year.

In the consequences related to prevention of IDD, the benefit accrued due to preventing manangement of endemic cretinism and visible goitre person year was calculated. The same assumption were made as in the previous estimate for India. The cost was estimated at Rs. 7,919,000 for NPP, Rs. 4,704,000 for IOP and Rs. 3,839,000 for ISP.

This means that the cost averted in management of IDD by ISP would be Rs. 4,080,000 in one generation while in IOP it would be Rs. 3,214,600.

Similiarly as in the previous study, production losses due to IDD was estimated. It totalled to Rs. 20,326,000. Which was constituted by productivity loss due to (a) endemic cretinism (42.6 %)(b) mild motor and mental impairment 11.6% and 46% for those healthy persons who look after the severly affected endemic cretins.

The total resource saving due to ISP was Rs. 24,406,000 (20,326,000 + 4,080,000) and due to IOP was Rs. 23,540,600 (Rs.20,326,600 + 3,214,600). In NPP none of the IDD is averted, therefore there are no resource savings. The difference in resource saving between ISP & IOP was Rs. 865,400 and this was largely contrributed by management of goitre. The cost of ISP for a generation is (17,669,400 - 13,717,000) i.e. Rs. 3,902,400 more than the cost of IOP. Thus IOP seems to have much more overall benefit than ISP. The unit cost of IDD averted were also less for IOP.

Thus the study concluded that IOP both in terms of cost effectiveness of irreversible and reversible IDD as well as with respect to resource savings is preferred.

Conclusion

Economic analyses should be an important theme in IDD control. They can be used to select the most resource efficient approaches to assessment and iodine prophylaxis through cost-effectiveness analyses. They can be used to establish priorities for iodine monitoring and control through cost-benefit analyses.

Economic efficiency is only one of the factors which influences choices between competing interventions. It may not even be the most important factor: concerns about equity, for example, may take priority at times. However, if economics is ignored and resources are used inefficiently, some people who could be receiving health care under existing resource constraints will be deprived of the benefits. Therefore, it is important that information about the economic impact of planned intervention is available to decision makers before the decision is made.

There are problems for which the solution is a matter of knowledge and there are problems for which the solution is a matter of will. IDD is a good example of a major nutritional disorder for which the techniques of prevention and control are available and should be affordable. All it takes is a strong will, wider awareness, and cooperation among those who hold a key to the solution of this problem. The need for additional information and research issues should not delay the implementation of intervention.

It is evident on the basis of economic evaluation that elimination of IDD confers an overwhelming benefit for human development and social well-being.

References

Acharya, S. 'Policy Conference on Ending Hidden Hunger'. Montreal-1991.

Correa, H. 1980. 'A Cost-Benefit study of iodine supplementation programmes for the prevention of endemic goitre and cretinism'. In Stanbury, J.B. and B.S. Hetzel eds *Endemic Goitre and Endemic Cretinism*. New York: Wiley.567-587.

Gutekunst, R. 'Costs and Benefits of Goiter prevention' Germany 1990. *Report of the Federal Association of Company Sick Funds*. Germany.

Hershman, J.M., G.A., Melnick and R., Kastner, 1986. 'Economic consequences of endemic goitre'. In Dunn, J.T., E.A., Pretell, C.H., Daza and F.E., Viteri eds. *Towards the eradication of endemic goitre, cretinism, and iodine deficiency*. Washington: PAHO Sci Pub 502. 96-106.

Hetzel, B.S. 1987. 'An overview of the Prevention and Control of Iodine Deficiency Disorders'. In Hetzel, B.S., J.T. Dunn, J.B. Stanbury eds. *The Prevention and Control of Iodine Deficiency Disorders*. Amsterdam: Elsevier. pp. 7-31. 1987.

Hetzel, B.S. 1988. *The Prevention and Control of Iodine Deficiency Disorders*. 'ACC/SCN State of the Art Series, Nutrition Policy Discussion Paper No. 3., Administrative Committee on Coordination. Sub-committee on Nutrition'.

Levin, H.M., E., Pollitt, R., Galloway and J., McGuire 1991. 'Population, Health and Nutrition Division HSPR-19'. Washington: World Bank.

McMichael, A.J., J.D, Potter and B.S., Hetzel 1980. 'Iodine deficiency, thyroid function and reproductive failure'. In Stanbury, J.B. and B.S. Hetzel eds. *Endemic goitre and endemic cretinism*. New York: Wiley. 445-460.

Pandav, C.S., J., Hurley, 1991. 'Economic evaluation of Iodine Deficiency Disorders Control Programme in Sikkim'. Thesis submitted for M.Sc. (Health Sciences), Canada: McMaster University, Hamilton.

Pfannenstiel, 1985. 'Direct and indirect costs caused by continuous iodine deficiency'. In Hall, R. and J. Kobberling eds. *Thyroid disorders associated with iodine deficiency and excess*. New York: Raven. 447.

Pharoah, P.O.D., I.H., Buttfield and B.S., Hetzel 1971. 'Neurological damage to the foetus resulting from severe iodine deficiency during pregnancy'. *Lancet* 1:308-10.

Sankar, R., T., Pulger, R., Bimal, S., Gomath, C.S., Pandav, 1993. 'Epidemiology of endemic cretinism in Sikkim'. *Paper presented at XV International Congress of Nutrition*. Australia: Adelaide.

Sankar, R., T., Pulger, R., Bimal, T.R., Gyatso, C.S., Pandav 1993. *Prevalence of endemic goitre in South Sikkim, India*. Paper presented at XV International Congress of Nutrition. Australia: Adelaide.

Sooch, S.S. and V., Ramalingawami 1965. 'Preliminary reports of an experiment in Kangra Valley for the prevention of Himalayan Endemic Goitre with Iodized Salt'. *Bull WHO*. 32: 299-315.

Sooch, S.S., M.G., Deo, M.G., Karmarkar, N., Kochupillai, K., Ramachandran and V., Ramalingaswami, 1973. 'Prevention of endemic goitre with iodized salt'. Bull WHO 49:307-312.

Thilly, C.H., F., Delange, R., Lagasse, P., Bourdoux, L., Ramioul, H., Berquist and A., Ermans, 1978.' Fetal hypothyroidism and maternal thyroid status in severe endemic goitre'. *J Clin Endocrinol Metab* 47: 354-60.

Thilly, C., R., Lagasse, G., Roger, P., Bourdoux and A.M., Ermans 1980. 'Impaired fetal and postnatal development and high perinatal death rate in severe iodine deficient area'. In Stockigt, J.R. and S., Nagataki eds. *Thyroid Research VIII*. Canberra: Australian Academy of Science. 20:386-389.

WHO/South East Asia Regional Office (SEARO) 1985. Iodine Deficiency Disorders in Southeast Asia. *Regional Health Paper No. 10*, New Delhi.

8

From Knowledge to Policy to Practice

David P. Haxton

One of the most frequently asked questions on IDD elimination is, "If David Marine was right in 1923, what has taken so long to get the task accomplished?". In the last decade of the 20th century, why is iodine deficiency still affecting the mental and physical development of 50 million children when the problem can be totally prevented at affordable cost?

The reasons simply stated are :

(A) Weak or absent political commitment to undertake the task;

(B) Those that could act were not informed of the problem and the means of prevention;

(C) Iodine deficiency never achieved an elevated position on the national public health agenda in most countries because health authorities failed to see the multi-sectoral, multi-professional dimensions of prevention;

In some countries economic development brought mass production and consumption of foods fortified with micronutrients some with iodine. When the connection between the reduction of iodine deficiency and the efficacy of fortification of common salt with potassium iodate was made, national programmes increased. Later advances in technology revealed the effectiveness of protection with iodinated oil injections, but that was post World War II. But even then, scientists and other promoters of good nutrition were not able to focus political attention on the problem and encourage application of national resources to interventions which would alleviate the situation.

In sum, knowledge of the problem was not wide spread in the 1930's or 1940's. During the 1950's and 1960's other national needs commanded attention in development despite resolutions of the World Health Organization and other agencies. Some countries began programmes with support from UNICEF and WHO, but few were sustained . The critical connection between knowledge, policy and practice was not made.

Serious efforts were undertaken in various parts of the world in the 1970's, but in a brief period, they languished. Evaluations of those results seem to teach us that the programmes failed principally because:
- there was not a political commitment to succeed;
- the knowledge about iodine deficiency and genetic potential was kept within limited professional groups;
- the consequences of IDD were not revealed widely to the governments or the public;
- those that knew did not understand how to address a public health issue in political and industrial terms; and,
- the role of communications was overlooked or understated.
- there was not a permanent quality assurance system

The concept of arguing that "good health" makes for "good politics" is not new. What is new is the strategy of sharing by the public health sector with other professionals. Gunnar Myrdal made this point eloquently in his "Asian Drama" some decades ago.

The concept of using conventional and modern media for communication of a good message is common in the private sector, but not in the public.

What is new is the awareness that national advocacy planning is required to combine political commitment; scientific support; communications strategy; and creation of public demand into a cohesive whole. This approach is what is responsible in good part for the success achieved in the past decade of elevating the discussion of the problems of IDD from internal scientific gatherings to national political significance and commitment.

Efforts to draw attention to IDD as a problem with significant ramifications had serious competition for attention from other issues made more understandable. Most of the attempts were undertaken by governments with support from UN Agencies, like UNICEF and

WHO. This had some success, but actions were limited because the key partners in any successful national endeavor were not the principal targets of the advocacy work : (a) the producers and traders of salt; (b) the food processing industry; (c) the ministries of agriculture, education, trade and commerce; (d) the communications networks of every country; and, (e) the public consumers. Moreover, the need to pull the producers together with the policy makers and the publishers of information was not recognized.

In face of reluctance of governments and private sector leaders to meet on public nutrition issues; and the hesitant communications links between scientists and other professional groups, the connections between public policy and political practice thus became challenges to overcome.

Review of Social Developments

A review of social development in the past decade revealed a number of significant experiences to indicate the potential of associating political leaders publicly and actively with specific social development issues.

- In Indonesia, the family planning programme had promised villages which became "acceptors" that additional activities to support social development would be delivered when the number of villages accepting family planning was raised. When the rate of accepting such services exceeded expectations, village leaders were impatient to obtain additional social investments. The National Planning Board (BAPPENAS) and the National Family Planning Organization (BKKBN) accepted the proposal of a "package" of nutrition interventions designed by national authorities and officials from UNICEF comprised of : baby weighing and growth monitoring; protection of breast feeding; supplementary targeted feeding; female education; immunizations; diarrhoeas management. Following training this primary health care "package" was to be managed by the village team with replacement of expendables a mutually shared responsibility. A key element in the expansion of this village based effort, was the simultaneous advocacy plan to attract political attention to nutrition (not malnutrition) and make it popular as an issue at the highest level. In addition to the Minister of Health, the Minister of Religious Affairs and the Minister of Home Affairs saw the value of the programme and this lead to the intervention of the President of the Republic to provide political and financial support directly to the effort by passing normal bureaucratic channels.

- Harnessing the influence of the "First Ladies" of the States of Brazil with the 4th largest Television Network in the World (Rede TV Globo) on issues of nutrition, particularly the protection of breast feeding, mobilized the entire gamut of development agencies, NGOs, and the public. The advocacy network created is generally given credit for reversing the trend to bottle feeding and for reforms in infant feeding practices. The alliance created with the powerful television network offered the opportunity to reach a large population with positive and clear messages daily on issues affecting their lives and at very low cost. The response created increased demand on public (as well as private) health services. The power of communications planning and execution was demonstrated as a new form of national nutrition programming. Prolonged breast feeding and improved infant feeding practices were the result.

These and other successful national endeavors gave encouragement to international organizations to "go public" on major development issues. Confidence was built through a growing awareness of the power of mass communications and the increasing number of international meetings on issues like: family planning; women's rights. Gradually, the value of social communications to aid in merging public policy and private action was seen as a vital under: used resource. The General Assembly of the United Nations in 1980 adopted a "Decade Development Plan" with specific targets in it. This gave the opportunity to conduct global sessions on specific issues and bring together the various local, national and international actors to design cohesive and practical actions.

UNICEF was the first major UN Agency to seize the idea of "advocacy for children" and to do so on a grand scale globally. The annual "State of the World's Children" gave all interested parties a technically sound, well written, succinct position to advocate. In 1982, successful efforts were made to present the report in formal ways to Heads of Government and State for endorsement of the principles and support to the actions outlined. Among the first to make this political commitment was the Prime Minister of India, Indira Gandhi, and H. M. The King of Bhutan. Other leaders quickly followed. The presentation of the SOWC to Heads of Government became a regular event in most countries.

This offered opportunities to bring together political leaders, and public leaders, organizations and legislators to review progress on the status of children in each country. It also demonstrated how a United Nations publication, appropriately designed and skillfully written, aimed at mobilizing political support for a cause could command attention and become a "standard". It became the most read United Nations Publication.

The idea of national advocacy events for specific issues in social development began to take shape. While there is a long record of national meetings of specifically interested parties on national issues of one kind or another. The idea of pulling a range of professions together with both public and private development sector including industry and commerce and political and social communicators as equals was largely untried.

Efforts in Colombia, Peru, India, the US and Brazil provided insights on the planning and communication needs of such ventures. Most were sessions of "interested parties", government officials from one sector, and led by a senior officers with a point to make and a budget to defend.

But even with a good number of instruments available, action in national programming lagged behind the potential. In 1986, the first ever Regional Political gathering on children met in New Delhi, India. The SAARC met at the Ministerial level to discuss major problems of: The Child and the Law; The Child and Health; The Child and Nutrition; The Child and Learning; The Child and its Environment. Each delegation had government officials and representatives of the public in it. Among the major results of the meeting was the recognition that social goals set by political leadership had a positive impact on development planning in the sectoral ministries; political leaders would dedicate the time and energy to social development issues when presented with proposals which made good sense and good politics; nutrition was elevated on the priority list and among the "doable" efforts, it was agreed that IDD be eliminated before the end of the century.

The SAARC meeting was a clear demonstration of the value of pulling together the forces of science, technology, politics, development, communications, public and private sectors on social development. It also demonstrated that positive and practical results could be obtained if the organizers persisted with appropriate follow up activities and proposals and if they understood the political processes within which social development takes place. It also showed that information for political leaders must be designed to meet their needs, and not the needs as perceived by others.

The lessons learned at the SAARC meeting led in part to the Global Summit. Both demonstrated that the convergence of good science, good policies, and good politics could be made to work. It also demonstrated that the marriage of good ideas with political support could create public enthusiasm for implementation by using the modern and expanding communications networks in each country.

The subsequent conference in Montreal to "End Hidden Hunger" was a further call to action. It indicated the need to pursue the incorporation of private sector food producers into the national plans to eliminate MNM. Vistas of opportunities for wider efforts at food fortification; for the use of powerful communications networks to effect dietary change; for improved fortification and promotion of consumption of supplements were reviewed. Although these offered both scientists and governments powerful instruments for development, acceptance of the challenge was slow.

Decades of development practice had not revealed to government planners or agency officials effective ways in which to deal with private industry and commerce in public health ventures. Equally, private industry was reluctant to approach social development problems for a range of valid reasons. Progress toward the understanding of mutually beneficial results of interventions in micronutrient malnutrition elimination was slow and hesitant.

Since World War II (and in good part due to the "cold war"), development policy makers and agencies put prime emphasis on the role of governments in a range of economic, social and development activities. There are noticeable shifts in that approach all around the globe. These shifts seem to be : (a) attempts to "privatize" holdings in infrastructure like mining, transport, real estate, banking, manufacturing; (b) in some places there is a shift from the centrally planned activities to market driven priorities;. (c) attempts to shift responsibility and management of basic services in education, health, agriculture, from government completely to a shared support of public and private resources. A major supporting reason is a growing awareness that public health and improved basic services are good investments for a healthy and productive population.

While this shifting may mean disruption or continuity in some cases, it supports the notion that too much was asked of a governing system that could not innovate in timely fashion and which was (perhaps) not designed for some of the requests made of it. A healthy population is good for business and good for politics.

National Advocacy Meetings

A review of the progress of putting knowledge of IDD into policy and into practice showed the following :

a. a reluctance by authorities to accept that IDD elimination could not be undertaken successfully by the Ministry of Health alone;
b. a lapse in understanding that it was producers who owned and traded in salt, not governments or international agencies;
c. a lack of advocacy planning and social communications. "Advocacy" was seen as an event; communications as "advertising"; neither were seen as processes. Thus political will and public demand were left unstimulated.

d. a need to understand how to insert a good policy idea into political discussion and into practice.

During the early 1980's, a series of workshops and seminars kept the idea of elimination of IDD on the agenda of development planning, but generated little additional interest in improved programme preparation. It became evident that the vital mutually supportive link between industry, government and science needed to be made before rapid progress good be expected.

A catalytic agent was needed. The idea of "National Advocacy Meetings" took shape to reach the goal of elimination by 2000. The basic idea was to bring together the scientists, the communicators, the food producers, the government officials (health, agriculture, education, trade, tax, commerce) for a short period:

    (a) to recognize the consequences of IDD in the country;
    (b) to recognize the roles each needed to play to eliminate them;
    (c) to assure adequate legal and regulatory procedures;
    (d) to establish intermediate targets in human resource development, quality assurance procedures, production capacity, communications, raw material supply assurance and,
    (e) to promote demand creation.

In addition, National Advocacy Meetings were seen as channels through which wider social changes could be made by understanding mass application of advances in technology, communications, and economic growth. It is now (virtually) possible through modern communications technologies to bring the benefits of scientific and technological progress to every community in every country. With the rise in literacy, wide application of the transistor battery, and the penetration of television, there is an equal rise in awareness that advances in nutrition, health, and the social condition are possible and that it is no longer necessary for millions to suffer problems which can be eliminated ..... like IDD.

National advocacy meetings are vehicles to enhance the communications between groups that use difference "languages" to communicate. The scientific community addresses and describes issues in language not conducive to public communications or to stimulate change. The commercial community addresses questions with a business plan and organizes itself with specific objectives in mind, one of which is creating profit (which allows it to stay in business and pay taxes!) It is not patient with the perceived ponderous methods of government. Government has its own language which is often obscured by bureaucratic terminology, legislative lingo and judicial language.

The World Declaration and Plan of Action of the Global Summit on Children, clearly called for action by the government departments, development agencies, and private businesses, citizens groups, and communities. The question regarding IDD, therefore, came to be: how to put policy to practice? how to make good policy good politics? how to make good politics, good business?

It is a challenging task to reduce the mutual suspicion of groups not accustomed to face each other as equal partners. National Advocacy Meetings are one way of beginning that effort.

The idea of meetings between government and industry; or between industry and science; or between science and government are not new. There is (practically) a cottage industry of such gatherings and a good number of people make reputations attending them.

A national advocacy meeting to eliminate IDD needs to take into account is that governments have the responsibility to protect the populace which implies the need for guidelines on food production and processing. But the requirements need to have enthusiastic support of industry to make them work. Governments have the responsibility to finance themselves mostly through taxes and fees, but this power also provides the authority for tax relief and incentives. What kind and how much needs mutually to be sorted out in each country.

Private industry cannot be expected to produce fortified food for every citizen (as desirable as that may be), but if the private market reaches the vast majority of consumers, the burden left for the public health sector is reduced and every one benefits. Private industry needs to be profitable and government agents need to understand that profit making is not an evil.

The range of talents in science, in market research, in sales promotion, in research and development, and management skills in the private sector when applied to micronutrient malnutrition efforts can make the significant difference between pronouncing a good idea in the public arena, and making a difference in the general public welfare. The role of industry in effecting dietary change, in food fortification, and in market reach of nutrient supplements has yet to be explored for national planning.

The planning of such meetings requires knowledge of the political situation in each case and of how processes are undertaken. The planning of each venture demands careful selection of participants to assure appropriate and balanced attendance from : groups which have the knowledge; groups which can apply the knowledge; and groups which can assure that knowledge is shared with those that need it. Planning demands balance between those that have been prominent in IDD work; those in other professions; those in government service; those in profit making businesses; those in political life; those in the general public.

Outcomes of such meetings were expected to be :

Political commitment to the goal of elimination of IDD renewed, with pledges to meet intermediate targets, with the understanding that elimination IDD must be permanent;

Economic commitment on the parts of government, industry, consumers, communicators, and development agencies both national and international.

Putting these prospects into practice called for an advocacy plan on the parts of many : UN Agencies; ICCIDD; PAMM; MI; Governments: Alliances needed to be created or re-enforced. National leaders needed to be convinced to take the lead and to make micronutrient malnutrition elimination "good politics".

In 1992, a meeting was arranged in Atlanta by ILSI, PAMM, and the USCDC and food producers, food processors and the packaging industry. A major conclusion was that mutually supportive alliances in countries with MNM could be productive. Governments would need to establish standards acceptable to industry and to create a level playing field for those who fortify foods. Industry could use its power in market strategies, communications advertising, research and development to fortify common foods with iodine, vitamin A or iron and promote their consumption.

The potential of national meetings called by political leaders was demonstrated in The Americas in the early 1970's when President Carlos Lleras Restrepo called a national conference on children comprised of government, non government, private industry, religious, labor and other leaders and groups. This resulted in elevated priorities for social development and created the Institute Colombiano de Bienestar Familiar built around the National Institute of Nutrition. It pulled all of the elements of government dealing with children into one comprehensive undertaking.

A meeting of all the Governors and First Ladies of the States of Brazil in 1979, the International Year of the Child, indicated the potential of mobilizing disparate political forces for a good cause.... the improvement of the quality of life of children.... and simultaneously to decentralize the process

ICCIDD saw early in its history that a major function of the organization was to the advocate of the idea that IDD could be eliminated. It moved aggressively with development agencies and began to work with some governments. Relationships with industry were slow to build. A first attempt was made at the Quadrennial Meeting of Salt Producers and while this resulted in some contacts and set up the potential for national collaboration, follow up was tentative and slow.

UNICEF, among UN Agencies, had a good track record of political advocacy and gradually built up activities relating to IDD elimination. But even with the vast experience of UNICEF, the essential idea of working with private industry and government simultaneously was for the most part a new and untested arrangement. Moreover the Agency was still feeling the stress of working with some private corporations on questions relating to the protection of breast feeding and the unfair market and sales practices of some infant formula products.

PAMM, the center offering multi-professional and cross sectoral training for national team capacity in MNM elimination began to incorporate special emphasis on advocacy techniques as parts of the training courses. A good number of national events either arose from those efforts, or benefitted from national trained personnel in their execution.

In the mid 1980's in South Asia, the time was ripe for a political meeting on questions of children. Under the leadership of the President Ershad of Bangladesh, the Chairperson of SAARC in 1986, the First Conference on Children was held in 1986 in New Delhi. It was attended by delegations at the Ministerial level representing all sectors of government and public institutions. The results were fed into the Summit Meeting of SAARC held later in Bangalore. Among the principle proposals was to eliminate IDD in this century through the medium of access to iodized salt in every country. The success of this venture led in good part to the idea that a global summit meeting could attract strategic political attention.

The 1990's saw a growing acceptance of the essential idea of such National Advocacy Meetings to plan elimination of IDD. In Botswana a meeting between salt producers, scientists, government officials, international agencies, communicators and non governmental organizations from 9 countries tested the potential for collaboration. The results were positive and again demonstrated that private industry appropriately approached with a practical proposal was positive in its response. It also indicated ways in which governments could relieve themselves of some burdens by sharing responsibilities with private industry for the common good.

President Ramos of the Republic of the Philippines called a meeting at Malacanang Palace in June 1993 to plan to eliminate hidden hunger from the country. It brought together government, private food producers, private food processors, non governmental organizations, scientific organizations, communicators, political leaders from the Congress, the Senate and the Provinces. It resulted in a decision by him that the elimination of IDD was a national political priority demanding the full collaboration of all Departments of the Executive Branch. The successful iodization of all alimentary salt and its sale and distribution throughout the country offered the prospect that a public health menace could be eliminated which would be paid for substantially by the public which buys and consumes salt.

The meeting was preceded by supporting activities including studies to demonstrate the magnitude of the problem in the country, (including urban areas), and the consequences to national development of continued inaction. Since the meeting, private industry has responded ; all municipalities have pledged support; communication strategies to sustain progress have been developed in both public and private channels.

Good progress had been made toward elimination of IDD in China over many years of hard work but efforts successfully to design and to implement a multi-sectoral programme reaching all provinces supported by significant national political leadership and the full participation of the massive salt industry had not borne fruit. It was clear in 1992 that the goal of elimination by 2000 would remain illusive unless dramatic steps were taken in management of the programme, its focus and objectives, and its financial and technical support.

In June 1993, the Government and UN Agencies agreed that : (a) the national commitment by the Government of China to the goals of the Global Summit on Children to eliminate IDD was a political priority; (b) The State Council would be host to a meeting in the Great Hall of the People to announce a new plan for elimination of IDD; (c) the Plan of Action to would be multi sectoral; (d) all Governors, all producers of salt, all scientific groups and other organs public and private were to be involved in its execution.

The decision to use consumption of appropriately iodized salt as the principle delivery vehicle meant that the major issues were the implications of those decisions on the Ministries and organs of government; the Party; and in particular, the Offices of the Governors of the Provinces in their critical roles in all development issues in China. The World Bank agree to a loan to renovate the massive salt industry.

For decades there have been attempts to eliminate IDD in Pakistan. While the problem was pronounced as serious the communication of that problem to the political leaders did not produce visible support. Moreover, the resources of private industry, which produce a good bit of the salt in the country, were not tapped. A general tendency of the scientific community to be cautious resulted in continued efforts to focus on study of the problem.

A high level political meeting to discuss the elimination of IDD was proposed to the Prime Minister with participation from a range of government agencies and sectors, scientific and technical groups, and private food producers. UNICEF agreed to co sponsor the event. Studies were compiled to indicate the magnitude of the problem and plans were drafted to show what could be done with the talent and resources available in the country.

The meeting in February 1994 in Islamabad sparked a series of activities :

(a) it showed that government and private industry could harmonize efforts. The Government officially invited the participation of industry in the design of the programme and in the discussions to draft new laws and regulations governing the fortification of salt.

(b) it demonstrated that there was a demand for protection from IDD once the public became aware of the terrible consequences ;

(c) the supply of essential raw materials could be put into place quickly and efficiently at low cost;

(d) the elimination of IDD was a good idea and good politics and popular policy.

ECO and UNICEF meeting of the States Members was held in Ashgabad, Turkmenistan, in June 1994 to discuss how to eliminate IDD in this decade. Studies in many of the countries with the problem of IDD and on the salt situation were completed. In others, existing information and data showed a serious public health problem of national significance obviating the need for time consuming additional surveys.

A more complete analysis of the process and the meeting is contained in Chapter 15 of this book.

Moving from study, to policy, to political commitment and action is difficult but possible. Many issues in social development cry out for more attention. Some will require more imaginative approaches to political commitment than others.

Conclusions

The general conclusions that can be reached in the entire process are :

a. political commitment will be offered when evidence is clear and understandable that a problem is significant, has an understandable solution, and to attack and eliminate it is good politics;

b. industrial commitment will be offered when evidence is clear that the productive capacity of private industry can make a significant contribution at a profit and enjoy competition with a level playing field;

c. planning the process for national advocacy events requires skills in political understanding, communications, and ability to pull disparate forces together into a cohesive union;

d. most of the problems of social development are multi sectoral in nature and governments must learn to create an atmosphere of collaboration with mutual support;

e. scientific groups need to improve skills at communicating what they know to those that can apply it for the public good and to those that need it in their lives;

A major conclusion of these experiences, and one endorsed by ICCIDD is that a National Advocacy Meeting must be seen as an event within a process.... and not an end in itself. The results of such an event should build a stronger process leading not only to eliminate IDD but to a national commitment to sustain that elimination once achieved.

History reminds us that to sustain the achievement requires constant vigilance. This implies a continuing advocacy strategy to assure transition over generations; over changes in leadership, over changes in national development priority and to assure the more rapid application of knowledge than in the past. To sustain IDD elimination much is required. One of the major elements is that of assurance that the dangers of iodine deficiency are taught in medical school as well as to nutritionists.

It is also clear that sustaining achievements is not without cost. Failure to sustain will not be blamed on science but on management.

To sustain IDD elimination the major requirements are

    (a)   a continued political commitment;

    (b)   a permanent quality control system to assure quality of the product, of the process and of the progress in human development;

    (c)   a sustained public commitment to elimination; and

    (d)   a communications/advocacy strategy to underpin all.

References

'Children First' A Report on the First SAARC Conference on Children, UNICEF and SAARC, 1986.

ECO : Economic Cooperation Organization, comprised of Afghanistan, Azairbaijan, Kazakhstan, Kygryhstan, Pakistan, Turkey, Turkmenistan, and Uzbekistan.

'Ending Hidden Hunger', October 1991. A Policy Conference on Micronutrient Malnutrition, Montreal, Quebec, Canada.

Hetzel, B.S. 1992. *The Story of Iodine Deficiency*, Oxford University Press.

Heyward, E.J.R. June 15, 1992. 'The United Nations System and Nutrition'. In the 5th Annual Martin Forman Memorial Lecture.

Haxton, D.P. March, 1993. 'Public Health and Private Industry', an environment for creative alliances in nutrition, Atlanta.

ISLI, 'International Life Sciences Institute' Washington DC, USA; USCDC, United States Centers for Disease Control, Atlanta, Georgia, USA.

Ibid.; and Haxton, D.P., personal records and reviews of national programmes in 15 countries.

Informe Final, 1968. 'Reunion Nacional de Planificaciion Social Para la Familia en Colombia', Bogota..

Marine, David, PhD, who said in 1929 at the University of Michigan, 'iodine deficiency can be prevented any time we want to do it'.

Plan of Action for Implementing the World Declaration on the Survival, Protection and Development of Children in the 1990's, paragraph 34.

PAMM, 'Programme Against Micronutrient Malnutrition', Atlanta, Georgia, USA; MI, 'Micronutrient Initiative', Ottawa, Canada.

Report on the National Advocacy Meeting in The Philippines, 1993; Report on the National Advocacy Meeting in Pakistan in 1994; Report on the National Advocacy Meeting in China in 1993.

So far as the author is aware, no regional political group in the world had met exclusively on issues of children until the SAARC Regional Meeting in 1986.

SAARC : South Asian Association for Regional Cooperation, comprised of Bangladesh, Bhutan, India, Maldives, Nepal and Pakistan, and Sri Lanka.

Scrimshaw, Nevin S. 1993. 'The Challenge of Global Malnutrition to the Food Industry'. In Haxton, D.P., opcit *Food Technology* in February.

'The Global Summit on Children', United Nations, New York, 30 September 1990.

UNICEF, Annual Report of the Representative to Indonesia, 1977. 'The mix of interventions was later promoted globally as GOBI-FFF'.

UNICEF, Annual Report of the Representative to Brazil, 1979

UNICEF, *opcit*.

9
The Process of Communicating the Message

David P. Haxton

Introduction

A fundamental lesson learned over the past few decades in national endeavours to eliminate IDD was that a communications strategy must be an essential component of the endeavour from the beginning. The absence of planned communications has been a significant factor in the waning support and sagging political will for the work.

For years it has been said that of all the malnutrition problems, IDD was perhaps the easiest to prevent. Why then is it still a global problem?

The principal reason is that the ideas were not communicated to those who controlled the capacity to act whether in government or in private industry. Moreover, the science that was known was not communicated to those that could consider it and act upon it. When attempts were made to share they were often cautious and limited.

Communications between professional circles were restrained. The idea that representatives of medicine, health, education, agriculture, industry, communications, management, and mining could share information and plans for the national good did not come into vogue until recently.

The absence of adequate communications is directly responsible for setbacks in the elimination programmes in a number of countries. In one South American country, a senior government official proposed a budget reduction for the IDD programme because of the absence of visible goitres. By the time the decision had been implemented, it was too late to resurrect the programme because only a few minor officials were aware of the consequences of IDD. After further damage to public health and at increased cost, the programme has recently begun again. In a European country, the lack of adequate communication on the interrelated management issues have caused efforts towards the iodization of salt to collapse. Absence of demand creation and lack of quality control of the product assured failure.

More than a decade ago, impressive starts to eliminate IDD were under way in all Central American countries. Yet, today the situation in each country ranges from highly endemic to mildly affected. Surveillance systems have failed to develop. Communications to inform people of the magnitude of human damage and to create and sustain a political commitment to elimination were not aggressively pursued.

In other places the programme planners are still grappling with the idea that communication is a process that conditions and permeates to effect all development action be it public or private. In order to sustain political commitment, it is required that community interest is sustained and progress is measured and sustained. Posting a good idea on the airwaves alone is not good communication. Social communication is more than just dropping a letter in the mail system; sending a periodic newsletter; or sharing a document.

Lessons Learnt

In the planning of communications it is necessary to understand that to possess information is power. Lack of information is a facet of under-development. Sometimes there is a reluctance to share information since it means sharing power.

Communication is still confused with media transmission of information; or public education campaigns, or project support activities. All of these are useful methods of supporting a project with materials and visual aids to describe a good thing we are about to do for people. Communication includes and uses all of those tactics in a strategic comprehensive plan to inform of the problems and dangers; of the prospects for progress; of actions to be taken; of the methods of measuring progress. It requires communication horizontally between and among professional groups, government agencies, private industry, and communicators. It requires communication between each of these and other actors in the process. It requires vertical communication from people to progamme managers through Knowledge, Attitude and Practices (KAP) studies and demand for good health and good products as well as vertical communications in ministries and private industry to satisfy public demand.

Communication is a resource equal to finance, physical inputs and manpower. The decade of the 1990s should be a lesson to us of the power to alter behavioural patterns due to the relentless advertising communications assailing people to change. Significant changes in political structure and management have been the results. Personal health management changes, such as the reduction in smoking and the increase in exercise are due to persistent communication.

In what are considered to be remote communities, products not essential to survival or to life are available and purchased as a result of effective communication.

The accelerated expansion of communications in recent years is awesome to behold. The challenge for development planners is to seek ways to apply these existing communication networks in each nation to the new technologies for life improvement such as the elimination of IDD. CP Snow sadly predicted that a good portion of the world would sit comfortably in homes watching others suffer of starvation on television. This is all too frequent. But radio, television, the print media and traditional media, can all be sensitively and creatively cultivated as allies in the task of eliminating the stealthy scourge of IDD.

The message of IDD elimination must become as ubiquitous as the transistor radio and the video tape. (Fig. 9.1, Fig. 9.2, Fig. 9.3)

Over the past few decades marked progress is evident but in large part, the full potential for development has not been real- ized. The prospect that this might largely be due to the lack of social communications in development plans must be pondered.

As the concept of social communications began to be considered, it was evident that a reluctance to consider social marketing as a public health measure remained. This scepticism was partly understandable. Marketing was a process considered a negative without social conscience. Women were seen buying packaged foods for infants and

IODINE DEFICIENCY IS PREVENTABLE

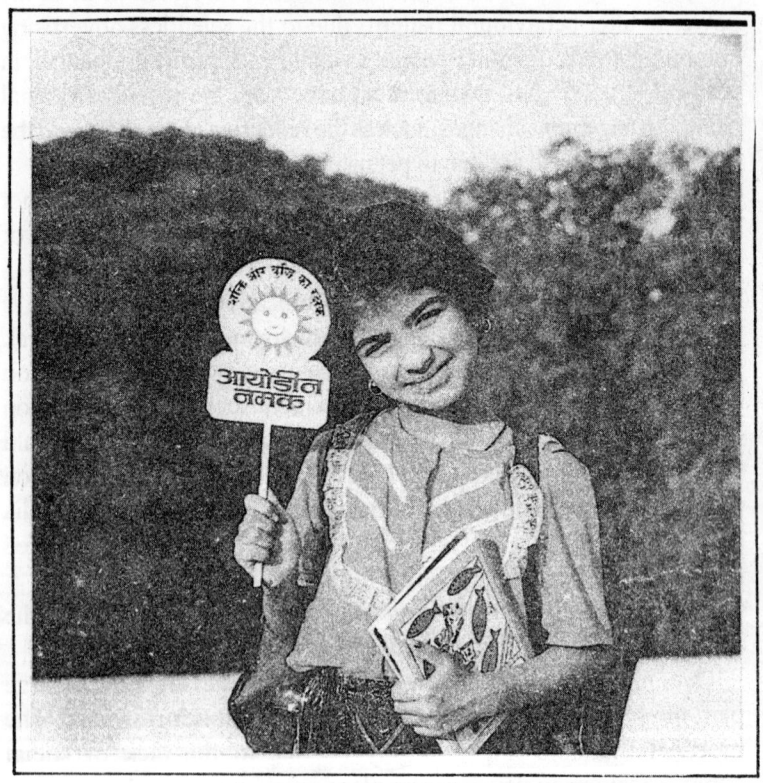

Consume only iodised salt

Fig. 9.1 Message of use of iodized salt being promoted through school children in India.

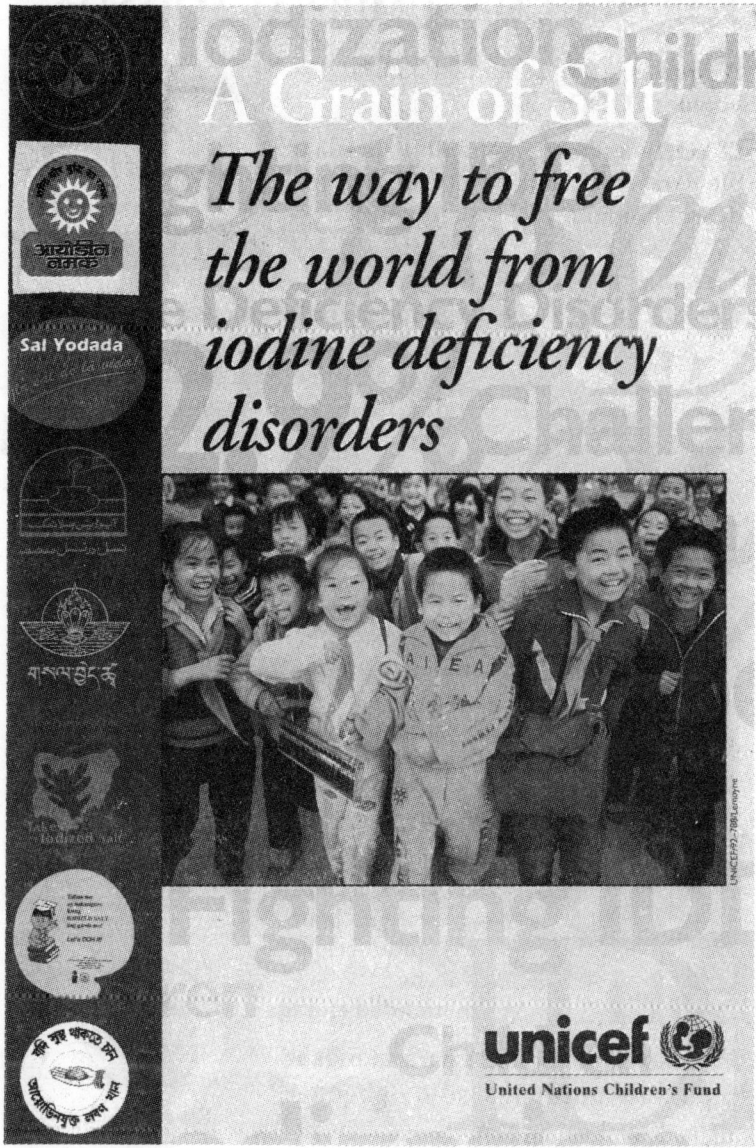

Fig. 9.2 A grain of salt-The way to free the world from iodine deficiency disorders a UNICEF publication. The cover border of which shows iodization logos and symbols from Bangladesh, Bhutan, Bolivia, India, Nigeria, Pakistan, Peru and the Philippines.

POR QUE CONSUMIR SAL YODADA

Porque es la mejor manera natural de obtener YODO.

El YODO es un elemento indispensable para el desarrollo y el crecimiento del ser humano y de los animales.

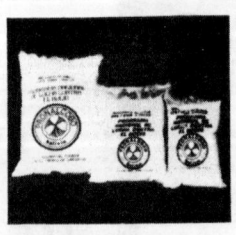

(•) Cantones con bajo consumo de SAL YODADA y con alto riesgo a contraer enfermedades por falta de yodo en 1991.

La falta de YODO en el organismo puede causar:

en los humanos:
- - bocio o k'oto
- - hijos opas
- - sordera
- - tartamudez
- - falta de atención y memoria
- - cansancio en el trabajo diario

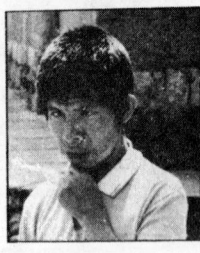

en los animales:
- - abortos frecuentes
- - crecimiento lento
- - baja producción de leche
- - mortalidad elevada

Por eso para cocinar, para la mesa y para los animales, sólo debemos usar SAL YODADA.

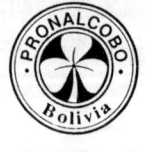

sello de Garantía

Programa Nacional de Lucha Contra los Desórdenes por deficiencia de Yodo-Bolivia Ministerio de Previsión Social y Salud Pública - Dirección General de Salud OPS/OMS - UNICEF

Fig. 9.3 A poster for spreading messages about IDD in Spain.

mixing them inappropriately as a result of pressure from marketing techniques.

A good marketing effort such as a good development programme should never ask people to incur a transaction with a higher performance cost than they are prepared for or can be persuaded to pay. ICCIDD and others can formulate the basic information and promote the essentials, but each country must transform that information into a comprehensive communication plan.

Work on the communication plan should proceed in step with the preparation of other elements. First, because it is accepted that prevention is better than cure; second, plans are required to prevent negative approaches to the IDD plan; third, because it puts communications into the right perspective for dealing with a range of essential issues.

Assessment of the national magnitude of the IDD problem should include assessment of the resources available to address the problem. A major element is communications.

Communications are integral to all actions: to ensure understanding of the problem; to understand the role of each agency; to understand the need for constant quality control and assurance procedures, processes and products; to sustain the need for financial and other support once begun.

Ignorance of the magnitude of the problem on the part of Governments was a serious problem due to poor communication between them and those who had the knowledge and information. A stimulus to assess the problem was also lacking. Essential health information is made needlessly complicated and even mysterious due to poor communication. This is indeed a serious problem.

The need to depend upon professional communicators for the work from the beginning of the situation analysis to the application of the intervention and to the monitoring of results is another lesson learned. Public officials and many scientists are not yet fully comfortable working with communicators, especially in the public sector. But all the evidence shows the value of each collaboration once the roles are understood and mutual professional respect is attained.

Modern print media communications are a problem where illiteracy is high, but traditional communications systems abound in every society. These need to be explored and exploited as parallel supportive channels. Such channels are folk dances; street dramas; puppet shows; person to person communication; radio drama; and traditional art forms. There is a range of people that people listen to and from whom they seek advice and information. A good Communications plan would include priests, imams, village leaders, tribal leaders and sports personalities properly oriented to the problem.

Professional communicators can best assist in stating objectives in communications and in selecting the strategy, developing and testing of messages, developing training techniques and testing them, redesigning, and monitoring.

Imaginative social communications plans have achieved significant results in a variety of situations. A case in point refers to: **Infant feeding practices in India.** There were two major communications problems for the protection of breast feeding and the promotion of improved infant feeding. On the one hand, the vast majority of rural women breast feed, but do so exclusively for up to two years, with little or no supplementation. On the other hand, the pervasive advertising and marketing of 'substitutes' had seriously changed ideas made serious in roads on the concept of breast feeding among the urban middle class and the elite. UNICEF and the Government agreed to a contract with a private sector advertising agency, after careful screening to assure no conflict of interest. A promotional campaign was designed and tested over some months. After the public communications campaign began, the office was flooded with over 4,000 letters a month from interested people around the country. A task force comprising NGOs, government and other representatives was formed to assure responses to all queries for more information. A panel of doctors and nutritionists was set up to effect professional, accurate and prompt communications. Side by side a campaign was launched to secure a ban on publicity for bottle feeding and this led to the adoption by the Government of India of a code of practice for improved infant feeding practices, in many ways more stringent than the WHO recommendations.

An approach in Nepal to promote oral rehydration therapy shows how a blend of traditional and modern channels of communications brought success. Recognizing that diarrhoea related illness was the largest single cause of infant and child deaths, the Government requested assistance for the preparation of a communications strategy as part of the long term solution to provide education, drinking water, sanitation, and for community development. Interim measures were required to improve conditions while the long term efforts were continuing. The communications strategy was aimed at the 400,000 faith healers to whom villagers looked for help since the national population of 17 million had only 600 doctors. The strategy included visual literacy research to reveal how visual messages were received and perceived and how to improve them. Radio personalities, comedians and others added ORT messages to their performances as did puppet masters. Video tapes were made and distributed. Retiring Gurkha soldiers returning to their villages, who had learned sanitation during military service, were enlisted to teach sanitation. Fabric was designed with messages and sold for use as curtains, mattress covers, shirts, uniforms, vests, umbrellas and hats. Comic strips were used. These efforts continued over three years.

In **Ecuador,** the Roman Catholic Church magazine, 'Ser Familia', published a range of suggestions on health and nutrition. This started monitoring and almost culminated into a national movement. Over 300 enterprises of the Chamber of Commerce were motivated to distribute messages through every thing printed by each company. Radio and television co-operated by assuring at least one report each month on basic issues. Students at medical and nursing colleges were motivated into volunteering to perform services in the community. Artists, communicators with great significance, were mobilized, and they created a circus showing with humour, music and vitality the basic health and nutrition issues. They travelled widely in the neighbourhoods which were at risk. What was instilled by a campaign became a public education venture.

Forming grand alliances for IDD elimination. A communication plan and strategy for any national endeavour should begin with the recognition that the success of the venture is not dependent upon the

Ministry of Health alone. Success requires the full participation of a range of organizations both public and private. Various governmental departments including Health, Education, Industry, Finance, Planning, Agriculture and Commerce will require the support of the Executive, Legislature and Judiciary. In the private sector it would include the salt industry, the packaging industry, communication outlets, the visual, audio and print media. In addition, the traditional forms of communication should be enlisted for support. Men's and women's organizations are key elements in success. Organizations like the Kiwanis Clubs are excellent allies. Religious leaders should be approached for collaboration.

There are examples of alliances that have been formed for social development in countries on every continent. In China, the All China Women's Association reaches out to the media and has country and village membership with an impressive outreach capacity of 50 million persons. In Ecuador, over the past few years, the IDD programme has worked schoolteachers, town leaders and government personnel as promotion agents who organized education sessions, discussion groups and public events to support the purchase and consumption of iodized salt. These were in turn bolstered by 40,000 bilingual radio messages aimed at the population at risk. (These were determined by a market survey in advance.) The messages gradually altered from those that promoted the consumption of iodized salt for health and nutrition reasons alone, to include those stressing the better product which was clean, easy to transport and store and which had status and prestige.

National action is the key to success. International support, whether through official development agencies or through the private sector is marginal at best compared to the national resources which must be applied persistently in IDD elimination schemes.

The World Summit for Children which set the goal of elimination of IDD in this decade and the Montreal Meeting on 'Ending Hidden Hunger' which looked at strategies and tactics to achieve the goals comprised national leaders. Now there are political, scientific and professional leaders in all countries which have accepted the challenge. In both these global gatherings of senior leadership, the role of communications was recognized. In fact, it was the role of communicators which helped to foster the composition and substance of the conferences. Governments and private industries approach development problems in different ways. But in the case of IDD elimination, there is much of mutual interest. It is difficult for government officials and officials of industry to work together, but this is also due in part to the lack of practice at doing so and in part to lack of agreement on mutually supportive roles. For IDD elimination, it is vital that these alliances be created. An effective communications plan will help to assure that.

Industry is the arm of society which processes, packages and sells food and has the professional marketing experience to create and sustain a public demand for iodized salt and for the elimination of IDD.

In preparation for the initial attempt to look at the IDD problem in the country and to quantify and analyse it, it is important to have an analysis of the potential and capacity of social communications. It should not be assumed that the planners know what others know or what is not known by others.

A communication plan as part of the whole endeavour, will also include strategies which encourage change. The application of power alone is not enough, since quality assurance is still required, and ingenuity will find escape routes. Logic will be part of the strategy using the facts of IDD and the consequences of poor action. A strategy of appeal will generate emotion and cause reactions perhaps favourable. Incentives can be used to assure a product which is of consistently good quality. Above all the communications plan will attempt to address questions before they become problems (i.e. be preventive in nature), and to facilitate matters by removing obstacles to the success of the programme.

The essence of the communications plan; in fact the entire enterprise is persistence. IDD elimination is a permanent endeavour, not a campaign which can be allowed to wax and wane.

The best marketing over time of commercial products has demonstrated that it is essential to get a good message and repeat it time and again. Everyone recognizes that this technique could be successful.

The plan must also have the built-in dynamic capacity for adaptation as circumstances require. In creating demand, for example, for iodized salt, it must be assured that the supply is sufficient. In addition to creating the demand, caution must be exercised to avoid creating fears among people, industries, or government officials. There is no room for complacency or rigidity if communication is to succeed. Neither is there room for intellectual or professional snobbery.

It must be clear that communications not only put people in touch with each other, but builds partnerships of trust which share equally the essential information in ways which are mutually beneficial. Communication efforts are the bridge between people's knowledge, on awareness of needs, and the benefit of the proposed change.

10

Planning and Managing National Programmes for Elimination of Iodine Deficiency Disorders

Africa
K.V. Bailey

The World Food Conference in 1974 adopted a Resolution aiming at the acceleration of programmes for the elimination of hunger and malnutrition, including vitamin and mineral deficiencies. Iodine deficiency figures in the latter category. The World Food Council, an inter-agency body of the United Nations, was then set up in 1975 and it made concerted efforts towards stimulating coordinated action towards those goals. Among other plans, a ten-year plan for the control of 'endemic goitre' was drawn up in 1977. Another plan was presented to the ACC Sub-Committee on Nutrition in 1987.

The African Region of WHO–which corresponds roughly to sub–Saharan Africa–was spurred on by the World Food Council initiative and contacted a dozen countries in 1978, the ones having the most severe problem of iodine deficiency. Those which responded were Ethiopia, Tanzania, Senegal and Mali, all of them with a view to developing salt iodization programmes.

At this time Kenya was the only country in the Region having a national programme for the control of IDD. This was thanks to initiatives of the Medical Research Centre in Nairobi, whose Director (Dr Hanegraaf) was mainly responsible, not only for but also for securing the co-operation of the government and the private sector so that much of the salt produced in the country was iodized, since the early 1970's. The only other active programme for the control of IDD was in Zaire, where an initial research project using iodized oil had been undertaken in Idjwi Island; from 1976 a mass programme of distribution of iodized oil was launched in the northern region of the country, supported by the Government and the Belgian Co-operation.

Africa was thus far behind other continents in both the assessment and the control of IDD, for historical reasons. But the following pages suggest that Africa is rapidly catching up, and the African Region provides the best barometer of progress towards the global elimination of IDD.

Resulting from the initiatives of some leading endocrinologists of the Region, including Professor Edpechi, the Organization of African Unity convened in 1980 a Symposium on Endemic goitre whose recommendations gave further impetus to national efforts for the control of IDD. But Ministries of Health were not yet ready to give much priority to this problem.

In 1986 the Nutrition Co-operation group in Eastern Central and Southern Africa (ECSA) carried out a review of the IDD situation in 9 countries of eastern and southern Africa. Also in 1986, the newly created ICCIDD contacted the Regional Directors of WHO and UNICEF with a view to organizing a regional seminar on IDD and its control, and this was organized by WHO and held as a joint WHO/UNICEF/ICCIDD bilingual meetings, attended by a total of 22 countries; these were highly productive in generating broader and deeper awareness of the IDD problem and in mapping out strategies for their control.

Immediately after the Yaounde meeting the African Task Force on IDD was set up, comprising representatives of the 3 organizations, and representatives of countries to the extent feasible. The ICCIDD representatives on this Task Force included both the Regional Co-ordinator, and the three sub-regional, co-ordinators, corresponding to the western, central and eastern/southern African regions of WHO. Inclusion of country representatives posed two problems:

that of funds for their attendance, and that of language; about half the affected countries being anglophone and most of the rest francophone. In 1990 an IDD Sub-regional Working group was set up in each of the three sub-regions, comprising the national programme managers from each country. All these groups now meet if possible annually to review problems, progress and new programme proposals.

Most of the countries needed more detailed or updated IDD surveys before being able to formulate comprehensive national control programmes and action plans. Areas of high endemicity were mostly known from surveys of earlier decades, as reported in the WHO Monograph (1960), Endemic Goitre. But the true extent of ID in the countries was commonly unknown and underestimated. The earlier data was mostly inadequate for the purpose of problem definition an subsequent monitoring and evaluation. Usually only goitre surveys were available, often without clear indication from the published reports, whether total goitre rates or visible goitre rates were being referred to. In some countries, such as Rwanda and Burundi, it was hardly possible to decide whether a localized oil prophylaxis would be sufficient or whether a national salt iodization programme would be required. In some countries major problems have recently been discovered where previous reports suggested only a minor problem (e.g. Burkina Faso) or none at all (e.g. Uganda). there are now 40 countries (out of 45 in the WHO African Region) which are identified as having an IDD problem of public health dimensions; in about 20 of them, over 25% of the population are at risk, and this is considered as a criterion of a major IDD problem.

Most of the earlier surveys, especially the larger ones, had little or no biochemical component-urinary iodine or thyroid-related hormone assays. There is now a consensus among national authorities and the supporting agencies that instituting a sound monitoring and evaluation system, including a biochemical component, is one of the best ways of ensuring sustainability of national control programmes.

Especially since 1987 therefore, a series of technical co-operation visits has been made by IDD experts, mostly the ICCIDD regional and sub-regional co-ordinators or other experts in the Region, to stimulate and support national efforts to draw up comprehensive plans for the assessment and control of IDD, including monitoring and evaluation systems. These countries included, in West Africa–Senegal, Gambia, Mali, Burkina Faso, Guinea, Guinea Bissau, Sierra Leone, Ghana and Nigeria; in Central Africa–Cameroon, Central African Republic, Chad, Congo, Zaire, Burundi, Rwanda; in Eastern and Southern Africa–Ethiopia, Kenya, Tanzania, Zambia, Zimbabwe, Malawi, Lesotho, Botswana, Namibia and Madagascar. Many of these dealt with the formulation of national programmes along standard lines such as indicated in Table 10.1, including an assessment of the necessity and feasibility of salt iodization or iodized oil programmes.

A considerable number of missions were concerned solely or mainly with assessment of the feasibility, and organization of salt iodization programmes. These include: Senegal, Mali, Guinea, Guinea Bissau, Burkina Faso, Ghana, Nigeria, Cameroon, Zaire, Rwanda, Burundi, Ethiopia, Kenya, Tanzania, Malawi, Zambia, Botswana, Lesotho, Mozambique, and South Africa.

A remarkable feature of the Africa story is the current impetus towards salt iodization. In 1987 salt iodization was going on only in Algeria and Kenya. By the end of 1993 about 28 countries have a full or partial national salt iodization programme, using iodized salt produced or imported in the country (Table 10.2).

Apart from Ethiopia, all the salt industries mentioned are privately owned. With the separation of Eritrea from Ethiopia the salt iodization plants, now in Eritrea, are for the moment non-operative. The response of the private sector in several countries (Kenya, Cameroon, Botswana, Namibia) to requests to iodize their salt, has been very gratifying, once the issues have been clearly explained. The main producers in Kenya, Botswana and Cameroon have produced iodized salt basically at their own expense; all that was needed was initial encouragement and legislation, to protect them against uniodized salt producers or importers. The production of iodized salt has even preceded the adoption of formal legislation in some cases. Only in Senegal, for commercial reasons, the willingness to iodize was long delayed, but, it is now on track; again at the company's own volition.

A new feature of the Africa programme was the organization in 1992 by ICCIDD/UNICEF/WHO, with the support of the Canadian International Development Agency, of two inter-country workshops on salt iodization; one in Botswana for 8 countries of southern Africa, and one in Senegal for 11 countries of west and central Africa. These workshops brought together the government, IDD programme managers, those in charge of the salt sector (production or importation, and marketing) and personnel of the information sector, as well as representatives of most of the major salt producers or importers concerned. The workshops were highly productive in terms of exchange of information and problems and in generating co-operation and joint commitment, between the government and salt sector, to the iodization of salt and its systematic and effective use for control of IDD.

A particular difficulty in promoting iodized salt has been of course the slight increase in cost (normally up to 10%) which iodization implies. Governments were reluctant to legislate for iodized salt unless it could be at competitive prices obtained on the market; and on the other hand some salt producers were unwilling to iodize unless there was a demand for the iodized product. A truly vicious circle! This was particularly the problem in West Africa. In 1993 there is still a large amount of uniodized salt being produced in Ghana and circumstances have only just become favourable for iodization, thanks to reorganisation of the small producer co-operatives involved in Ghana's coastal lagoon areas. Multiple small-scale producers also constitute a problem in Tanzania, Mozambique, Guinea Bissau and Senegal. With time, and a lot of sensitization in the salt sector, it is expected that all these problems can be overcome; certainly before the turn of the century. Indeed the only major producers yet to be convinced about the need to iodize are in Angola and Mozambique; a feasibility study has already been undertaken in Mozambique and procedures are expected to be under way there in the near future.

Table 10.1 *Outline of National IDD Control Programme*

Title:
Duration:
Institution responsible:

Situation Analysis
    IDD situation
    Justification
    Policy basis
    Institutional framework
    Expected benefits
    Links with national development plans

Objectives
    General
    Specific/operational
    Impact

Strategies
Control methods: iodized salt
                     iodized oil
                     others

Plan of Action
    Baseline IDD survey
    Baseline salt survey: feasibility and modalities of iodization
        relevant Legislation
    Oil: mode of administration
        populations to be covered

Monitoring and Evaluation
    of activities
    of epidemiological situation (goitre rates; biochemical)

Supporting Activities
    Training
    Advocacy and social communications
    Operational research

Management System
    National Council for Control of IDD
    Role of specialized Institutions
    Programme manager
Budget
Calendar of Activities

Table 10.2 *Countries with national programme of iodized salt*

Region	Local production	Importation
Western Africa	Algeria Nigeria (Senegal - 1993)	Nigeria (Mali - 1993)
Central Africa	Cameroon	Burundi Central African Republic Chad Congo Equatorial Guinea Rwanda Zaire
Eastern/Southern Africa	(Ethiopia)* Kenya Namibia Tanzania (Botswana)	Malawi Zambia Zimbabwe

* Production ceased when the factory site became part of Eritrea.

Another problem has been the setting of appropriate levels for the iodization of salt. Some producers were using iodide rather than the recommended iodate. In most of the IDD-affected areas in Africa, the consumption of salt is relatively low (3-10 g per person per day). Also the long distances traversed between the salt producer and the consumer results in severe exposure and the losses during cooking. Because of these, the levels of iodine recommended in Africa are between 50 and 100 parts per million; generally, 100 ppm.

It is fitting to place on record here a tribute to the work of Mr Venkatesh Mannar who, as ICCIDD Board Member and Consultant for ICCIDD, WHO, and UNICEF or the World Bank has visited nearly all of these countries. Appropriate standards and technology for iodized salt were spelt out in most of these countries, and they are being progressively implemented. Draft legislation was provided where there was none; or recommendations for the revision of existing but inadequate legislation.

Countries in which national or local iodized oil programmes are under way, pending adequate salt iodization, include Mali, Burkina Faso, Ghana, the Central African Republic, Zaire, Rwanda, Burundi, Ethiopia, Tanzania, Namibia, and Mozambique. Water iodination is also being done in parts of Mali and the Central African Republic. Thus approximately 30 of the 40 affected countries now have some form of IDD control under way.

Those countries which have not yet (1993) embarked on any intervention include Guinea, Guinea Bissau, Togo, Cote d'Ivoire, Liberia, Niger, Angola, Uganda, Swaziland, Comores, and Madagascar; but interventions are being planned in most of these countries and are likely to be under way in some, by the time this publication appears.

Part of the reason for the successful development of IDD programmes in Africa has been the IDD Task Force and Working Groups which have reviewed the progress annually since 1987, with opportunities to share information, problems encountered and solutions arrived at. The Task Force meeting in Abidjan in 1989 included practical work in the formulation of national control programmes. In addition two training workshops in the management of IDD control programmes were organized in Burveli, 1992, one at Dar es Salaam (anglophone) and one at Yaounde (francophone), with the help of ICCIDD, UNICEF and WHO, with resource persons almost entirely from the Region. A further course in French was organized in Burundi, 1992 by the Belgian co-operation with support from the usual three partners. These three workshops provided a quite comprehensive discussion and guidelines on steps in the development and management of IDD control programmes. The national programmes are now essentially managed by trained and committed national officers with an adequate grasp of the principles and practical realities of programme management. In the past two years, several African countries have sent multidisciplinary teams for in-depth training at Atlanta, Georgia, in the USA (Programme Against Micronutrient Malnutrition).

An area in which strengthening of facilities in the Region was needed was in the laboratory assessment of iodine and thyroid status. The technologies require considerable investment in terms of laboratory infrastructure and training. It is gratifying that with help from several sources, there are now at least 11 operational IDD laboratories capable of urinary iodine and/or thyroid-related hormones, for their own or other countries, in Algeria, Burkina Faso, Ghana, Nigera (Ibadan), Cameroon, Ethiopia, Tanzania, Zimbabwe, Namibia, Madagascar and South Africa. This will greatly facilitate effective and continuous biological monitoring of the impact of the national programmes.

One area in which most programmes remain rather inadequate is that of social communications and advocacy; even though there is some degree of national commitment, Some locally-adapted advocacy materials are available and activities are under way in most countries. There is need for much more effective communication, both at the level of national policy and decision-making as well as the salt sector and to the public through mass media. It is also essential in communities to ensure continuing commitment to and participation in IDD control. In most countries the salt and information sectors are not informed well enough about IDD issues and on the other hand, IDD programme personnel are not specially skilled in the area of communications and advocacy. More training workshops, both inter-country and national, are planned on these aspects. Overall in the Region, national programmes have mostly passed through the first phase of baseline (re)-assessment of IDD problems, and a second phase of national programme

Table 10.3 *Regional strategy and plan of action for IDD control in the African region*

Activity	Number of countries		
	Existed (End 1986)	Target (End 1993)	Achieved (End 1993)
1. Survey	4	16	30*
2. Sensitization	4	16	31
3. National Programme Draft		16	16
4. National Programme Implemented		8	14
5. Salt surveys	4	16	25
6. Salt iodization	3	12	16
7. Iodized oil	2	8	12
8. IDD laboratory	1	6	12
9. Applied research	2	8	6
10. Trained staff	4	16	31

Note: This table is derived from Table 3 of the Regional Strategy and plan of Action, formulated in 1986 and adopted by the Regional Seminar on IDD, 1987. Table 3 was published on p. 129 of the Report of the Regional Seminar (WHO, Brazzaville, 1987; document AFR NUT 99). The targets were set by biennially, i.e. 1986/87; 1988/89; 1990/91; 1992/93; and the year 2000.

*Approximately 20 of these surveys are sufficient to serve as a basis for a national programme. Others are only partial.

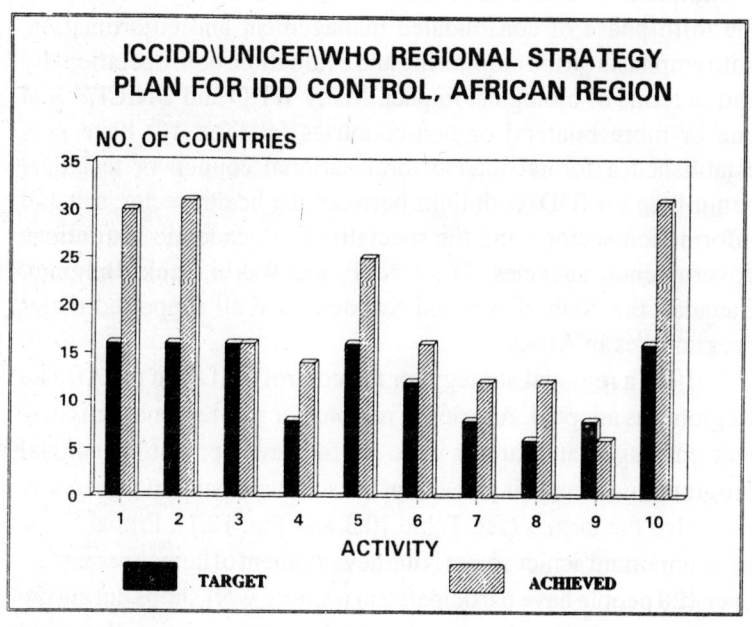

Fig. 10.1 Achievements in Relation to Targets (Dec, 1993)

KEY TO ACTIVITY COLUMNS:

1 = IDD SURVEYS*
2 = SENSITIZATIOJN
3 = NATIONAL PROGRAMME DRAFT
4 = NATIONAL PROGRAMME IMPLEMENTED
5 = SALT SURVEYS
6 = SALT IODIZATION
7 = IODIZED OIL
8 = IDD LABORATORY
9 = APPLIED RESEARCH
10 = TRAINED STAFF

* Approximately 20 of these surveys are sufficient to serve as basis for a national programme. Others are only partial.

formulation and implementation. Many of them are now entering the third phase of consolidated management and co-ordination, with emphasis on the monitoring and evaluation, both operationally and in terms of biological impact. Many WHO and UNICEF, and one or more bilateral or non-countries (at least 10) have now established a formal intersectoral national council or technical committee for IDD, with links between the health sector, salt and information sectors, and the specialized or academic institutions governmental agencies. The UNDP, the World Bank, Belgium, Canada, the Netherlands and Sweden have all supported major programmes in Africa.

In 1987 a regional strategy for the control of IDD in the African Region was adopted. A series of regional or sub-regional activities was envisaged and targets were set for development of national programmes. Analysis shows that the achievements have generally exceeded the targets (see Table 10.3 and Fig. 10.1). Probably the most important achievement is the development of human resources: over 120 people have participated in training workshops during the 6 year period; this is a vital condition for assuring the good management and sustainability of the programmes. Some allowance must be made for the fact that 40 countries are now recognized as having a significant IDD problem whereas at that time only 30 countries were included in the targets. However, it does appear that unless there are major unforeseen constraints (such as for the iodization of salt in Ghana), the processes should be under way leading to the substantial control of IDD in all countries of the African Region by the year 2000. If sufficient resources are mobilized and political stability is adequately maintained, the elimination of IDD on schedule should be feasible.

References

Benmiloud, M., H., Bachtarzi and M.B., Chaouki 1983. 'Public health and nutritional aspects of endemic goitre and cretinism in Africa'. In Delange F. and R., Ahluwalia eds. *Cassava toxicity and thyroid.* p.50 Ottawa: Research and public health issues, IDRC.

Kelly, F.C. and W.W., Snedden 1960. 'The prevalence and geographical distribution of endemic goitre'. In *Endemic goitre* pp.27-234. Geneva: World Health Organization.

World Health Organization 1987. Control of IDD in Africa. Regional Seminar, Yaounde, Cameroon, 23-25 March 1987. Report of Joint WHO/UNICEF/ICCIDD Regional Seminar. Congo: Brazzaville.

Asia
C.S. Pandav

> "*A centipede had arthritis. And he had it in all his hundred legs. So he went to the wise old owl for advice. The owl thought about it for a while then said, "the only remedy for you is to turn yourself into a man. With only two legs, you shall find that the pain is much easier to live with." So the centipede thanked him and went home. The next day, he came back to the wise owl. "Pardon me, Sir" he said, "I was so excited about your answer yesterday, I foolishly forgot to ask you how I should become a man". The owl looked at him sternly and said, "my dear young fellow, I only make policy decisions. It is up to you to implement them."*
>
> — Panchatantra, India.

This popular folklore from India best illustrates the chasm between policy formulation and its execution. The best of the programmes can be unsuccessful if at the stage of planning, proper thought has not been given to its implementation. Management concerns itself with precisely this problem of policy formulation and its implementation. Management has been defined in many ways. One which is more comprehensive defines it thus "Management is to make efficient use of resources and to get people to work harmoniously together in order to achieve objectives" (WHO 1980).

Traditionally, nutritional programmes have always been managed by nutritionists or health professionals. One of the reasons for the failure of the IDD control programmes is their "myopic" approach. IDD is an unique nutrition problem in which the most physiological, cost-effective and widely applicable solution, that of iodized salt, lies outside the domain of the Ministry of Public Health. Therefore there is a need to see "beyond the self" and step out of this frame of mind in order to get a new perspective.

Wherever IDD control activities started as projects, they were very successful. However, when the projects were scaled to the national level, the performance has not met with the same degree of success. For example, in India the Kangra Valley experiment (Sooch et.al, 1973) initiated in 1954 was highly successful in decreasing the prevalence of IDD through salt iodization. After five years of using iodized salt, the prevalence of goitre came down in the study areas from 38% to 19% compared to no decline in the control area. Eighteen years later, studies showed negligible prevalence of goitre in school children. But the performance of the National IDD control programme, launched in 1962 after the success of the Kangra valley experiments has yet to achieve the same degree of success. In Nepal also the iodized oil injections form a part of the Goitre and Cretinism Eradication Project (GCEP) and has been successful in achieving the objectives. The possible reasons may lie in the fact that in a small project setting it is easier to co-ordinate, supervise and intervene which may not be possible on a large scale.

For successful planning and management of a national IDD control programme the following three questions need to be asked.

(1)   What is the current situation regarding IDD prevalence, salt use and the salt industry?
(2)   Is the IDD programme being carried out as planned?
(3)   Has the purpose of the IDD programme been communicated to the community?

1. Information

The first step is to decide what information is needed and how to collect it. This depends on whether in the country the programme is vertical or integrated with the existing health system. In India, for example, it is a vertical programme but efforts are being made in the newly launched Child Survival and Safe Motherhood (CSSM) programme to integrate the IDD Control programme, especially the monitoring of salt, with the primary health care infrastructure. In Nepal, integration of the iodized oil programme with the immunization programme made it possible to reach remote and inaccessible areas. This played a major role in the success of the programme.

A vertical system is likely to be expensive and difficult to sustain. However, in most countries where IDD is a problem, the health information system or nutrition surveillance system is already overloaded; people who would collect, analyse and present the data are overworked, and budgets for monitoring as well as for programmes are strained. Consequently, there is a need to choose the data to be collected, the sample sizes and the frequency of collection so as to provide adequate, relevant information which can be assessed realistically and usefully applied .

This problem has been addressed in a joint WHO/UNICEF/ICCIDD Consultation in November 1992 on "Indicators for assessing iodine deficiency disorders and their control programmes" and a comprehensive list of indicators have been recommended. Also an easier and faster way of collecting this data by the "EPI 30 Cluster" method has been suggested. This approach has already been implemented by Bangladesh, Bhutan and Nepal to carry out their National IDD Prevalence surveys. India also proposes to use this methodology for future surveys.

Information regarding salt use and the salt industry is more difficult to get. In different countries, the responsibility of dealing with the salt trade rests with the Ministry of Industry, Trade, Commerce or Energy, Water, Minerals, etc. The concerned Ministry can provide valuable information on the availability of sources of common salt, trade practices, consumption patterns and preferences, family level purchase and storage habits, iodization equipment, iodine requirement, packaging facilities, transportation, distribution and storage facilities and so on.

On the basis of this information, a plan can be formulated, objectives fixed and carried out in order of priority. For example in the SEARO region of the WHO, the target is the universal iodization of salt by 1995 so that the goitre rate would be no more than 5 per cent by the year 2000.

2. Implementation

After the goals have been set, comes the stage of implementation. For this, the most important requirements are the resources:- money, material and manpower. For any government, money is always a scarce resource. Fortunately the cost of the universal iodization of salt is minimal: less than the cost of a cup of tea per person per year. The Indian subcontinent is self sufficient in salt production and manufacture of iodization plant. More research is being done to reduce the costs of the programme. An example of this are the salt testing kits developed by India and Bangladesh. If the programme is integrated with the existing health infrastructure, the amount of manpower needed will be limited. However there is certainly a need for orientation courses in IDD and its control, for stakeholders at all levels. It is also necessary to have technical personnel trained for the job.

It is however at the implementation stage that challenges lie. For example, in India, some of the reasons that have stalled the performance of the National IDD control programme can be summarized as (i) the absence with an agency of sufficient authority at the central and state level which could take an inter-sectoral view of the whole chain of operations involved in IDD control. (ii) lack of regular and periodic supervision and evaluation by the IDD cells in the state. (iii) lack of co-ordination between health, salt commissioner and civil supplies departments at the state/district level (Pandav et al, 1988).

The programme can be successful only if these points are given due and careful attention. For example, important reasons for the success of the programme in Nepal (Acharya, 1991) are that the programmes were included as a part of a periodic comprehensive five year development plan and the availability of core group of experts along with supervisory and managerial manpower.

3. Communication

The next important input for an effective IDD control programme is that of communication. This is a specialized discipline that requires special skills. Communication is concerned with target audiences that include the people, salt dealers, health professionals, decision-makers and government officials. Communication inputs should be incorporated into the project from its inception. The components of a good communication programme are:

(i) **communication research** among the public, with a view to gathering information regarding public awareness about IDD and its solution, i.e. public perception of these matters;

ii) **communication** with public health professionals and government officials at every level, in order to obtain their understanding and support in the planned effort;

iii) **the dissemination** of appropriate messages to the public, in order to educate and motivate them to accept the products and work towards achieving the objectives.

In S.E. Asia region, Communication has yet to receive due attention in the IDD control programmes. There have been some modest efforts towards better communication in this region. Though Bhutan has made efforts to use different media for community education, a recent survey did not show a satisfactory impact. Radio jingles were effectively used for the iodized oil programme in Nepal. In India, a professional advertising agency has created a comprehensive package and it will be implemented soon. In Bangladesh also an advertising agency has been commissioned to carry out the communication campaign.

Requirements for Success

An analysis of successful development programmes all over the world have identified four critical dimensions which have contributed to its success. They are:

(i) Political commitment
(ii) Administrative infrastructure
(iii) Scientific leadership, and
(iv) Monitoring and evaluation

i) Political commitment
In India, when the late Prime Minister Smt. Indira Gandhi was briefed by the researchers from the All India Institute of Medical Sciences, New Delhi and the Indian Council of Medical Research, with support from UNICEF on the results of the neonatal screening for hypothyroidism in iodine deficient areas and the serious consequences it could have on human development, she included "Goitre Control" in her '20-point programme'. She was also shown a film on IDD 'Will the Salt reach Padrauna'. She was very moved on seeing the plight of the people living in iodine deficient areas and the fact the all this was totally preventable at such a low cost. Similarly, in Bhutan, when His Majesty Jigme Singay Wangchuk was presented with the result of the first nation wide comprehensive survey on IDD in 1983 and also shown the film produced by UNICEF, on IDD in Bhutan, 'An end to an age old scourge', an immediate decision was taken to give high priority to the IDD Programme. In Thailand too, H.R.H. Princess Maha Chakri Sirindhon after being informed and convinced of the enormity of the problem graciously agreed to be the president of the National IDD Control Committee to help resolve the IDD problem.

ii) Administrative infrastructure

For proper administration, it is essential to have a nodal point for the programme. India has it as an Adviser (Nutrition) and Deputy Assistant Director General (Goitre). IDD cells are also being established at the state level to act as a nodal point for the respective states. Nepal has two departments involved: GCEP and the Salt trading Corporation. Bhutan, Thailand and Indonesia have also identified the nodal agencies for implementing and monitoring the IDD control activities. In Bangladesh, though the programme is doing extremely well, the nodal agency is yet to be identified. The nodal agency is essential for the sustainability of the programme. All the countries in this region have formed National IDD Co-ordination Committees. The composition of these have been multi-disciplinary. But the key issue is to have regular meetings and an action-oriented agenda. More work is required in this direction.

iii) Scientific leadership

In India, a series of state level workshops have been organized, starting with Himachal Pradesh in 1986. Later on a number of them were conducted for the states of Uttar Pradesh, Bihar, Madhya Pradesh, Maharashtra and the north-eastern states. The objective was to prepare a plan of action for the implementation of the programme with active participation from the different agencies involved, in the execution of the programme at the state level. A similar exercise was also carried out at the national level. However, the important aspect of these activities is their sustainability they have to be a regular annual feature. The same is also applicable at the regional level. The workshops provide an unique opportunity for an exchange of experiences-reviewing the progress, identifying the bottlenecks, learning from the success stories of other departments at the state level; from other states provinces at the national level and from other countries at the regional level. This has been an extremely rich and rewarding experience. The south east Asian region has taken the lead in organizing a series of such exercises: the IDD National Programme managers meeting in October 1990; the Tri-regional Workshop with site visits to India and Nepal in Nov-Dec 1991. Such exercises are to be actively promoted and ICCIDD is playing a catalytic role in making this happen.

iv) Monitoring and Evaluation

Monitoring and evaluation are an essential part of the programme. It is necessary to carry out concurrent and periodic evaluation of the programme, for both process and output (impact) indicators. Regular monitoring of salt iodine content is an essential measure for the success of the programme. Different countries in this region have different ways of doing this. India has a system of food inspectors for collecting the salt samples and sending them to laboratories for analysis. It is being proposed to hand over this activity to multipurpose health workers under the CSSM programme. An innovative approach of utilizing the non-governmental agencies for this purpose has been successfully tried out in India (Pandav, 1994) and this approach is being implemented in other countries as well. The current status of IDD control activities in different countries of south-east Asia is given in Table 10.4.

The elimination of IDD is a necessary condition but not sufficient in itself condition for the socio-economic transformation of the underdeveloped population living in iodine deficient areas (Pandav, 1986). The determined efforts of planners, administrators, and scientists have now been backed by political will in all countries of this region. This is reflected in most countries which already have a sound salt iodization programme and the countries that do not have one are to start it soon. It is hoped that with sustained political commitment and adequate financial resources, the presence of scientific leadership and the well organized primary health care infrastructure, these countries will jointly achieve the goal of reducing the prevalence of IDD to below 5 percent by the year 2000.

Table 10.4 *The status of IDD control activities in the WHO-SE Asian region*

Country	IDD Prevalence in endemic areas	Years of Survey	Current status of IDDCP
Bangladesh	> 40%	1993	Salt iodization programme (SIP), Iodized oil
Bhutan	18-46%	1991-2	SIP.
DPR Korea	Yes, but not documented		Comprehensive survey of IDD prevalence to be carried out.
India	>10%	1956-92	SIP.
Indonesia	>10%	1980-2	SIP. Iodized oil.
Maldives*	>20%	1995	SIP to be introduced
Myanmar	>10%	1982-86	SIP Iodized oil
Nepal	>10%	1986	SIP Iodized oil injection
Srilanka	>18%	1986-7	Plan to action for SIP to be developed
Thailand	10-30%	1987	SIP, Iodized oil. Iodized water.

* Survey of school age children

References

Acharya, S. 1991. 'Proceedings of Ending Hidden Hunger - A policy conference on micronutrient malnutrition'. Canada Montreal. October 1991:17.

Bhutan 1992. *Iodine deficiency disorders - The Bhutan Story*. Directorate of health services. Royal Government of Bhutan.

Pandav, C.S. 1986. 'Towards the eradication of iodine deficiency disorders in India'. *Indian journal of community medicine (editorial)* 1986;xi(4).

Pandav, C.S., M.G., Karmarkar, L.M., Nath, 1988. 'National goitre control programme, National Health Programme Series 5'. New Delhi: National Institute of Health and Family Welfare.

Pandav, C.S., S., Pandav, K., Anand, S.A., Wajih, S., Prakash, J., Singh, M.G., Karmarkar, 1994. 'Elimination of Iodine Deficiency Disorders: Role of NGOs in monitoring iodine content of salt in an endemic area of Northern India - A preliminary report'. (in press) Bull: WHO.

Sooch, S.S., M.G., Deo, M.G., Karmarkar, N., Kochupillai, K., Ramachandran, V., Ramlingaswamy. 1973. 'Prevention of endemic goitre with iodized salt'. *Bulletin of World Health Organization.* 49 : 307.

WHO 1980. *On being in charge, A guide for middle level managers in primary health care.* Geneva.

Latin America
Mauro Rivadeneira

Iodine Deficiency Disorders (IDD) as a public health problem have been reported in Latin America since 1830, or even before. More recently since 1960, research groups have been working in several countries. Their studies have provided a much better knowledge of the situation and the geographical distribution of the problem (Dunn et al 1986).

In short, it has been established that IDD severely affects the five Andean countries located in the north of South America, i.e. Venezuela, Colombia, Ecuador, Peru and Bolivia.

Chile, probably due to its large coast is not seriously affected, and the same is true of Uruguay.

Argentina has had an effective programme since 1970 which covered 99% of the population. Brazil is a big country which should be considered as a whole, because of the variety of ecological conditions. IDD is present in certain areas, but in others is not a serious problem. However, IDD control has now been achieved with a good salt iodization programme (Medeiros Neto 1988). Paraguay is also among the seriously affected areas.

In Central America several studies have been carried out. Despite the fact that most countries have large coastal areas, IDD is still a public health problem.

This situation was virtually unchanged until recently in spite of the fact that almost every country passed a law making compulsory the use of iodized salt for human consumption. This occurred between 1965 and 1970. Most of the laws established that salt should have a high concentration of iodine between 50 and 100 ppm.

Unfortunately mechanisms to ensure enforcement of the law were not implemented. Colombia was the single exception. A careful control of iodization produced a dramatic reduction in goitre prevalence within a short period. Later Guatemala had similar success.

After the initial success, neither Colombia nor Guatemala maintained a strict control system with the result that IDD reappeared in both countries. This experience, which was not detected for some time, called attention to the importance of a well designed surveillance system.

Research done in several countries has led to a better knowledge of the causes and consequences of IDD. Iodized oil as a preventive measure has been studied in Peru and Ecuador and a great deal of the present knowledge on the social consequences of IDD, mainly mental retardation, has come from research in Latin America.

However, the practical approach provided by public health and epidemiology in determining the best way to apply the knowledge gained from investigation, was lacking. During the last few years, thanks to important financial support from the governments of Italy and Belgium, through multilateral and bilateral co-operation, various programmes have been developed successfully. Special attention will be given here to Ecuador, Bolivia and Peru.

The application of the action research methods accompanied by efficient management, free of any bureaucratic obstacles, has permitted the development of an efficient and low cost intervention, particularly in the case of the Ecuador programme.

Indicators have been developed that permit identification of the areas of highest risk in a short period of time and at minimum cost. An indirect indicator has been developed using "type of salt consumed" in order to establish the risk levels. More precise indicators, such as levels of urinary iodine have also been used in high risk communities. In this way the operational costs have been reduced. The system of establishing levels of risk, permits the application of corrective measures of different intensity, resulting in reduction of costs. The intervention is accompanied by a careful control of the quality of iodized salt, and permanent pressure on the manufacturers to secure a good product.

The setback to the programmes in Colombia and Guatemala has led to special attention been paid to the epidemiological surveillance system.

The Ecuador experience has shown remarkable success in IDD reduction, and has helped to establish a programme for the Andean sub-region with a methodology that other countries may adopt since it has proved effective in Ecuador. It has been assumed that administrative conditions are similar in the countries of the Region, and that the problems and behaviour and attitude of the populations are the same. This suggests that the same methodology with slight adaptions can be applied with consequent saving of time and resources.

Since 1991 a sub-regional programme has been developed. The changes observed in these two years are important. Bolivia has already adjusted the methodology to its special situation and has succeeded in remarkably accelerating IDD control. Peru is following the same pattern, even though the solution of the problem is more difficult due to the greater area of the country. Colombia and Venezuela, even if they do not have national programmes of control, have established working groups; first, in order to have a better diagnosis in the short term, and then, to design faster and effective intervention measures.

Paraguay, due to its special situation, as a country that does not produce salt, requires a different strategy as it totally depends on salt imported from Argentina or Brazil.

In Central America a strong task force, similar to the Andean region should be established, and Mexico has the human and technical potential to eliminate the problem as soon as the political decision is taken.

In conclusion, Latin America is currently providing evidence that permits us to be optimistic with regard to IDD control. By political commitment, perseverance and especially with motivated people, the virtual elimination of these disorders that have caused so much social damage, may be reached before the turn of the century.

References

Dunn, J.T., et al ed. 1986. 'Towards the eradication of endemic goitre, cretinism and iodine deficiency'. Washington: Scientific Publication No. 502, PAHO.

Medeiros-Neto, G.A., 1988. 'Towards the eradication of iodine-deficiency disorders in Brazil through a salt iodination programme'. *Bulletin of the World Health Organization* 66(5): 637-642.

11
The Role of the International Agencies

UNICEF
P. Greaves and D. Alnwick

The United Nations Children's Fund is the part of the system with a special mandate to improve the welfare of children and women. It differs from the Specialized Agencies (FAO, WHO, UNESCO, ILO) in two important respects. The World Health Organization, for example, has responsibility in its own specialist sector, Health, to promote optimum health in all its aspects for all people. UNICEF, by contrast, has responsibility to a sector of society, children–and more so to women–for all of whose needs it has a legitimate concern.

The second respect in which UNICEF differs from the Specialized Agencies is with regard to its structure and mode of operation. UNICEF is perhaps the most decentralized part of the UN system: some 80 per cent of its staff of about 5,000 are in the field. UNICEF works in about 130 countries, and maintains 210 country and sub-country offices. The UNICEF representative in each country is given the responsibility and the authority to negotiate with the government a proposed programme of co-operation which addresses the priority needs perceived by the country within the framework of UNICEF policies as established by its Executive Board. The representative can do this within the limits of a financial allocation from UNICEF's general resources, issued by Headquarters, supplemented if necessary by additional funds to be sought for specific purposes. The proposed programme, after scrutiny by Headquarters, is then submitted to the Board for its approval.

Over the years, UNICEF has evolved a country programme process intended to ensure that UNICEF support relates to the needs of children and women in each country, reflects government policies as well as those of UNICEF, is fully integrated into the government programme, and is complementary to assistance provided by other multilateral and bilateral agencies. Thus, if WHO is primarily concerned with the establishment of norms and standards which have a universal validity, UNICEF is chiefly concerned with the translation of those precepts into practical action in particular countries. The two agencies are essentially complementary. Their respective governing bodies many years ago established a Joint Committee on Health Policy (JCHP) to facilitate harmonization.

Assistance provided by UNICEF to a country for the control of IDD has to fit within this context and within a broad UNICEF policy of support to improve nutrition with respect to both macronutrients and micronutrients. Support can extend from advocacy, through assistance for programme development (including provision of consultants, and support for surveys), to various aspects of programme implementation (for training, strengthening legislation and regulation, communications and development of communications materials, supplies, for example of potassium iodate and iodized oil, equipment for salt iodization and for laboratories) and to monitoring and evaluation. But UNICEF is also mindful of the larger context that enables country programmes to begin and to develop, and consequently has provided financial and other support to international advocacy events, international and regional training courses, expert meetings convened by WHO, operational research conducted by ICCIDD, and indeed core costs of ICCIDD itself. Some of these activities will be further elaborated.

UNICEF was aware of the importance of iodine deficiency from its earliest days. The advisory report on child nutrition prepared in 1947 by FAO and the WHO Interim Commission at the request of the (then) International Children's Emergency Fund, pointed out that 'in areas where soil and water are deficient in iodine, iodized salt needs to be provided,' and the use of iodized salt in school meals was recommended. UNICEF was active in providing consultants and salt iodization equipment to countries in Asia and South America in the sixties and an engineer with experience in such matters was based in the Food Conservation Division in New York for many years. However, the impact was limited. Maggie Black in her history of UNICEF, The Children and the Nations (Black, 1986), noted that 'adding iodine to salt was not a very efficient remedy in a country with no mass food marketing and distribution systems. In most such countries, salt mining was a cottage industry outside the reach of governmental control, and few people in the countryside bought their supply in a packet from a shop. Trying to solve nutritional problems by the processing of foodstuffs had in built limitations, therefore. People's nutritional conditions could not be invisibly 'fixed'. A health education campaign was needed to help people understand the need to protect themselves by buying the 'improved' version.

This perceptive passage identifies several important issues.

Firstly, the strategy of salt iodization is dependent for its success less on technical details related to the process of adding iodine to salt (these are relatively simple, and well understood) than to organizational matters related to the operation of the salt industry itself. A comprehensive understanding of that industry where the salt comes from; who handles it, how, and where; how it moves around a country; who purchases which forms of it, and at what price must be obtained before there is any need to be concerned with the business of fortification as such.

Secondly, there may well be groups for whom fortification of salt with iodine is not, at any rate for the time being, the most appropriate strategy: administration of iodized oil, which only became available later, could be much more suitable. For example, while salt iodization is being established (a process that may take some time, with equipment and supplies to be ordered and installed, and training to be designed and completed), the worst effects of iodine deficiency can be prevented by providing high risk groups (particularly women of childbearing age) with oral doses of iodized oil; and for people living in isolated villages with ready access to salt from natural deposits it will take a long time for salt iodization to become an effective strategy; meanwhile an alternative means of supplying iodine will have to be identified.

Thirdly, availability of iodized salt is one thing, but usage is most decidedly something else: hence the need for an informed and motivated public and the value of iodizing all edible salt.

It is true that in Britain during World War II the main architect of the government's food and nutrition policy, Sir Jack Drummond, referred to the practice of fortification of basic foodstuff in the words of Alexander Pope as 'doing good by stealth': people did not need to know, in order to obtain the benefit. But the conditions that made that policy practicable--a government in complete control of the movement of food, with adequate resources for inspection and enforcement, and by and large a co-operative population--are hardly the norm in most of the world today. Experience has confirmed again and again the need for communication at the core of a programme, to inform and to motivate not just the public, but those responsible for framing policy and also those having to carry it out.

Slowly the lesson was learnt. Mr Henry Labouisse, UNICEF Executive Director at the time, declared to the International Union of Nutritional Sciences at Rio de Janeiro in 1978: 'Iodine deficiency is so easy to prevent that it is a crime to let a single child be born mentally handicapped for that reason.' And Mr James P Grant, addressing the inaugural meeting of ICCIDD at Kathmandu in 1986, after he had become Executive Director of UNICEF, said: 'IDD is a good example of a major nutritional disorder for which the techniques of treatment, control and prevention are easily available and affordable. All it takes is a strong will, wider awareness, and co-operation among those who hold a key to the solution of the problem.' He went on to ask: 'why has progress not been broader and more effective? The most probable answer is that the policy making bodies in many countries were not fully aware of its health and development significance. The salt industry did not have sufficient incentives to co-operate; and the public did not know the root of the problem, its health hazards and the ease of preventing it.

So, renewed emphasis was given to advocacy at all levels. At the start of a paper prepared for presentation in January 1989 to the Committee on Health Policy UNICEF/WHO (JCHP 1989) a summary of proposed appropriate actions at country level and at global level concluded with the following paragraph:

'If little of this appears new, that is no cause of disappointment. The purpose is not necessarily to be innovative, but to be effective. This requires clarity of concept, strong motivation, thorough training and systematic supervision. Practical support is critical. The reason why past efforts have so often not been successful is that one or more of these requirements were lacking. Things don't have to be different. What matters is that they be done, and done properly. The chief reason to set targets is to motivate people to get things done. Targets may not be reached, but they must be approached.'

And one of the targets proposed for the nineties was 'the elimination of iodine deficiency disorders.'

The next year saw this process much advanced. In April 1990 the UNICEF Executive Board adopted a number of goals for the year 2000, including 'the virtual elimination of IDD.' In May the World Health Assembly adopted the goal of 'eliminating IDD as a major public health problem' (meaning the same thing). And in September this goal (amongst a range of others) was endorsed by the World Summit for Children, the largest gathering of Heads of State and government in history (71, with representatives of 88 others). Although the Summit had been suggested by Mr Grant in his State of the World's Children report for 1989, 'to discuss and prepare for action on the great opportunities now available for protecting today's children--and tomorrow's world,' and UNICEF provided the secretariat, it was not specifically a UNICEF affair: the Summit was convened by six Heads of government, and held under the auspices of the United Nations.

The Children's Summit was followed a year later by an international policy conference (convened by WHO and UNICEF, with support from FAO, UNDP, IBRD, USAID and CIDA) in Montreal in October 1991, on how to achieve the three micronutrient goals endorsed by the Summit. The conference was called 'Ending Hidden Hunger,' and a video of the same name, sponsored by UNICEF and WHO with support from USAID and IDRC, was made in 1992 and first shown at the

International Conference on Nutrition in Rome in December. The video illustrates the nature of the problems of iodine, vitamin A and iron deficiencies and how they are being addressed around the world through location shooting in Bangladesh, Ecuador, Tanzania and Zimbabwe. Available in English, French and Spanish it shows what needs to be done to achieve the Summit goals, and is particularly suitable for viewing by busy political leaders and executives in business and government, as well as by the general public. It can be used to introduce the topic for further discussion at a meeting or for broadcast on television.

Agencies of the United Nations system work of course through governments, and it is governments that ultimately set the pace. Therefore, a strategy aimed at obtaining their commitment, which reached its zenith at the World Summit for Children, goes to the heart of the matter. The world leaders agreed that their countries should prepare national plans of action, detailing how they were to achieve the goals, and that progress should be monitored.

Since the World Summit for Children, a series of high level Regional Consultations have taken place with governments in most parts of the world: of SAARC countries in Colombo and of African countries in Dakar in 1992, of countries of east Asia and the Pacific in Manila in September 1993, and of Latin American countries in Mexico City in October 1993. At each of these consultations, it was agreed that some of the actions required to reach the goal of the World Summit were so important and so eminently feasible and affordable that they should be reached by the middle of the decade--the end of 1995. Ensuring that all salt consumed by both people and animals in all countries with a problem of public health significance-the Universal Iodization of Salt-was one of these 'mid-decade goals'.

During 1993, rapid progress has been made towards the achievement of universal iodization of salt in many countries. Most salt consumed in Latin America is already iodized, and in Ecuador and Bolivia, IDD is close to being eliminated as a public health problem. In Africa, where much salt is traded between countries, emphasis is being placed on ensuring that all salt imported to countries is adequately iodized and that the major salt exporting nations, including Ghana, Senegal, Kenya, Tanzania, Namibia and Botswana, export only iodized salt. In India, efforts have concentrated on tightening existing controls on production and movements of uniodized salt, and expanding the control to all States and Union Territories. Bangladesh is equipping over 200 salt producers with iodization machinery and a supply of potassium iodate, and is providing the salt producers with the necessary training. In China, the country with the greatest number of people affected by iodine deficiency disorders, the government has called for all salt to be iodized before the end of 1996, and UNICEF is working with the World Bank to ensure that the necessary funds are available for this ambitious undertaking. It has already been proved that it is possible for salt to be effectively iodized in some of the world's poorest countries. No country is too poor to ensure that all of its citizens consume adequately iodized salt. The achievement of Universal Salt Iodization is not so much a matter of political will as political choice--a government can either decide to iodize salt or not to. The difficulty of ensuring that all salt is iodized in a country where salt production is a cottage industry remains. In order to ensure that salt is iodized in such countries, some modernization and investment in the salt industry will be required. This investment is likely to be considerably less than that required to develop a new airport, or even a major road, but its long term impact on human development is likely to be far greater. UNICEF is not generally able to provide such investment itself, but, as has been the case in China, has been able to assist countries in developing plans and proposals that can be funded by other agencies such as the World Bank.

UNICEF stands ready to help countries in such endeavours, through the country programming process referred to earlier. Other UN agencies in a position to provide substantial financial support are UNDP and IBRD (the World Bank), with both of which UNICEF has a close working relationship.

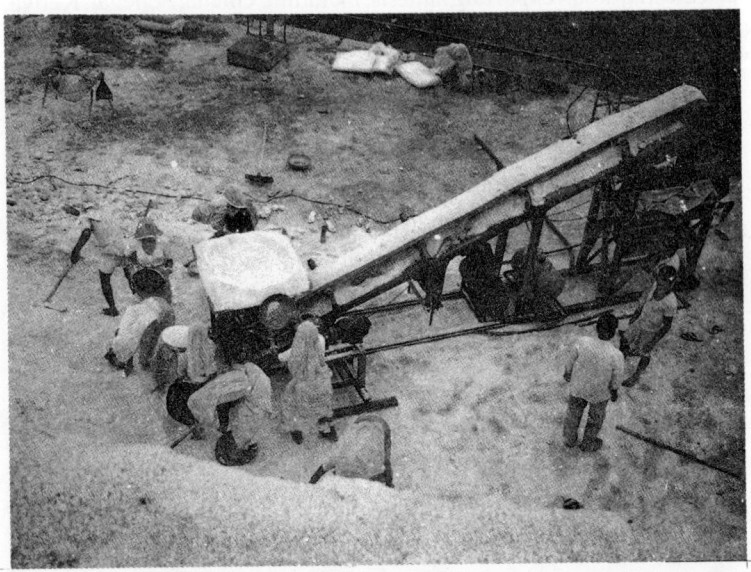

Fig. 11.1 Iodizing salt at the Great Sambhar Lake Salt Works in Rajasthan, India, where UNICEF provided the first iodization plant (much more massive than this one) in 1992 (photograph J P Greaves 1993).

Kiwanis International, a worldwide service organization, has agreed to make the elimination of IDD one of its top priorities. Kiwanis International has agreed to work with UNICEF to raise funds to help countries achieve the Universal Iodization of Salt as noted elsewhere in this book. At the beginning of the nineties UNICEF was supporting activities towards the elimination of IDD in thirty or more countries; by the end of 1993 UNICEF was actively involved in assisting, or planning to assist, salt iodization in at least 60 countries (Fig. 11.1 and Fig.11.2).

UNICEF estimated that the total need for iodine for salt fortification in all developing countries in Asia, Africa and Latin America is some 500 tonnes per year (approximately 5 percent of Japan's production), valued at current prices at about US$ 10 million. UNICEF provides some potassium iodate to countries, as part of its programme of co-operation, and has advised that it is prepared to procure supplies on behalf of countries, which are then able to benefit from favourable prices consequent on bulk orders. Such arrangements may be useful for a limited initial period while a more sustainable system of procurement is established.

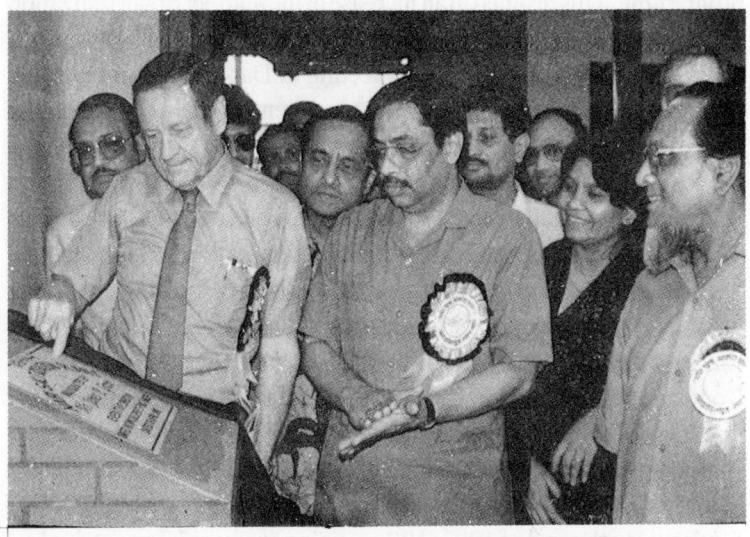

Fig. 11.2 Mr James P Grant, Executive Director, UNICEF inaugurates a salt iodization plant at Keraniganj, Dhaka, Bangladesh; on 29 April 1992, in the presence of the Honourable Minister of Health and Family Welfare, Mr Chowdhury Kamal Ibne Yusuf. (Photo Baquer. M-UNICEF Dhaka.) This is the first of 200 plants provided by UNICEF. The last is planned for June 1994.

In the long term the cost of fortification including the cost of iodate must be absorbed by the industry and passed to the consumer--and the sooner this can be done the better. This cost-recovery feature is an overriding advantage of salt iodization compared to other methods of providing iodine. People after all do buy salt, and the extra cost associated with iodization is very small.

UNICEF's experience of iodized oil is that demand has increased and that oral doses are increasingly being favoured as against injections.

For example, UNICEF supplied 4.8 million capsules in 1990 and over twice as many–10.9 million–in 1991. The immediate effect of iodized oil can create a demand for a programme sustainable for a longer term, usually based on salt fortification. For example, in a UNICEF programme in Vietnam in the latter part of the eighties, iodized oil brought about a significant reduction in the size and frequency of goitres, which stimulated a local demand for a permanent control programme. This resulted in an increase in the number of salt iodization plants.

Following an ICCIDD Board meeting in Dar-es-Salaam in March 1990 at which 'monitoring' and 'management' were identified as key issues requiring priority attention, UNICEF invited a proposal on how the experiences of the China-Australian Technical Co-operation on control of IDD could be extended and applied elsewhere. This led to the establishment in January 1991 of the International Training and Support Programme for the control of IDD (IPCIDD), involving exemplary collaboration between three Atlanta-based organizations: Emory University School of Public Health, the Centers for Disease Control, and the Task Force for Child Survival and Development of the President Carter Centre. Prompted by the Montreal Conference on 'Ending Hidden Hunger', this evolved into the Programme against Micronutrient Malnutrition (PAMM) with additional sources of funding. By the end of 1993, 100 participants from 22 countries had been trained.

An idea which excited several people in UNICEF was the thought that it might be possible (should be possible) to determine from a single spot of blood, dried on a filter paper the nutritional status of the individual with respect not just to iodine, but also to iron and vitamin A. This would enormously simplify the problem of tracking progress with respect to the micronutrient Summit goals--and of checking that there is no backsliding afterwards. In fact, the potential of blood-spot technology is even greater than this, and PAMM is actively working on its development though problems are more intractable than had been anticipated.

The question of backsliding is very important. It is no accident that the international agencies speak of the elimination of IDD, not of its eradication. The distinction is deliberate, and crucial. WHO's great achievement was the eradication of small-pox: the root cause of the disease, dreaded for thousands of years, was completely blotted out, so that small-pox can never come back. It is impossible for IDD to be eradicated in this sense. If for any reason the supply of iodine is interrupted, IDD will recur. Therefore, there is the need for continued vigilance and mechanisms to ensure sustainability. (see Chapters 2 and 3). The threat is not theoretical. As noted elsewhere in this work there is evidence (for example in Colombia and in former East Germany) that the IDD situation has worsened in recent years as uniodized salt has become available.

At the time of writing, the future shape of the United Nations and its agencies is under active consideration. One cannot tell what the future may hold for any of its organs, including UNICEF. But one can confidently hope that UNICEF's experience and traditions will survive and indeed be strengthened as they continue to be deployed in the service of the underprivileged, wherever in the world they may be. Recognition is not so important as that the work be done. Lao-Tsu (c. 600 BC) writing about leaders, said:

'But of the best, when their task is accomplished,
their work done,
The people all remark, 'We have done it ourselves.'

References

Black., Maggie 1986. *The Children and the Nations*. New York: UNICEF.

Joint WHO/UNICEF Committee on Health Policy 1989. JC27/UNICEF-WHO 89.4.

WHO

G.A. Clugston and K.V. Bailey

Global Historical Developments

WHO's first role in relation to IDD–then known simply as endemic goitre-goes back to the very earliest years of WHO's existence, when WHO made great efforts to define the national and global magnitude of iodine deficiency. The first WHO Nutrition Officers in Geneva set about documenting the extent of goitre in the world and methods of controlling it, culminating in the publication of a veritable mine of information on the subject in the WHO Monograph, Endemic Goitre, in 1960.

Since then WHO concentrated initially on more thorough assessments of IDD, refining the classification of goitre and extending surveys to part of nearly all countries of the world by the end of 1960's. At the same time efforts were made to develop IDD control especially through the iodization of salt, in co-operation with UNICEF: initially in Latin America but soon in Asia and eventually Africa.

The World Food Conference in 1975 stimulated a renewed emphasis on efforts to prevent micronutrient deficiencies including that of iodine. But only a few countries in Asia, Africa and the Middle East responded with serious efforts, until about the mid-1980's with the holding of a symposium on endemic goitre in Southeast Asia at the Fourth Asian Congress of Nutrition in 1983, where the term 'IDD' proposed by Dr Hetzel, was first adopted. There followed, in 1985, a historic Joint WHO/UNICEF Intercountry Workshop on the Control of IDD in South-east Asia held at WHO's South East Asia Regional office, New Delhi, India and it was there that the International Council for control of Iodine Deficiency Disorders (ICCIDD) was also proposed by Dr. Hetzel, and it was formally inaugurated in Kathmandu the following year. (see Chapter 2)

While these events were occurring, global advocacy efforts were continuing elsewhere on the world stage. However, it is probably fair to say that IDD really came on stage globally with the adoption in 1986 of the World Health Assembly resolution (Resolution WHA 39.31) on the prevention and control of IDD. Through this forum, all member States collectively recognized iodine deficiency disorders as a high priority, preventable cause of brain damage and mental impairment affecting millions worldwide.

With this acceleration in global momentum, it was recognized, around 1989, that with an extraordinary effort by all IDD affected countries, IDD could be actually eliminated from the face of the earth by the year 2000. Such an achievement would be another global triumph, ranking with the eradication of smallpox and poliomyelitis.

Thus in 1990 an enthusiastic World Health Assembly heard and debated the current world IDD situation, and passed a historic resolution (Resolution WHA 43.2) deciding that 'WHO shall aim at eliminating IDD as a major public health problem in all countries by the year 2000'.

This was followed the same year by the World Summit for Children, which endorsed as one of its decade goals the "virtual elimination of IDD".

This global momentum of IDD awareness and accelerating action continued, and the following year in October 1991, WHO and UNICEF convened a historic conference 'Ending Hidden Hunger: a Policy Conference on Micronutrient Malnutrition', which brought together over 300 people-ministers, policy leaders and scientists from all over the world. This conference encouraged many countries into initiating or reinforcing IDD control programmes as a national priority.

The World Declaration and Plan of Action for Nutrition, endorsed by almost all countries of the world, at the International Conference on Nutrition, organized by WHO and FAO in Rome in 1992, further emphasized the feasibility and commitment of the world community to eliminating IDD by the year 2000, and provided pragmatic guidelines on how this can be achieved.

In essence, WHO's particular role in relation to world health issues, including IDD, has three main dimensions: its co-ordinating and regulatory role in international health; its normative role in scientific aspects; and technical co-operation with and among Member States. The following paragraphs illustrate how this mandate is being exercised in respect of IDD. Furthermore, from 1986 onwards, it would be rather invidious to talk about WHO and UNICEF partnership without bringing in the third partner, ICCIDD, which has done so much to reinforce and even to spearhead, jointly with WHO and UNICEF, the efforts for advocacy and prevention of IDD at global, regional and national levels.

Regional Programme

The second half of the 1980's saw an acceleration of activity firstly in the African and South East Asian Regions and then other Regions with meetings being held in each of the six world's Regions between 1987 and 1994 (see Table 11.1). Resolutions on prevention, control

Table 11.1 *Joint regional meetings WHO/UNICEF/ICCIDD*

1. With AFRO	:	Joint Regional Meeting on Control of IDD in Africa Yaounde, 1987.
2. With SEARO	:	Joint Meeting on control of Idd in SE Asia New Delhi, 1989.
3. With AFRO	:	Joint Meeting on control on in Eastern & Southern Africa-Dar es Salaam, 1991
4. With EURO	:	Joint Regional Meeting on IDD in Europe-a Continuing Concern, Brussels, 1992.
5. With WPRO	:	Joint Regional Workshop on a Regional Strategy Manila, 1992.
6. With EMRO	:	Joint Regional Meeting on IDD in the Middle East Alexandria, 1993.
7. With AMRO	:	Joint Regional Meeting on Elimination of IDD Quito, 1994.
8. With MI,CIDA	:	In Co-operation with THE GOVERNMENT OF BANGLADESH : Partnership to End Hidden Hunger, Meeting on Sustaining Elimination of Iodine Deficiency Disorders - Collaboration of Stakeholders in Mangaging Success, Dhaka, Bangladesh, 1995.

and elimination of IDD have been adopted by most Regions, indicating clearly a certain priority given by countries to this programme in the last decade. Through the close collaborative efforts of WHO, UNICEF and ICCIDD, Regional IDD working groups have been set up in each Region of the world, involving the three agencies as well as bilateral, non-governmental or other organizations wishing to participate.

These working groups generally meet annually together with the responsible officers of national programmes for control of iodine deficiency disorders as far as possible, for review of the programmes and exchange of experiences. The groups have proved themselves useful in encouraging and guiding the generation and implementation of national programmes. All these Resolutions and working groups have greatly supported and stimulated action in countries.

Training Programmes and Capacity-building

While advocacy could and did reach and sensitize a good number of key administrators and some political leaders, especially in the field of health, and much could be done through consultative services to countries, there was a great need to build technical capacity in the countries themselves, for IDD assessment and programme management. So increasingly the triumvirate galvanized itself for action in supporting this area. Initially this was tackled on a global basis with the holding of two "PEG" courses in Belgium, in 1988 and 1990, organized by the Belgian group (Prof. A.Evmans and colleagues) but with again the same tripartite collaboration. This was followed through with a series of regional training workshops as shown in Table 11.2. For instance in the African region it was estimated that there was only a handful of IDD experts in 1987 but by 1991 well over 100 persons were trained in 26 countries, in the main principles of management of IDD programmes.

National Programme Implementation

So by now some programme implementation, of varying comprehensiveness, is under way in the great majority of IDD affected countries. Certainly, advocacy, training and "triumvirate" support have done much to accelerate this action. We are reaping today the benefits of a well-orchestrated capacity-building support to countries, and it is gratifying to see the enormous efforts and motivation of the national officers responsible for IDD control in spite of innumerable and at times almost intolerable constraints!

Table 11.2 *Joint training workshops on IDD: WHO-organized or with WHO participation together with ICCIDD & UNICEF*

1. Programme for Eradication of Goitre (PEG) Course*, Brussels, (1987)
2. PEG Course,* Brussels, 1990
3. Training Workshop on IDD management (Anglophone African countries) Dar es Salaam 1991
4. Training Workshop on IDD management (Francophone African countries) Yaounde 1991
5. Tri-regional seminar (WHO/ICCIDD): Management and monitoring of IDD (South-east Asia, Western Pacific and Eastern Mediterranean) New Delhi, November, 1991
6. PEG Course* (francophone African countries) Bujumbura, Burundi, January 1992
7. Course on IDD management (Hispanophone) 1992
8. Laboratory methods, Damascus, (Eastern Mediterranean) 1992

* Also supported by Belgian Co-operation Fund.

Iodized oil. The use of iodized oil enjoyed a great popularity especially in the early days of programme development in many countries with major logistical or technical constraints to salt iodization, and particularly in areas of severe deficiency. This intervention in some cases helped to stimulate national concern and action on a broader front. The difficulty is of course the relatively high cost and low sustainability, with little possibility of cost-sharing by the communities. WHO provided technical support in the early stages of virtually all the completed or currently on-going iodized oil programmes.

Salt iodization. Salt iodization, the preferred long-term and sustainable solution to IDD control, is on the other hand a more cross-sectoral strategy which is very demanding in terms of co-operation between sectors of government and especially these days involving heavily the private sector.

WHO's role in salt iodization includes main types of activity:

-Advocacy: with the Ministry of Health initially, and then with other ministries concerned e.g. Ministry of industry, trade, etc.;

-Encouraging establishment of intersectoral IDD Technical Committees including the salt sector for management of IDD control programmes;

-Support in drawing up appropriate standards, regulations and enforcement measures for salt iodization, including guidance on desirable levels of iodine in salt;

-Workshops with salt producers/importers: The tripartite alliance initiated jointly, and with the special support of CIDA, a series of workshops bringing together national IDD programme managers with the main salt producers or importers in various sub-regions. The first such workshop was held in Botswana in April 1990 for 8 southern African countries, and the second in Senegal, September 1992. A further such workshop was held in Guatemala in 1993. WHO has also recently urged the rehabilitation of salt iodization facilities in eastern European countries;

-Emphasis on monitoring, both of the salt iodization process to ensure iodization is regularly up to standard; and epidemiological monitoring of IDD (especially urinary iodine levels) to verify that adequate iodine status is actually achieved and maintained.

Monitoring, Evaluation and Information Systems

It was recognized a decade ago that failure to develop adequate monitoring systems, both of iodine status and of programme implementation including salt iodization, was a major cause of breakdown of several national IDD control programmes, especially in Latin America. To avoid repeating this type of reversal, and hopefully to ensure permanent sustainability in the future of the whole programme, WHO has made much effort to foster the development of adequate monitoring and information systems for IDD.

Practically all national programmes are currently implemented against a backdrop of some baseline information; but often that baseline was quite weak due to technical difficulties or the non-availability or costliness of adequate laboratory facilities or personnel; or simply, lack of awareness of the importance of this aspect of the programme.

Consequently, and also in view of Resolutions WHA 43.2 (1990) and WHA 45.44 which charged both the countries and WHO with the monitoring thereof, WHO has been particularly concerned with two main developments:

1. The Micronutrient Deficiency Information System (MDIS), (Fig. 11.3) one component of which-and the best developed-is for IDD. The main originality of this system is that it includes data not only on IDD prevalence (various parameters-clinical and biochemical, and at various levels of disaggregation) but also a summary of programme implementation information.

Table 11.3 *Micronutrient Deficiency Information System–IDD Summary of data contained, and outputs*

Type of data	Format	Level of disaggregation

Clinical
  Goitre rates
  Thyroid volume
   (ultrasound)
	Maps	Global

Biochemical
  Urinary iodine
  Hormones-TSH
	Tables	Regional

Programmatic
  Salt iodization
  Iodized oil etc.
	Text	National

References	Text	Global

MICRONUTRIENT DEFICIENCY INFORMATION SYSTEM

WORLD HEALTH ORGANIZATION

MDIS Working Paper # 1

GLOBAL PREVALENCE OF IODINE DEFICIENCY DISORDERS

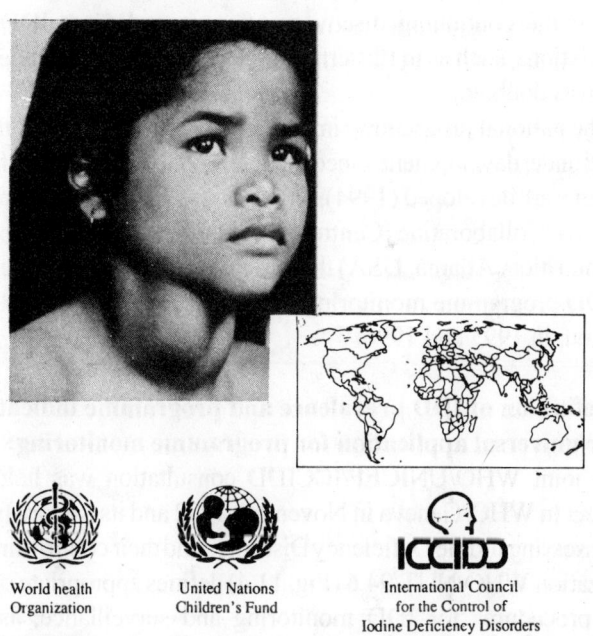

World health Organization

United Nations Children's Fund

International Council for the Control of Iodine Deficiency Disorders

Fig. 11.3 Micronutrient Deficiency Information System. a joint effort by WHO/UNICEF/ICCIDD for promoting information about Vitamin A, Iron and Iodine Deficiency Disorders.

A picture of the whole information assembled in MDIS is given in Table 11.3. Currently the whole global/regional system is established and available in the form of a multiple directory electronic data-bank.

A summary of the IDD prevalence data with brief programme notes is available in the document Global prevalence of IDD-MDIS (document # 1, 1993). This publication is the product of an exhaustive review of the most recent data, country by country.

It was found that the earlier (1990) estimate of 1005 million subjects at risk of IDD had to be increased to 1571 million, and the numbers affected by goitre, from 200 million to 686 million. This increase is partly due to the expert consultation's decision that goitre rates exceeding 5% (rather than 10% as adopted formerly) should be considered indicative of a public health problem. But it is also partly due to the continuing discovery of more and more IDD-affected populations, such as in Eastern Europe where the number identified at risk was doubled.

The national programme implementation component of the MDIS is still under development. Once suitable models for national information systems are developed (1994), it is envisaged to organize, through and with its Collaborating Centre (Programme Against Micronutrient Malnutrition, Atlanta, USA) the systematic training of national teams in IDD programme monitoring and information systems, Region by Region, in 1995 and 1996.

2. Definition of IDD prevalence and programme indicators, and their universal application for programme monitoring:

A joint WHO/UNICEF/ICCIDD consultation was held on this subject in WHO/Geneva in November 1992 and its Report-Indicators for assessing Iodine Deficiency Disorders and their control through salt iodization WHO/NUT/94.6 (Fig. 11.4) defines appropriate objectives and procedures for IDD monitoring and surveillance, as well as epidemiological and programme or process indicators in various circumstances, including those suitable for tracking progress towards the elimination of IDD (Table 11.4). This same consultation also dealt with desirable levels of salt iodization (Table 11.5) and indicators for salt iodization (Table 11.6). Criteria (both epidemiological and process criteria) have been drafted, and also an outline of the procedures envisaged.

Conclusion

WHO considers it a privilege to have UNICEF, ICCIDD and other partners working closely with its secretariat and Member countries towards the elimination of IDD—one of the most exciting prospects in the field of nutrition for a big success story in the next 5 years.

Table 11.4 *Criteria for tracking progress towards the World Health Assembly/World Summit goals: elimination of IDD as a public health problem*

Indicator	Goal
1. Salt iodization Proportion of households consuming effectively iodized salt	>90%
2. Urinary iodine Proportion below 100 µg/l Proportion below 50 µg/l	<50% <20%
3. Thyroid size In school children 6-12 years of age: Proportion with enlarged thyroid, by palpation or ultrasound	<5%
4. Neonatal TSH Proportion with levels > 5mU/l whole blood	<3%

Source: Indicators for assessing Iodine Deficiency Disorders and their control through salt iodization. Report of a Joint WHO/UNICEF/ ICCIDD Consultation, 3-5 November 1992, WHO, Geneva. Document WHO/NUT/94.6.

Indicators for Assessment of Iodine Deficiency Disorders and their control through salt iodization

Report of a Joint WHO/UNICEF/ICCIDD Consultation

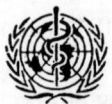 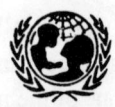 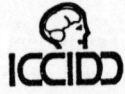

World Health Organization   United Nations Children's Fund   International Council for the Control of Iodine Deficiency Disorders

Fig. 11.4 Joint WHO/UNICEF/ICCIDD consultation on indicators for assessment of IDD and their control through salt iodization.

Table 11.6 *Criteria for assessing adequacy of salt iodization programmes*

Process Indicator	Criterion of Adequacy
A. Factory or importer level	
1. Percent of food grade salt claimed to be iodized	100%
2. Percent of food grade salt effectively iodized	≥ 90%
3. Adequacy of internal monitoring process*	≥ 90%
4. Adequacy of external monitoring process	10-12 monthly checks per producer/importer per year
B. Consumer and district level	
1. Percent of monitoring sites with adequately iodized salt i) households (or schools) ii) district headquarters (including major markets)	
2. Adequacy of monitoring process** Adequate in 90% of samples	90% or more

*Corrective action systematically taken with 3 hours in 90% of cases, using the lot quality assurance (LQAS) methodology
**Monitoring undertaken in 90% of districts in each province, at both household and district level

Source: Same as for Table 11.4

Table 11.5 ICCIDD-UNICEF-WHO recommended levels of iodine in salt

Climate and daily salt consumption (g/person)	Requirement at factory outside the country		Requirement at factory inside the country		Requirement at retail sale (shop/market)		Requirement at household level
	Bulk (sack)	Retail pack (<2 kg)	Bulk (sack)	Retail pack (<2 kg)	Bulk (sack)	Retail pack (<2 kg)	
Warm moist							
5g	100	80	90	70	80	60	50
10g	50	40	45	35	40	30	25
Warm dry or cool moist							
5g	90	70	80	60	70	50	45
10g	45	35	40	30	35	25	22.5
Cool dry							
5g	80	60	70	50	60	45	40
10g	40	30	35	25	30	22.5	20

Sources: Adapted from World Summit for Children-mid-decade goal; iodine deficiency disorders. Geneva, 1994. UNICEF-WHO Joint Committee on Health Policy, document JCHPSS/94/2.7, document WHO/NUT/93.1 and document WHO/NUT/94.6.

N.B. 168.6 mg of KIO_3 contains 100 mg of iodine.
N.B. These are indicative initial levels, which should be adjusted in the light of urinary iodine measurement.

In summary, the areas in which WHO has a particular role in this essentially national process, with full tripartite support, would be:

- The development of national monitoring, surveillance and information systems for both iodine status and programme implementation especially salt iodization.
- National, regional and global advocacy, making powerful use of the epidemiological and programme data assembled in the data banks at each level:
- Human resource development at each level, now, in most countries, emphasis on monitoring/evaluation and information system development (national MDIS):
- Systematic development of salt monitoring through technical support where necessary to installation of iodized salt production or importation systems, including appropriate regulations/legislation and enforcement measures, and encouragement of alliances of salt producers and importers committed to iodization, at national, regional and global levels:
- Development of the global systems for verification of sustainable elimination of IDD:
- Mobilization of resources necessary at each level for implementation of the above.

References

WHO/UNICEF/ICCIDD November, 1992. 'Indicators for assessing Iodine Deficiency Disorders and their control through salt iodization'. *Report of a Joint Consultation.* 3-5. WHO, Geneva. Document WHO/NUT/94.6.

WHO/UNICEF/ICCIDD, 1993. 'Micronutrient Deficiency Information system MDIS working paper # 1. Global prevalence of Iodine Deficiency Disorders'.

12

The role of Kiwanis International

W. Blechman

Kiwanis International, dating from 1916, consists of all chartered Local Kiwanis Clubs made up of Kiwanis members. The official motto is 'We Build'. Its objectives are:

(1) to give primacy to the human and spiritual, rather than to the material values of life.

(2) to encourage the daily living of the Golden Rule.

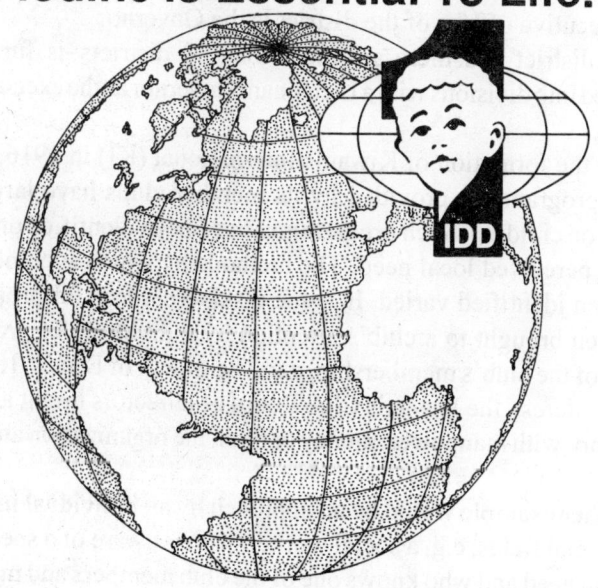

(3) the promotion of higher social, business and professional standards.

(4) to develop, by precept and example, a more intelligent, aggressive and serviceable citizenship.

(5) to provide, through Kiwanis clubs, a practical means of forming enduring friendships, rendering altruistic service, and building better communities.

(6) to co-operate in creating and maintaining sound public opinion and a sense of idealism which would make possible the increase of righteousness, justice, patriotism, and goodwill.

There are over 9,000 Kiwanis clubs in more than 70 countries or geographic areas with a total membership in excess of 320,000.

The Kiwanis International Board of Trustees has full administrative authority over all activities. The International Office is in Indianapolis, Indiana, U.S.A.

Kiwanis International is usually organized into districts–with territorial boundaries established by the International Board. Each Kiwanis club within that territory is a member of the district. The chief executive officer of the district is the Governor.

Each district and there are more than 40 districts–is further organized into divisions with a Lieutenant Governor as the executive officer.

Since the formation of Kiwanis International (KI) in 1916, the service programmes provided by its member clubs have largely focused on children. Such programmes have been identified on the basis of perceived local need. The methods by which such needs have been identified varied. In some instances, ideas for projects have been brought to a club's attention by individuals or groups outside of the club's membership, e.g. The March of Dimes. If this created interest, the Kiwanis Club Board of Directors might agree to support, with manpower, money or both, the organization and its efforts.

Another example would be an approach by an individual in one of the social fields, e.g. a social worker, who is aware of a specific family in need and who knows one of the club members and makes a personal contact. The social worker either presents the problem to the member who carries it to the club or perhaps is asked to speak directly to the club. The club can then accept a responsibility to participate in a suggested effort on behalf of the family, or it may decline to do so.

Another source of projects has come from KI itself. Until 1990, all Kiwanis clubs were encouraged to participate in programmes organized annually by the staff at Kiwanis International. The broad topic from which these suggested programmes were developed came from an idea or point of interest put forward by the individual who was to be the President of Kiwanis International that year. Though KI would promote this particular group of programmes strongly throughout the year, it was recognized that only a minority of clubs would actually participate, and most of these were within North America.

By the beginning of October 1990, however, in response to recognition that promotion of annual programmes was neither cost efficient nor effective, KI developed a pilot three year programme entitled, 'Young Children: Priority One.' The thrust of 'Young Children: Priority One' is towards the age group 0-5, a group that arguably has the weakest safety nets throughout the world. 'Young Children: Priority One' also had two facets that were basically new to Kiwanis: it encouraged an increased emphasis on projects aimed at prevention and early intervention and it promoted partnership and coalition development to allow Kiwanis Clubs to put better leverage on their efforts.

Within one year, it was so apparent that Kiwanians in many parts of the world were moving into projects affecting the 0-5 age group that the Kiwanis International Board removed the three year pilot status and made 'Young Children: Priority One' its primary worldwide service programme for an indefinite period of time.

The development of 'Young Children: Priority One' was aided through the support of many other organizations. Indeed, there remains a formal advisory council with members composed of 33 organizations from the United States. Additional advisory councils are planned for other regions of the world in the future.

Contacts with additional organizations interested in children's issues have also been maintained, and it was through one such contact (with the Task Force for Child Development and Survival at the Carter Center in Atlanta) that a recommendation was made for Kiwanis to be represented at two meetings held in Montreal beginning on October 9, 1991. These meetings, 'Protecting the World's Children: Keeping the Promise" and 'Ending Hidden Hunger" brought to Kiwanis leadership a new vision of potential service activity. Over a period of several months, following these meetings, KI developed a relationship with UNICEF that has since developed into a partnership. Taking goals presented during the World Summit for Children, UNICEF prepared a set of programmes for potential involvement by the Kiwanis. Following an extensive evaluation and discussion, the Kiwanis International Board chose to join UNICEF in an effort to virtually eradicate iodine deficiency disorders in the developing world by the year 2000.

While the Kiwanis role is primarily fund-raising, the ultimate goal is to help with the development of iodized salt plants in those countries where iodine has been leached from the soil, resulting in an iodine-deficient diet. It is recognized that part of the programme also requires the educating of both government leaders and average citizens to be willing to promote, pay for and use the 'new" salt, which will cost a small amount more. The Kiwanis-UNICEF partnership hopes to add 1000 of these new salt plants throughout the iodine-deficient parts of the world.

The programme was formally announced during the Kiwanis International Convention held in Nice, France on June 30, 1993 and it is planned to begin with pilot projects in several Kiwanis regions with eventual expansion to all Kiwanis countries. Money will be raised through the Kiwanis International Foundation, which is the fund raising arm of KI.

The International Council for Control of Iodine Deficiency Disorders has already assisted Kiwanis International in the development of its education programme throughout the world and the Executive Director has been appointed Senior Advisor to the Campaign Cabinet.

PART III

Stories from the Countries

13

IDD in Africa
IDD in Eastern and Southern Africa

F.P. Kavishe

Introduction

The Eastern and Southern African countries forming the Sub-regional Working Group on the control of IDD are Botswana, Ethiopia, Kenya, Lesotho, Malawi, Mauritius, Mozambique, Namibia, Seychelles, Swaziland, Tanzania, Uganda, Zambia, and Zimbabwe. (Fig. 13.1)

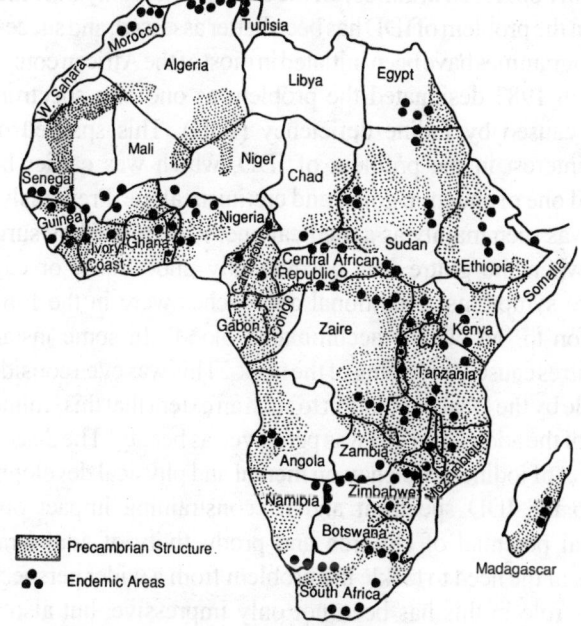

Fig. 13.1 Map showing distribution of IDD in Africa.
Source: Modified from Benmiloud, M., Bachtarzi, H., and Chaouki, M.B. (1983). Public health and nutritional aspects of endemic goitre and cretinism in Africa. In Cassava toxicity and thyroid (eds. F. Delange and R. Ahluwalia) p.50 Research and public health issues, IDRC, Ottawa.

The countries are of varying sizes and populations, ranging from 455 sq. km. (Seychelles) to over 1,000,000 sq.km. (Ethiopia) and populations of about 70,000 (Seychelles) to more than 50,000,000 (Ethiopia). With the exception of Mauritius and Seychelles, IDD is a problem of public health significance in all the remaining countries, but with varying degrees of severity.

A Historical Perspective

Before the 1980's, there was only scanty information on the problem of IDD in these countries. The earliest recorded accounts are described in Ethiopia where travellers were reported to have seen people affected by goitre as early as 1904. Although IDD manifested as goitre was subsequently observed in almost all the countries it is only over the last decade that the problem of IDD has been better assessed, and successful control programmes have been initiated in most of the African countries.

Hetzel in 1983 designated the problem as one of a spectrum of disorders caused by iodine deficiency (IDD), This sparked off a renewed interest in the problem of IDD, which was earlier being considered one of endemic goitre and cretinism alone. Previously, the problem was seen mainly as a medical one; to be treated by surgical removal when the goitre was cosmetically undesirable or caused obstructive symptoms. Traditional approaches were in the form of scarification to 'let out the accumulated blood'. In some instances visible goitres caused 'rounding of the neck.' This was even considered as desirable by the local population to such an extent that this 'rounding the neck' of the adolescent girl was perceived as beauty! The discovery of the effect of iodine deficiency on mental and physical development leading to the IDD spectrum and its constraining impact on the educational potential of children and productivity of adults raised awareness of the need to tackle the problem from a wider perspective. ICCIDD's role in this has been not only impressive, but also very successful. No wonder that the acceleration of IDD control in the Eastern, Central and Southern Africa (ECSA) region is traced back to the formation of ICCIDD in 1985 and especially after its inauguration in 1986.

Intercountry co-operation in the control of IDD in the ECSA, subregion started on 20th November 1986, when a one-day symposium was held as part of the annual consultations of the ECSA nutrition experts who comprise the heads of nutrition units or institutions in those countries. It is important to note that the symposium was moderated by Drs Fritz van der Haar and F P Kavishe, both ICCIDD Board members, who had attended the inauguration of ICCIDD in Kathmandu, Nepal, in March 1986. The ECSA co-operation in nutrition was the result of the Fifth Commonwealth Health Ministers Conference which was held in Wellington, New Zealand, in 1977, and it requested the Commonwealth Regional Health Secretariat in Arusha, Tanzania, to examine the nutrition problems and their solutions in the Commonwealth countries of Eastern and Southern Africa. A meeting of the nutrition experts consisting of the heads of nutrition units or institutions in the relevant countries was convened in 1979 and formulated an Eastern, Central and Southern Africa (ECSA) co-operation in nutrition. Since then annual meetings of the nutrition experts have been held under the sponsorship of the Regional Commonwealth Health Secretariat, initially under the Tanzania Food and Nutrition Centre (TFNC) as a provincial co-ordinator, but since 1992 under a full time co-ordinator based at its offices in Arusha, Tanzania.

The Need for an Institutional Framework

The 1986 IDD symposium was sponsored by the Netherlands Government, the United Nations University (UNU), the ICCIDD, and the Tanzania Food and Nutrition Centre (TFNC). An ECSA-IDD working group consisting of Ethiopia, Malawi, Tanzania (chair), and Zimbabwe was formed and in January 1987 formulated a regional approach to the control of IDD. This was the organizational framework which was used by the ICCIDD sub-regional co-ordinator when later in 1987, ICCIDD formulated an IDD Task Force for Africa and designated sub-regional co-ordinators for four sub-regions (North, West, Central and Eastern and Southern Africa) following the first WHO/UNICEF/ICCIDD Africa regional IDD meeting in Yaounde,

Cameroon. It was because of the existence of the ECSA nutrition co-operation that the control of IDD in the Eastern and Southern African region has achieved spectacular success. Experience gained so far indicates that an institutional framework is not only necessary at the sub-regional level, but also at the national level. The most successful country programmes are in those countries where one competent lead agency has been designated to catalyze and harmonize IDD control. Examples are the Tanzania Food and Nutrition Centre (TFNC), the Department of Nutrition of Zimbabwe, and the Ethiopian Nutrition Institute (ENI).

The Severity of the IDD Problem

In contrast to Central Africa, where the problem of IDD is severe in large parts of the affected countries, in Eastern and Southern Africa, the problem can be described as of generally mild to moderate severity. In South Africa the problem of IDD has not been reviewed, but is expected to be mild or absent because of the long history of using iodized salt. There are of course pockets of severe IDD in individual countries such as Ethiopia, Uganda, Tanzania, Malawi and Mozambique, where visible goitre rates of more than 60 per cent have been found with extremely low urinary iodine excretion and the prevalence of endemic cretinism approaching 10 per cent. The moderate and severe IDD endemicities seem to follow a rather clear geographical pattern which is seen as an 'IDD belt'.

The IDD Belt

In Eastern and Southern Africa, the highest IDD endemias are described in the highlands of the Great Rift Valley, as it descends southwards from Ethiopia, divides into an eastern and western arm in northern Tanzania which descend separately to unite again at Lake Nyasa. This 'IDD belt' extends further southwards to the northern parts of Mozambique, Malawi and Zambia and westwards to Uganda, Rwanda and Burundi. The 'IDD belt' is characterized by relatively recent volcanic activity; high soil fertility supporting high population densities and economies self-sufficient in food. These characteristics make it unlikely that the problem of IDD can be addressed through the economics of food movements, making it necessary to use the combined strategies of salt iodization and iodized oil distribution in some countries.

IDD Programmes

Activities to control IDD have been initiated in all the countries where IDD is a problem of public health significance. Most countries have in fact formulated national IDD control programmes. The most advanced programmes are in Tanzania and Zimbabwe, with Ethiopia, Kenya and Malawi having made considerable progress. All the programmes use two main strategies:- salt iodization alone or a combination of salt iodization and iodized oil. These are supported by IEC activities.

The level of salt iodization used varies from 50 to 100 ppm with the lower level being used in the more temperate countries of the region. A regional strategy for salt iodization has been advocated and its implementation is slowly taking shape. The strategy envisages the iodization of export salt by the salt producing countries. Already, the Sua Pan Soda Ash Company in Botswana expected to produce over 600,000 metric tonnes of salt at full capacity has started to iodize its salt at a level of 50 ppm. This company can satisfy all the iodized salt requirements in the region at full capacity. Presently this salt is available in Malawi, Zambia and Zimbabwe. Iodized salt is also produced in Kenya (exported to Tanzania and Uganda), Namibia (exported mainly to Botswana, Lesotho, Malawi, Swaziland, Zambia and Zimbabwe) and Tanzania (exported mainly to Burundi, Rwanda and Zaire). Iodized salt is also expected to be produced in Mozambique and resumed in Eritrea where production had already started when it was a region of Ethiopia.

Large scale iodized oil programmes are being implemented in Ethiopia, Malawi, Tanzania and Zimbabwe in severely affected regions where the visible goitre rate is more than 10 per cent, as a short-term stop gap measure. During the early 1980's, the iodized oil was given by intramuscular injections, but this was later switched to the oral route due to the potential risk of spreading HIV/AIDS and hepatitis inherent in mass injections.

The major constraints to the IDD programmes in the region are related to low human resource development, low institutional capacity in management, monitoring and evaluation and the lack of a clear IEC strategy. The relevant international organizations (ICCIDD, UNICEF and WHO) have recognized these problems and are now working in partnership with the relevant governments to address them.

It is perhaps in the field of IDD control in the ECSA countries that a unique model partnership between governments, bilaterals, multilaterals and NGOs has been forged. It is particularly satisfying to note, among other organizations, the co-operation of UNICEF, WHO, ICCIDD, World Bank, SIDA, and the Netherlands Government in providing both financial and technical support to the control of IDD in the region.

The Future Challenge

While great progress is noted in the control of IDD in the ECSA region, a great challenge lies ahead. Great expectations in achieving the goal of eliminating IDD by the year 2000 calls for the strengthening of networks, advocacy and technical support systems at all levels – global, regional and especially at the national level. Our targeting needs to be more sharply focused and more efforts need to be put into crucial areas where big gaps in action and capacity exist, in order to increase the synergy and cascade effect of our efforts. Large gaps still exist in IEC, human resource development, programme management, monitoring and institutional capacity building. ICCIDD has rightly been focusing on these areas and perhaps a more multi-disciplinary and multi-institutional perspective and involvement is now required. I believe that the issue is not merely one of resource (financial, human and organizational) constraints, but one of prioritization of resource allocation since 'to plan is to choose'.

Conclusion

In conclusion, the great progress which has been made in the control of IDD in the Eastern and Southern African region only offer the promise for further success and not complacency.

Greater challenges lie ahead especially when it is considered that even if the goal for eliminating IDD were to be achieved ahead of schedule, strong vigilance will need to be maintained to prevent the recurrence of an 'eliminated' problem, otherwise resource diversion will lead to recurrence. It cannot be overemphasized that the control of IDD should be on the permanent developmental agenda of all countries.

IDD in Western and Central Africa

M. Benmiloud and D.N. Lantum

Most of the 22 French speaking countries are located in the western and central sub-regions of Africa (Fig. 13.1). At least 13 of these countries have sizeable IDD endemias which, in some cases, represent a severe public health problem. The affected population could be estimated at 50 million although the actual number is not known because of the scarcity of comprehensive data from national surveys.

Awareness of the problem of endemic goitre goes back to colonial times when military physicians conducted surveys in the late 19th and the early 20th century. Unfortunately preventive programmes have not followed and it is only after the revival of scientific interest during the sixties that some preventive actions were initiated in different countries.

However, it was only after the IDD meeting held in 1987 in Yaounde under the sponsorship of WHO, UNICEF and ICCIDD that a systematic approach produced rapid changes. During that meeting it was realized that there was insufficient data on IDD to decide on prevention programmes. An IDD Task Force was set up to impulse and monitor national programmes in the different countries.

We shall present four countries: Algeria, Cameroon, Mali and Zaire which all have an important IDD problem. There has been enough progress in these countries to initiate national programmes. Because of the various contexts with regard to alimentary salt distribution the preventive strategies were different.

Algeria

The first written reports on endemic goitre in Algeria date from the late 19th century. Successive maps of the endemia were drawn from heterogeneous data. The main endemia involved a quadrangle in the mountains east and west of the capital Algiers, with smaller pockets at the north-western and north-eastern borders. Excluding the large cities the population at risk is about 5 million (1/5 of the population) and the goitre prevalence varied from 10-70% until the seventies.

From 1970 to 1990 a team of endocrinologists from the medical school of Algiers investigated the etiological factors. Iodine deficiency is the predominant factor aggravated by a higher thiocyanate intake from Cruciferae vegetables and by pollution of the drinking water. When endemia was severe (urinary iodine <20 µg/litre) other manifestations of iodine deficiency were detected: endemic cretinism, neonatal hypothyroidism, increased rate of abortions, prematurity and perinatal deaths.

Political will to solve the problem was demonstrated as early as 1967 when a legislation on iodized salt was adopted (10-15 ppm), to be implemented in the affected districts. Unfortunately this laudable initiative could not be enforced. The production of iodized salt was insufficient in quantity and quality. Furthermore, it did not reach the isolated areas where it was most needed. This situation prevailed until 1983 when a modern plant started to produce a large quantity of iodized salt, but the iodization level remained too low.

Small scale preventive programmes using oral iodized oil were launched in two severely deficient areas with positive results. The extension of the programme was difficult because of the lack of a national survey which was mandatory for selecting the locations of severe IDD where women and children should be treated. It was evident that more could be accomplished by strengthening the iodized salt programme. Several years of advocacy by the university group were necessary to obtain the creation of an intersectoral committee including industry, economy and health, the first task of which was to modify the legislation: the level of iodization was increased to 30-50 ppm and the implementation of the regulation was extended to the whole country (1990).

To avoid a relapse of iodine deficiency, a monitoring system was set up by the National Institute of Public Health. Clinical and biological evaluations (goitre prevalence and urinary iodine) were effected through the primary schools health system. The 1991 survey confirmed the previous map with a new pocket in the Atlas mountains. Also the severity of the endemia has decreased as judged by goitre prevalence.

Furthermore the urinary iodine concentrations were in general much higher (100-200 µg/l) with the exception of a few mountainous villages where the population still consumed local salt. A preliminary salt survey indicated that 89% of the samples are within the specified limits of 30-50 ppm.

Cameroon

Endemic goitre was reported in the eastern region of Cameroon in 1955. Successive investigations demonstrated other endemias in the north and north-west. The 1991 survey by the team from the University Health Center of Yaounde has shown a global prevalence of 26% in the 8 provinces (range 5-57%) with only the coastal region spared. The population at risk is 6 million, more than half of the inhabitants. Iodine deficiency was recognized from the low iodine content in urine and water. Some of the population used cassava as a staple food with a consequently high thiocyanate intake.

A pilot experiment with oral iodized oil was conducted, swiftly followed in 1991 by a national programme based on iodized salt. The disadvantage of nonexistent salt production in Cameroon was offset by the existence of a single port of entry for all imported salt (Douala). The energetic leader of the university team (Professor D Lantum, ICCIDD Sub-regional Co-ordinator) succeeded in convincing the Ministry of Health to impose a 100 ppm iodine level in all alimentary salt distributed in the country. The main salt refinery agreed to instal an iodization unit which could supply not only Cameroon but also neighbouring countries such as Chad and the Central African Republic (Fig 13.1). It is producing 47,000 tonnes well above the 36,000 tonnes needed for national consumption. According to a 1993 survey 95% of the salt samples were iodized between 10 and 50 ppm.

Goiter prevalence and urinary iodine concentrations have improved in most of the 17 sentinel sites. However, cassava still widely used as a staple food brings about high thiocyanates in some areas. Lipiodol is still used in some hyperendemic rural enclaves, where juvenile hypothyroidism could be as high as 4-20%. IEC has been developed in parallel to improve awareness of the population as well as their nutritional practices with respect to salt and cassava.

Cameroon has the advantage of trained personnel and competent leaders. It has developed a small laboratory for hormones and iodine assays. Thus Cameroon should be a success story in Africa thanks to the strong involvement of nationals.

The interventions of WHO, UNICEF and ICCIDD through the seminar and workshop held in Yaounde were important. They had a very positive effect on advocacy and manpower training. It has enhanced the resolve of the university team. External help is still needed to consolidate the laboratory support and complete the monitoring network. Cameroon will be a catalyst for neighbouring countries.

Mali

In the past 40 years, different studies conducted by teams from ORANA (Dakar), the Medical School of Bamako and the National Institute of Research in Public Health of Mali have confirmed the existence of severe to moderate goitre endemias in the five southern provinces. At least half of the 7 million population is affected. Following the recommendation of the IDD task force for Africa, a national programme was drafted at the end of 1988, by an IDD technical committee. However, it was not formalized at the country level. Then with the financial support of the Joint Nutrition Support Programme of WHO and UNICEF a regional programme of prevention using oral iodized oil was implemented in a severely iodine deficient area (Cercle de Tominian). A mid-term evaluation conducted in 1991 demonstrated that it was generally successful.

In addition a limited but interesting study of water iodization was conducted by the Rhone Poulenc Foundation using a silicone polymer matrix to release iodine in bore wells. It was demonstrated that an adequate supply of iodine could thus be made available to the village population over a twelve month period. (Fisch et al 1993). The extension of this programme through a World Bank project is under way for 200 wells.

With the help of WHO, a study was conducted on salt production and commercialization. Although rock salt can be found in the Taoudenit mines of northern Mali it supplies only 10% of the needs. The remaining 30,000 tonnes are mostly imported from Senegal. A project for a small iodization unit is presently backed by UNICEF, to cover the Bamako area.

In conclusion, it can be seen that in Mali, a country with a severe IDD public health problem, combined international help and national will has resulted in a successful core programme. The impact was good with regard to training and information. However indecision in the strategy and inadequate funding hampered a more extensive implementation.

Zaire

Zaire is known as the most severe IDD-endemic region in Africa since the report of several Belgian investigators during the 1930's and the 1950's. At least 4 million people are at risk, the goitre prevalence is very high (80%) and the percentage of endemic cretinism in the northern provinces is one of the highest in the world.

The classic research work conducted by Belgian teams from the universities of Brussels and Louvain in the 1960's and 1970's confirmed the existence of iodine deficiency complicated by a high intake of thiocyanate contained in the staple food cassava (Ermans et al 1980).

Zaire was also one of the first countries where iodized oil injections were used on a large scale with very good results. Therefore, it is not surprising that it was singled out as a top priority for a control programme during the 1987 meeting in Yaounde. On the recommendation of the IDD task force a national workshop was convened in Kinshasa in 1988, the outcome of which was a national programme draft which was finalized the following year. This proposal received financial support from UNDP and the Belgian Co-operation Programme. In a systematic approach, a National IDD Bureau was created with IDD units in the most severely affected areas (Gemena in South Ubangi, Gbadolite in Northern Ubangi, Rota in Lower Uele, Isiro in Higher Uele and Goma in Kivu).

The main objective was the reactivation and extension of the preventive programme with iodized oil: mostly by injection but also by oral administration. A study of alimentary salt distribution was conducted to pave the way for a long term programme. A legislation on iodized salt was gazetted in October 1993 with by-laws regulating production, marketing, consumption and control of iodized salt. The extension of the national survey to other regions revealed new sites of iodine deficiency.

The programme in Zaire was a model for other French speaking countries. There was training at national and local levels, IEC production was effective and the National Bureau was setting up its laboratory in Kinshasa when political upheaval stopped the momentum.

The diplomatic cooling off between Belgium and Zaire resulted in the suppression of financial support, which of course decreased the possibilities of intervention. The Kinshasa riots in 1991 totally destroyed the IDD Bureau of Kinshasa including records and equipment, and only the regional units were able to continue their work.

In Zaire we have a typical example of a well thought out programme which offered a systematic approach to eradicate, with international help, a very severe public health problem. The intermediate prevention programme was based on iodized oil injections because of the difficulty in controlling imported salt entry from several different countries, in addition to the main imports from Namibia and South Africa. Political interference, unfortunately all too frequent in Africa, has now paralysed the programme and new efforts are necessary to make up for the losses.

All the four countries which have been presented here have different socio-economic profiles. Algeria and Cameroon have a higher per capita income and were able to reach a higher level of self sufficiency. The former is a salt producer and should be able to entirely control its iodized salt production. Both have a legislation which should help to sustain the programme. However the monitoring systems for iodized salt have still to prove their efficiency. Zaire on the other hand, a potentially rich country, has seen its programme inhibited by interference. Its mid-term strategy with iodized oil will require more continuous external support until a master plan for salt iodization in Africa is adopted. Among the four countries Mali has the lowest income per capita and therefore is even more dependent on external help. Potentially it could produce iodized salt but it may still have difficulty in controlling imports from other countries and therefore would profit from a master plan for Africa.

These four countries are among the more successful and give by no means the full picture of the African continent. The development of their IDD programmes emphasize the persistent need for international co-operation in this domain.

References

Benmiloud, M., H., Bachtarzi, and M.B., Chaouki, 1983. 'Public health and nutritional aspects of endemic goitre and cretinism in Africa'. In Delange, F., and R. Ahluwalia eds. *Cassava toxicity and thyroid* p.50 Research and public health issues, IDRC, Ottawa.

Ermans, A.M., N.M., Mbulamako, F., Delange, and R., Ahluwalia, 1980. eds *Role of cassava in the etiology of endemic goitre and cretinism*. IDRC, Ottawa.

Fisch, A., E., Pichard, T., Przauck, et al. 1993. 'A new approach to combatting iodine deficiency in developing countries: the controlled release of iodine in water by a silicone elastomer'. *Am J Public Health.* 83:540-5.

IDD in Nigeria

O.L. Ekpechi

Nigeria is a federation of 30 States with an army President as the Head of State. It is rich in human and natural resources including petroleum products. Many of the small countries of Africa look up to Nigeria for leadership. The population of Nigeria estimated at 110 million in 1990 is the same as that of 31 smaller African countries; one out of every four Africans is a Nigerian. Nigeria's IDD problem is, therefore, immense and diverse.

The IDD Situation in Nigeria

Between 1960 and 1986, Wilson in 1954, Nwokolo and Ekpechi in 1960-65, the US Nutritional Team from the Department of Health, Welfare and Education in 1965, Olurin in 1970-74, Udeozo and Agharanya in 1975, Isichei and his team (1985-87) carried out goitre surveys in different parts of Nigeria. Table 13.1 represents the goitre distribution as reconstructed by Ekpechi. In 1991, in Edo State, Dr I. Lubere, and C.P. Longe, reported a visible goitre rate of 13.8% amongst school children in Ekpedo, 17.6% amongst women of childbearing age in Igarra, and 16% in women attending a child welfare clinic in Igarra with identification of more than five cretins.

Analysis of work carried out by the various authors shows a mean visible goitre rate of 26% in 5 of the states in Zone A; a mean total goitre rate of 21% in 6 States in Zone B; 12% total goitre rate in Plateau State. In 12 Local Government Authorities (L.G.A.), an intervention measure was rated as critical; urgent in 22 other L.G.As and important in over 30.

There is thus a population of approximately 41 million people living in the areas of the country with very severe to moderately severe IDD prevalence and 38.7 million living in areas with mild to moderately severe IDD prevalence.

Table 13.1 *IDD prevalence rates in the states*

A. In 8 States with adequate sampling techniques

State	No. of LGA sampled	Mean visible goitre rate.	Total Goitre rate	No. of villages sampled	Intervention rating
Anambra (Anambra & Enugu)	5	36	-	28	Critical
Cross River (AQ. IBOM & X River)	2	32	-	8	Critical
Benue (Benue & KOGI)	4	26	-	5	Critical
Oyo (Oyo & Oshun)	4		24.2	10	Urgent
Ondo	2		26	9	Urgent
Bendel (Edo & Delta)	5		26	9	Critical
Lagos			11		Urgent
Plateau	14		17		Urgent (Critical ILGA)

Population-41 million

B. In 7 States with inadequate sampling techniques

State	No. of LGA Sampled	Total Goitre Rate	Intervention Rating
Bornu (Bornu S Yobe)	38	21	Important
Kano (Kano & Jigawa)	96	18.7	Important
Niger	65	7.7	Important
Kaduna / Zaire	96	10.4	Important
Sokoto / Kebbi	Notstated		Important
Bauchi / Katsina	Not stated		Important
Kwarka	Not stated		Important

Population of 11 States=38 Million

C. 7 States with no report or any survey

ABIA   IMO   RIVERS   OGUN   ADAMAWA   TARIBE
and FEDERAL CAPITAL TERRITORY ABUJA
Population - 16.7 million

Cretinism

In the course of the IDD survey in Bassa in Pankshin L.G.A, Isichei detected a number of cretins, deaf mutes and mentally retarded persons. Cretins were sighted by Nwokolo and Ekpechi in Anambra State, in Obudu L.G.A in Cross Rivers State and Okpukwu L.G.A in Benue State. Table 13.2 shows IDD prevalence, the total population, the population at risk in the 4 L.G.As where cretins have been sighted or reported. Cretins have been reported in 1991, in Akokoedo L.G.A in Edo State.

Table 13.2 *Local governments with critical goitre rate*

LGA	State	Visible Goitre	Populatiion of the LGA	Population at risk	Population of Pregnant women
BASSA	Plateau	24%	113,000	60,000	5,700
Obudu	Cross River	33%	103,000	55,000	5,200
Uzouwani	Anambra/Eugu	28%	163,000	86,000	8,200
Okpokwu	Benue	36%	225,000	119,000	11,300

Food Goitrogens

These have been demonstrated by Ekpechi in Uzo-Uwani and Igbo-Eze L.G.As, in the former Anambra State, and in Okpokwu L.G.A in Benue State, where Cassava and Okoho are the staple food and vegetables.

Intervention with Salt Iodization

Recommendations in 1974 by the Salt Iodization Committee set up by the Government and again in 1989 and 1991 by the WHO Salt Consultant, Mr Mannar, and by the National IDD Workshop respectively confirm the feasibility of salt iodization as a cheap and effective method of delivering iodine to the population on a national basis.

Salt is imported from nine overseas countries. Some of the imported salt is iodized at a low concentration level. Most of the salt importing companies are willing to co-operate. The percentage of the Nigerian population using either rock salt or salt brine is now known.

Conclusion

A visible goitre rate higher than 10% in the general population or a total goitre rate higher than 20% in the school population is indicative of a severe endemic.

In most of the Local Government Areas surveyed and reported on in Table 13.1, both the mean visible goitre rate and the mean total goitre rate is over 20%. A mean visible goitre rate of over 20%, and the daily consumption of goitrogenous foods as staple foods, suggests that IDD is an important public health problem in Nigeria.

National Policy on IDD

As of 1990, there was no firm Government policy on IDD control. Policies on IDD may be said to be in place only to the extent:

1. That over the period 1965-1991, the Federal Ministry of Health publicly made Statements of Support for the IDD Control programme.

2. That the Federal Minister for Health proposed a Resolution at the Regional Committee Meeting in 1987 in Bamako, Mali, supporting AFRO Regional action on IDD Control.

3. That the Federal Minister for Health seconded Resolution 39.31 at the World Health Assembly Meeting in Geneva 1986, supporting action for the global control of IDD.

4. That the Federal Ministry of Health on separate occasions has commissioned or sponsored:

(a) A project proposal for pilot intra-muscular iodized oil injections for one L.G.A. That proposal was approved of but then the offer was later withdrawn.

(b) The meeting of a Government Iodization Committee in 1974.
(c) The meeting of an IDD Expert Committee in Enugu in 1988.
(d) A National IDD Workshop in April 1991.

Recent developments in Government Policy on IDD Control

The creation of a National Committee for Food and Nutrition in 1990 under the Federal Ministry of Science and Technology represented a most welcome policy development on macro and micronutrient deficiency disorders including IDD. The membership of this Committee is drawn from:

The Federal Ministries: The Ministry of Health; The Ministry of Science and Technology (former)

The Universities: The University of Nigeria; The University of Ibadan; The University of Jos; The University of Benin

The Donor Agencies: The WHO; UNICEF; The World Bank; UNDP

A sub-committee of the National Committee for Food and Nutrition called 'The IDD Working Group' under the Chairmanship of Prof. O L Ekpechi has been formed and entrusted with the development of an IDD Project Proposal. This committee has met three times. A draft project proposal for IDD Control has been discussed with the World Bank and UNDP officials.

Constraints

National commitment in Nigeria

Failure to obtain a sustainable and firm political, moral, and logistic commitment from the Government at this stage, is the primary constraint to IDD control in Nigeria.

With an assured firm commitment, it would be easier and quicker to put into effect the recommendations of the IDD Expert Committee, the National Workshop on IDD and the WHO Salt Consultancy etc. The operational and management institutions for IDD Control could then be constituted and commissioned.

The failure to create and commission the National Council on IDD Control (NCCIDD), and consequently the IDD Control Unit at the National, State and L.G.A levels is to a large extent responsible for the slow take-off of the programme. At present, the development of strategies for the control of IDD remains stunted to the extent that it lacks the drive from the IDD Control Unit and the NCCIDD. The creation of these two functional organs depends on the Government's initiative. And without it, the following necessary control strategies cannot be fully activated-namely:

1. The organization of national surveys; 2. The development of the laboratories; 3. Information, education and communication; 4. Advocacy for the IDD programme; 5. The mobilization of internal and external resources; 6.The development of managerial competence.

The requirements of the IDD elimination programme for Nigeria are as follows –

1. To secure a FIRM NATIONAL COMMITMENT FROM THE POLICY MAKER

2. To organize an URGENT BASELINE RESURVEY IN 37 L.G.As in 12 STATES

3. To organize EMERGENCY INTERVENTION with iodized oil in all local Government areas with severe IDD such as: BASSA, OKPOKWU, OBUDU and UZOUWANI

4. To undertake a NATIONAL IDD SURVEY IN THE REST OF THE COUNTRY

5. To organize TRAINING PROGRAMMES locally with PAMM support

6. To secure Government support and approval of iodized salt as the most practical and the cheapest vehicle for the delivery of iodine to the community.

7. To discuss and finalize the Draft Proposal for IDD Control particularly involving the salt sector

8. To support the IDD work in PLATEAU STATE already at an advanced stage

9. To obtain financial sponsorship from DONOR AGENCIES in carrying out the above programme.

Summary

In the last 32 years, the Federal Government, either on its own, or in conjunction with UNICEF, has set up a number of committees to study and report on various aspects of IDD. After reviewing the IDD situation in Nigeria, the three committees namely: The Iodization Committee in 1974; the IDD Expert Committee in 1987; and the National IDD Workshop in 1991; individually and collectively and at different times called the Government's attention to the urgent need for the institution of urgent intervention measures to control IDD.

There is sufficiently reliable information on IDD to start some intervention measures.

14

IDD in Central Asia

Gregory Gerasimov and David P. Haxton

Background and Introduction

Member nations of the regional alliance called the Economic Co-operation Organization (ECO), with the support of UNICEF and the co-operation of WHO, convened an historic meeting in Ashkabad, Turkmenistan, in June 1994. It was the first of three meetings to discuss common social problems and to address solutions in each of the Member States. It is significant that the first subject was IDD.

The 10 member states of ECO thus joined the growing number of countries around the globe to endorse the goals of the Global Summit on Children, one of which is the elimination of IDD before 2000. ECO was created in 1992 by Turkey, Iran and Pakistan, as the successor to the Regional Cooperation for Development and continued the principal aims of increasing economic, technical and cultural co-operation among and between its members. The meeting in Ashkabad marked an important stage in the momentum towards global elimination and was the first time that a regional economic organization had put a vital public health and nutrition issue squarely on the agenda for implementation.

The idea for the meeting arose from a session of the Health Ministers of the ECO countries held in Tehran in January 1994 which produced a commitment by ECO, UNICEF and WHO to try to defuse the worst aspects of the growing crises in public health in the States members by identifying significant problems which have acceptable solutions. IDD met that criteria.

In preparation for the meeting each State Member was asked to review the situation of IDD in the country; the situation of salt production; and to prepare a position paper outlining the plans to be undertaken as a consequence of the reviews. The preparation for the conference took different forms in each country.

In some, national plans for the elimination of IDD, principally using improved iodization of alimentary salt, were already in place and operating. (Iran, Pakistan and Turkey). In others, the review of the salt industry indicated a need for modernization, but no further studies were required to move forward (Kazakhstan, Uzbekistan). Surveys were undertaken in Azerbaijan, Kyrgyzstan, Tajikistan. It was not possible to undertake new studies in Afghanistan.

This documentation showed that the States Members of ECO faced a diverse range of circumstances. In states of Central Asia formerly parts of the USSR, salt had been iodized or iodized salt had been imported and national programs had been in place for long periods. In recent times, however, political changes, economic and other reorganization and internal turmoil, hampered endeavors and the problems of iodine deficiency emerged again as a serious public health menace. In some countries serious shortages of fuel, of foreign exchange, and of modern packaging operations were revealed as difficulties.

Preparations for the meeting were complex and required the full collaboration of a range of interested parties and experts. The publication of the information and data which existed was in languages not usually used for international scientific meetings and needed to be translated and analyzed. Standards were often not comparable with UN publications. The design of the documentation for the meeting had to be acceptable to all States Members, some of which were meeting at an international conference on IDD for the first time. The review of the national situation in each country called for a team effort of national experts and foreign consultants. In addition, the planning for the meeting in June could not get underway until February.

Consultants were recruited from USSR, Pakistan, Denmark, India, Germany and the USA. In an innovative undertaking to support the meeting with qualified technical and scientific talent while expanding the roster of available consultants on IDD, the Micronutrient Initiative recruited and supported completely 5 associate consultants from Canada.

The meeting was held under the official patronage of His Excellency, the President of Turkmenistan, Saparmurad Turkmenbasi Niyazov, and the sessions were conducted by the Deputy Minister of the Council of Ministers of Turkmenistan, Madame Abat Rizaeva. Each delegation was led by a Minister and was comprised of representatives from education, salt industry, agriculture and health sectors.

Summary Review of National Situations

Afghanisthan

The endemic goitre areas are mainly in the northern parts of the country. Surveys performed in 1989-1992 show that 25-29% of adult females, 16-19% of school children have goitre. Cretinism was found in 1% of children.

There is no National IDD control program. Salt supply is from national sources; packaging and distribution is primitive. Local production amounts to 60,000 tons by three producers. Because local sources of salt do not suffice for the needs of the country, a good amount of pure table salt (uniodized) is imported from Pakistan. Since iodized salt is more expensive and because the Afghan community has not been educated about the need for iodine, nearly all imported salt is non-iodized. Modernization of the industry could eventually provide 312,000 tons of iodized salt per year in an efficient and profitable manner.

In 1992, capsules of iodized oil containing 200 mg of iodine each were provided by UNICEF for pregnant women, (one capsule for 6-12 month). Unfortunately, the results were not assessed.

Azerbaijan

Mild and moderate IDD is known in 23 of the 48 provinces of Azerbaijan. Goitre prevalence in these areas varies from 2% to 40%.

The limitation of the data available is due to unsystematic selection of persons and age groups studied. The figures are exclusively based on palpation using the former Soviet goitre grading system which is difficult to compare with WHO standards. No biochemical indicators have ever been applied.

At present, no law or decree exists to monitor IDD nor to regulate salt iodination. Before independence, 25% of alimentary salt was delivered from Russia, 25% from Ukraine and 50% from Kazakhstan. Less than 5% was produced within the country. Most of the salt was not iodized. At present most of salt is imported from Ukraine.

Azerbaijan was a producer of iodine and provided 45% of the needs of the former USSR. Russia now imports only a small fraction of the previous amount. The iodine stock in the country was found to be about 12,000 tons.

Iran

IDD was considered a public health problem in Iran. In 1989 a National prevalence survey conducted by the government showed in many regions a goitre rate in school children from 17 to 75%. In 20% of neonates in the Tehran region transient elevation of TSH was observed.

A national plan was prepared and is in full operation. Iran is self sufficient in salt. There are 26 registered factories which produce 70% of all salt. All have iodination capacity. The remaining salt factories are small and scattered throughout the country and are responsible for the other 30% of all salt, none of which is yet iodized. All salt used in the country is unrefined.

Potassium iodate is used for iodination. The level of iodination at the production site is 40 ppm using the spray method. It has been decided jointly by the Ministries of Health and Industry that all newly registered salt producing factories must produce only iodized salt. An Iodine Salt Production Union has been organized by all salt producers and is supported by Government.

The National IDD Committee supervises iodized salt production and has produced training manuals for doctors and mid-level health personnel and other communications.

Kazakhstan

There is extensive evidence that IDD exists as a public health problem. According to the new WHO/UNICEF/ICCIDD criteria, more than two thirds of the country is at risk of IDD. The regions with moderate iodine deficiency include mostly mountain and their foothill areas. The prevalence of goitre by palpation in most settlements is 35-40%. The iodine content of daily rations is below 100 µg/day in 78% and less than 50% in 42%. The latest survey in Eastern Kazakhstan shows high (63-90%) prevalence of thyroid enlargement (by ultrasonography) with moderate decrease of urinary iodine (3.2 µg/dl). In 33% of children thyroid hormone level was decreased. Neurological impairment by iodine deficiency was observed in isolated mountain areas.

Presently there is no National IDD control program. The country is self sufficient in salt with only one state owned salt producer located at the Aral sea. The total requirement of iodized salt is based on the average consumption of 5.5 kg per person per year. Assuming universal alimentary salt iodination, the total estimated requirement is 113,500 tons. In 1993, a total of 131,700 tons of iodized salt was produced of which 43,360 tons were exported to Uzbekistan, Kyrgyzstan, Tadjikistan and Russia. Since May 1994 salt has not been iodized due to lack of potassium iodide.

Potassium iodide was used and was procured from Azerbaijan (3000 kg per year). Only 10% of iodized salt was packed in polyethylene bags. Packaging is one of the major problems.

There is Government legislation for salt iodation. In certain endemic areas iodized bread was introduced in 1983. Bread iodination has been discontinued due to lack of potassium iodide. In 1993 a total of 6,000 capsules of iodized oil were administered to school children in Eastern Kazakhstan.

Kyrgyzstan

There is limited recent data on the prevalence of IDD. Surveys in 1991 demonstrated goitre rates in adults between 25 and 28% in three separate locales. Biological indicator studies have not been done due to limited laboratory capacity. Rapid assessment of school children in 1994 showed total goitre rate in various provinces between 33 and 46% indicating a serious problem. Biochemical indicator analysis was in process at the time of the meeting.

The main source of salt is from Kazakhstan. The quality of salt is poor. Another major problem is that the packaging is such that there is a loss of iodine during transportation and storage. Due to transportation costs other sources of salt are few. There are some locations in Kyrgyzstan where salt deposits are known to exist, but only 3 of these have been explored. Currently salt from these mines is used only for animals and industrial purposes. Dyrgyzstan has no production of iodine.

Pakistan

IDD was thought to be prevalent only in the northern part of the country. However, recent surveys have shown that it is prevalent throughout the country.

Early efforts, with the help of UNICEF, to treat this problem with the distribution of iodized oil injection and capsules proved to be impractical. The Government has recognized the importance of eliminating IDD and has recognized that the best way is through the widest possible use of iodized salt. An Iodized Salt Facility (ISF) has been set up in Islamabad by UNICEF and the Government to encourage, support, promote and sustain universal access to iodized salt in the country. The Prime Minister has directed the government to draft a bill for universal iodination of edible salt.

Tadjikistan

This is a mountain state with severe IDD. In 1930's surveys revealed that up to 5% of the population of some mountain valleys was represented by cretins. After the civil war (1991-1992) severe IDD reappeared and now contributes to major health problems of the country. A rapid assessment in 1994 showed by ultrasonography that the goitre rate in school children (by ultrasonography) is 42% in capital city Dushanbe and 86% in a village. Median urinary iodine concentration was 1.2 µg/dl in Dushanbe. In the village median urinary iodine was 0.0 µg/dl (less than 50% of all samples contained iodine).

There is currently no IDD control program in the country. Tadjikistan has large salt deposits. The quality of salt is rather low, production sites have primitive equipment. Part of salt is iodized by potassium iodide using the spray method to a level of 35 +/- 10 ppm. Salt is not packaged. Due to lack of fuel for trucks salt producers trade crude, low quality salt, which is cheaper than in state-owned shops. In mountain areas people use natural rock salt, which can be easily found. Tadjikistan has no production of iodine. Potassium iodide is delivered from Turkmenistan.

Turkey

IDD is a problem in almost all parts of Turkey. The data established is thought to be sufficient for the initiation of an iodine fortification and supplementation program. However, no prevalence data were published in the preliminary report nor was information on annual capacity of salt production and consumption provided to the meeting.

For more than 20 years the food law has allowed the iodination of salt with 50-70 ppm of potassium iodide. No iodine derivatives may be used except potassium iodide. At present only 17% of the salt is iodized. There is no laboratory in Turkey able to determine iodine in urine. A National IDD Elimination Program and Plan of Action are being finalized.

Turkmenistan

No information has ever been published in the scientific literature and no assessment has been done on the distribution and severity of IDD in this country. A rapid assessment in 1994 in Ashkabad (capital city) and Tashauz (oasis in Karakum desert) showed a goitre rate in Ashkabad (by ultrasonography) of 20% and in Tashauz of 64%. Median urinary iodine was significantly decreased in Tashauz

(3.7 µg/dl) and marginally low in Ashkabad (7.5 µg/dl). Theoretical estimation of iodine in the diet made on the basis of the study on food consumption shows intake of iodine is 2 to 4 times lower than the recommended daily requirement. Thus, the available information underline that Turkmenistan has an IDD problem and that iodine supplementation is necessary.

Salt is easily produced in the country and is concentrated at one place. No iodized salt is currently produced. Salt had been iodized for human consumption between 1976 and 1991 using potassium iodide solution dripping on the conveyor. The standard used for salt iodination (as always in the former USSR) requires addition of 25 +/- 10 ppm of potassium iodide. The salt industry interrupted the production of iodized salt in 1992 due to the lack of sodium thiosulfate, a reagent used to stabilize iodine in salt. There is no industry producing polyethylene bags in Turkmenistan. Therefore, paper packaging is used which is not appropriate and which contributes to increased losses of iodine.

Turkmenistan has its own production of iodine at the Cheliken chemical plant near the salt factory. Potassium iodide from this factory has never been used for salt iodination. The product seems to be of good quality. The Cheliken industry has a certificate allowing the production of potassium iodate for livestock but reports that no iodized salt has ever been given to animals.

Turkmenistan has a rare opportunity to implement an IDD elimination program since it has its own salt and iodine to solve the problem with minimal expenditures in a short period of time.

Uzbekistan

The problem of IDD is well known and relatively well described in Uzbekistan. Certain places, in particular in the Ferghana valley in the south eastern part of the country, have long been known as highly endemic goitre areas. The goitre rates (up to 30% in school children) clearly indicate that IDD remains a significant public health problem in most parts of the country. In addition to goitre surveys urinary iodine has been determined in selected population groups. For children in Tashkent (capital city) a mean urinary excretion of iodine of 35µg/24 hours has been reported. Recent information collected after independence by the Institute of Endocrinology in Tashkent shows that the prevalence of goitre is increasing.

Uzbekistan has considerable reserves of rock salt. Until independence in 1991, all edible salt was imported from Ukraine and Kazakhstan. Since 1991, because of financial constraints, the government has faced difficulties with imports. It has started production of salt for human and animal consumption at two plants, neither of which has any iodination equipment. The technology is not available and there is no experience with iodination in the country. The total requirement of salt for human and animal consumption is estimated at about 240,000 tones, of which 128,000 tones is imported from Turkmenistan and Ukraine. Packaging material is in short supply. Uzbekistan has no production of iodine for supplementation.

To summarize the above information, all countries attending the meeting have serious IDD problems. The most severe seem to be in Afghanistan and Tadjikistan, which also suffer from civil war and economic breakdowns.

The distribution and severity of IDD in several countries is not as well defined as might be desired. However, with the preliminary and partial studies available there is ample evidence to recommend urgent action. Future assessments of the effectiveness of iodized salt consumption should be conducted in accordance with the guideline of WHO/UNICEF/ICCIDD published in November, 1992.

Recommendations and Conclusions

Measures to address the problems revealed in the comprehensive country assessments were discussed. The meeting reviewed ways governments and the salt industry could adapt and expand technical and material capacities to iodize salt, as well as ways to create public demand for a good quality product. Such issues as laboratory and other quality control needs; potential legislation; and technical problems of salt iodination in each country were reviewed.

The meeting concluded with the unanimous adoption of the following 10 detailed recommendations:

1. The Governments and Institutions of ECO member countries should do all possible to ensure that the right of all people in ECO countries to be free from IDD is fulfilled.
2. All alimentary salt manufactured in or imported into ECO member countries should be appropriately iodized by the end of 1995.
3. Any ECO country which exports alimentary salt to any other ECO country should ensure that this salt is iodized to agreed standards before export.
4. A multi sectoral approach to ensuring that salt is iodized in member countries should be adopted, which recognizes the major contributions of the salt industry, the communications and marketing, education and agriculture sectors and the justice system as well as those of the health sector.
5. A standard for iodized salt should be established for use in each country in the region, based on a knowledge of minimum iodine requirements, the average quantity of salt consumed, and the quality and type of packaging used for salt. In establishing this standard the meeting recommended that the recommendations of the WHO/UNICEF/ICCIDD meeting on Indicators for assessing Iodine Deficiency Disorders and their control through salt iodization be followed.
6. Governments should assist the salt industry to assess its requirements and to obtain any necessary equipment and supplies to ensure that salt is properly iodized, recognizing that iodination is most likely to be sustainable when ongoing costs of supplies and depreciation of equipment are born by salt consumers.
7. Quality control and monitoring systems should be established to ensure that all iodized salt meets the specified standards.
8. Systems for regularly monitoring progress towards the goal of elimination IDD should be established.
9. Governments and institutions of ECO member countries should establish strategic incremental targets towards the 1995 goal of universal iodization of salt, such as:

By mid 1994	National priority to eliminate IDD to be declared.
By Sept 1994	National training plan designed and operational.
	Sources of supplies and raw materials identified and supplies ordered.
	National legislation drafted and ready.
	Marketing and demand creation plan ready.
By end 1994	At least 75 per cent of all salt producers should be iodizing salt.
	Salt packaging should be adequate.
	Reporting and monitoring mechanism to be in place.
By mid 1995	All salt factories must be equipped to the necessary minimum standards.
	National cluster survey to be undertaken to review progress in availability of iodized salt at household level.
	Plans to be adjusted accordingly.
By end 1995	All households consuming adequately iodized salt.

10. The ECO secretariat and those of UNICEF and WHO, and their Regional and National Offices, should work together with the Governments of ECO countries to assist these countries to prepare specific programs and projects to achieve the iodination of all alimentary salt, and ECO, UNICEF and WHO should approach the donor community for the necessary support required. It's co-operation between ECO member countries in establishing salt iodination programs an in establishing sources of the necessary supplies should also be encouraged.

This meeting again demonstrated the efficacy of bringing various professional and sectoral groups together to discuss the common national problem of IDD. When the decision is made to eliminate IDD, each must review the implications of that decision on all professional participants and in all sectors of government and the private sector. In addition to the formal and official recommendations approved by all governments in attendance, the following were the general conclusions of the participants:

-- it was agreed that all alimentary salt would be iodized with potassium iodate. This would assure elimination of competition with non iodized salt in the market and would provide sufficient iodine in the daily diet for humans and animals.

-- it was agreed that national training was important and that immediate steps would be undertaken to assure the creation of a critical core mass of professionals in management, communications, quality assurance, and food fortification would be a priority.

-- it was agreed that history had taught the valuable lesson that eternal vigilance is required to assure quality throughout the national effort: quality assurance of the product from the plant to the consumer; quality assurance of the process so that management is provided the information required to assure continued high level performance; and quality assurance that the levels of iodine in human consumption are adequate and are eliminating IDD in the population.

-- it was agreed that while iodization of salt is a low cost solution to this national health menace, it was not without cost. National plans will be drawn up to provide for national investment in improvement of the salt industry; in logistics and marketing; in quality assurance systems; monitoring and evaluation procedures and processes; and plans will be prepared to approach development organizations for financial, technical and other support.

-- it was agreed that new or revised legislation was required to assure compliance with the recommendations. In addition, regulations and guidelines will need to be prepared to support the legislation and licensing arrangements will be considered.

-- it was agreed that a range of issues lend themselves to mutual support and to regional cooperation: trade in iodized salt; trade in potassium iodate; trade in plastic packaging materials; trade in fortified foods (not those limited to fortification with iodine); exchanges of a technical, scientific and professional nature.

The elimination of IDD from ECO countries means that more than 200 million people living there will be free from this ancient stealthy scourge and that their children can be born with the assurance that they can reach their genetic potential.

References

Country report on Iodine Deficiency Disorders in Turkmenistan. Ibid.

ECO Member States are : The Islamic Republic of Afghanistan, the Republic of Azerbaijan, the Islamic Republic of Iran, the Republic of Kazakhstan, the Republic of Kyrgyzstan, the Islamic Republic of Pakistan, the Republic of Tajikistan, the Republic of Turkey, Turkmenistan, and the Republic of Uzbekistan.

ECO/UNICEF/WHO workshop on iodine deficiency disorders. Ashkabad, Turkmenistan, 15-16 June 1994. IDD in AFGHANISTAN.

ECO/UNICEF/WHO workshop on iodine deficiency disorders. Turkmenistan: Ashkabad. 15-16 June 1994. 'Draft country paper - Uzbekistan'.

ECO/UNICEF/WHO workshop on iodine deficiency disorders. Turkmenistan: Ashkabad. 15-16 June 1994. IDD in Republic of Kazakhstan.

Gerasimov, G. 1993. 'Update on IDD in the Former USSR'. *IDD Newsletter*. Vol. 9, Number 4, pp. 43-48.

Gerasimov, G. Iodine deficiency disorders (IDD) in Tadjikistan. Ibid.

Gutekunst, R. Report on IDD in Turkey. Ibid.

Gutekunst, R. A report on a visit to Azerbaijan. Ibid.

Houston, R., B., Rashid, J., Kalanzi. 'Rapid assessment of iodine deficiency in Kyrgyzstan'. Ibid.

Presentation on behalf of the Islamic Republic of Pakistan by H.E. Mr Tariq Oman Hyder, Ambassador. Ibid.

Situation of iodine deficiency disorders and activities for prevention in the Islamic Republic of Iran. Ibid.

Turakulov, Y. 1991. 'Iodine deficiency and iodine deficiency disorders: Iodine prophylaxis of endemic goitre in Uzbekistan. In: The elimination of iodine deficiency disorders'. *Abstracts of International Symposium, Tashkent*. pp. 25-34.

Zeltser, M. et al 1991. 'Iodine deficiency and its clinical manifestation in Kazakhstan. In : The elimination of iodine deficiency disorders'. *Abstracts of International Symposium, Tashkent*. pp. 25-34.

15

IDD in South-East Asia

C.S. Pandav

South-East Asia

The countries of Asia present a particularly urgent challenge for the control of IDD. Many countries in south-east Asia have iodine deficiency disorders as a significant health problem (Fig.15.1). There are more people in south-east Asia suffering and disabled by some form of IDD than in any other region of the world.

Regional control programmes for iodine deficiency disorders in south-east Asia have recently gained substantial momentum. WHO/SEARO in collaboration with UNICEF and the International Council for Control of Iodine Deficiency Disorders (ICCIDD), has been supporting these programmes through joint inter-country consultations and workshops, held in March 1985 and March 1989. A regional working group meeting was held at Delhi in October 1990 and a joint WHO-UNICEF-ICCIDD Tri-regional workshop on the Control of Iodine Deficiency Disorders was held in November and December 1991.

The commitment of the South Asian Association for Regional Cooperation (SAARC) to eliminate IDD by the year 2000 is reflected in the declaration of 'Universal Access to Iodized Salt by 1995' at the second SAARC conference held in Colombo, Sri Lanka in September 1992.

The targets for IDD control in the south-east Asian region are that by 1995, all countries with an IDD problem will have ongoing national IDD programmes and goitre rates will be below 20 percent. By the year 2000, the regional aim is to have goitre rates no more than 5 percent.

The current status of IDD control programmes in different countries is described below.

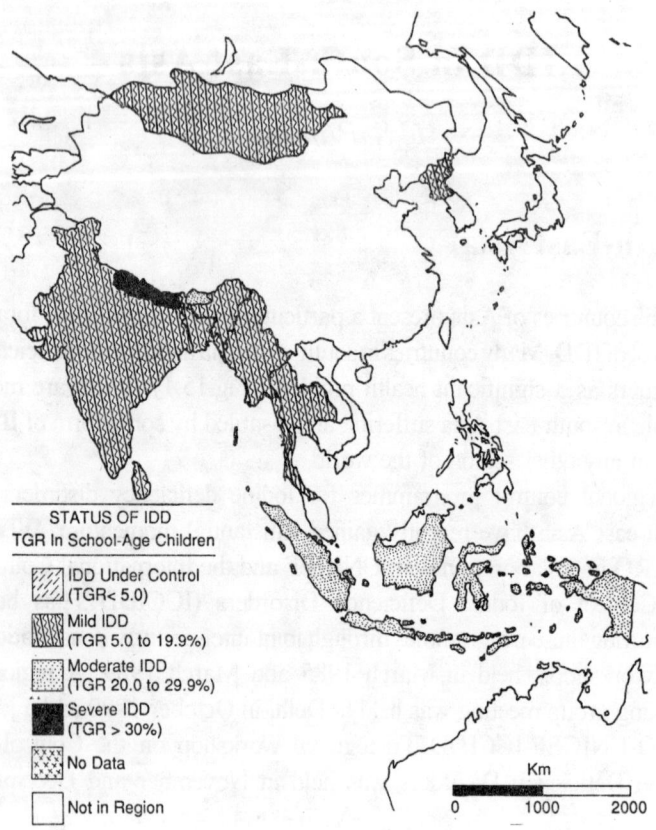

Fig. 15.1 Prevalence of iodine deficiency disorders in the south-east Asian Region. (Reprinted courtesy: Micronutrient Deficiency Information System, WHO MDIS working paper # 1, 1993).

Bangladesh

Bangladesh has a population of 115 million. The country is divided into 64 districts. The Ganges valley of the country is subjected to heavy and repeated flooding. In 1962-1964, a nutrition survey was carried out by Dhaka University. This survey revealed for the first time the high prevalence of endemic goitre in the country, particularly in some northern districts such as Rangpur, Dinajpur, Jamalpur and Mymensingh. A survey, conducted in rural Bangladesh later, also confirmed the existence of severe environmental iodine deficiency.

The first National Goitre Prevalence Study was conducted in 1981-82 by the Institute of Public Health and Nutrition, Dhaka with WHO and UNICEF collaboration, and covered 214,768 persons in 417 Upazillas in all the 64 districts of the country. The mean goitre prevalence found in the survey was 10.5 percent. The two most severely affected districts were Rangpur and Jamalpur. In these districts there were pockets of some Upazillas with a high goitre prevalence of between 50 percent and 70 percent. The results of the surveys indicate that 38.1 percent of the Bangladesh's population live in areas where the goitre prevalence exceeds 10 percent. These surveys also showed that goitre occurred in varying degrees of severity in almost every part of the country. The estimates from the Dulberg model (1985) were of 354,000 cretins and more than one million suffering some significant mental or other neurological handicap.

A national IDD prevalence survey was done in Bangladesh in 1993 by the Institute of Nutrition and Food Science, Departments of Biochemistry and Statistics of Dhaka University, with financial support from UNICEF Bangladesh and technical assistance from ICCIDD. The country was divided into three ecological zones: Hilly, Flood Prone and Plains. The "EPI 30 Cluster" methodology as recommended by WHO / UNICEF / ICCIDD in November 1992 and was used with the household as the ultimate sampling unit. A total of 7,517 households and 30,072 people were covered in all the three zones. The results of the IDD prevalence survey are shown in Table 15.1. From these figures, it is obvious that IDD is a severe problem in all the three zones of Bangladesh. Nearly 69% of the country's population have biochemical iodine deficiency (urinary iodine levels less than 10 $\mu g/dl$), 38.8% have palpable goitre and 8.8% have visible goitre (total goitre rate 47.1%).

In 1977 the Institute of Food Science and Nutrition carried out an iodized oil injection programme covering 95,000 people in hyperendemic areas while in 1983 a further 80,000 persons were injected with iodized oil in Rangpur district. In 1985, the 'Lipiodol Injection Campaign Project' in the northern and eastern districts of the country was launched. Under this programme, an estimated 3.2 million people have received iodized oil injections so far. The programme is presently in the last cycle of its implementation.

In 1988, the Bangladesh government took the decision for the universal iodization of salt and the programme is being implemented with assistance from Canadian International Development Agency (CIDA) and UNICEF. The total annual salt requirement is 600,000 tonnes. The Government through legislation has declared that from February, 1995 production and trading of non-iodized salt in the country is prohibited. Local fabrication and production of good quality of salt iodization plants (SIP) has been done. A total of 253 out of 265 salt refineries are now equipped with SIP. The indigenous capacity to manufacture and instal salt iodization plants has ensured technical sustainability. The cost of one plant is approximately US $ 12,500.

Simple and low cost kits have been developed for estimation of iodine in salt. Over 200,000 of these have been widely distributed including 40,000 primary schools. With the involvement of private professional agency, communication strategy has been developed that covers information package for mass media. As an interim measure, 3.5 million target population in 38 hyper-endemic areas has been covered with iodized oil injections. The production of iodized salt has been gradually increasing from 19% in December 1994 to 62% in June 1995. With the installation of SIP, Bangladesh is steadily moving towards reaching the mid-decade goal of Universal Salt Iodization.

Table 15.1 *IDD in Bangladesh (1993)*

Indicators	Hilly	Flood-Prone	Plains
Sample Size	7,320	11,445	11,307
Total Goitre Prevalence (%)	44.7	50.7	45.6
Prevalence of Cretinism(%)	0.8	0.5	0.3
Median Urinary Iodine(μg/dl)	3.4	5.1	7.4
Population with urinary iodine < 10 μg/dl	84.4%	67.1%	60.4%

Based on the results of a Knowledge, Attitude, Practice (KAP) survey on IDD a comprehensive social mobilization plan is being finalized with the help of a professional advertising agency. The orientation and training of key stakeholders-salt manufacturers and traders, school teachers, district health workers, journalists and doctors is being carried out systematically. Law governing universal salt iodization is already promulgated.

Based on the findings of the 1993 survey, the strategy for IDD control in Bangladesh will focus on advocacy and communication activities, management, inter-sectoral co-ordination, and strengthening of monitoring.

Bhutan

Bhutan is a small hilly country in the eastern Himalayas. The total population is 1.2 million. The people live in 4500 villages in an area of 47,000 km. A study conducted by Dr. Mahendra in 1975 in certain districts of Bhutan indicated a goitre prevalence of 47 to 68 percent in school children, and 50 to 53 percent in the community. Bhutan's first national IDD prevalence survey was carried out by a team of physicians from the All India Institute of Medical Sciences, New Delhi with WHO and UNICEF support in 1983. The survey was carried out in 11 of the then 18 districts and included school children as well as adult males and females. The results showed goitre to be present in all the districts of the country, with a national mean prevalence of 64.5 per cent. No district had less than 50 per cent prevalence. Cretinism was found in all the districts, reaching 10 per cent or higher in those districts most severely affected. Two smaller studies conducted in 1985 and 1987-1988 reported lower prevalence than the above, but they concluded that goitre was an important public health problem. A pilot neonatal screening programme using cord blood on filter paper revealed 10 percent of the 650 samples tested had neonatal chemical hypothyroidism. In summary, Bhutan's entire population of 1.2 million people is at risk of IDD, with some 64.5 percent of the population having goitre, and an estimated prevalence of 5.6 percent (i.e. 81,000) with cretinism and an additional 16.7 percent (242,000) with minor neurological impairment attributable to environmental iodine deficiency.

Bhutan has adopted a multi-pronged strategy for the control of IDD. In 1985, a salt iodization plant was commissioned with UNICEF assistance on Bhutan's southern border. All salt sold in Bhutan has to be processed at this plant. All salt importation and distribution is controlled by the government and legislation is in force to prevent the importation of salt which has not passed through the iodization plant. The Food Corporation of Bhutan is responsible for the storage and distribution of iodized salt throughout the country.

Table 15.2 *Summary of results of the National IDD Survey, Bhutan 1991-2*

	Northern Women (age 15-45 years)	Southern Women (age 15-45 years)	Northen Children (age 6-11 years)	Southern Children (age 6-11 years)
Total Goitre prevalence (%)	28.5 (1581)*	45.9 (988)	18.4 (1443)	32.5 (992)
Visible Goitre Prevalence (%)	3.8 (1581)	7.1 (988)	0.3 (1443)	1.0 (992)
Cretinism prevalence (%)	0.9 (1581)	0.8 (988)	0.4 (1443)	0.4 (992)
%With UIC < 10 µg/dl)	14.8 (893)	18.1 (878)	12.6 (864)	16.2 (871)
Median UIC (µg/dl)	23.90 (893)	23.35 (878)	28.30 (864)	24.40 (871)
% With TSH > 5 mU/l	10.79 (1548)	7.42 (984)	20.38 (1423)	22.34 (985)

* Figures in brackets are numbers of people examined or samples collected.

During 1988-91, iodized oil injections were administered to women of child bearing age in those border areas. In all 54,220 injections were administered. A nation-wide study was conducted in late 1991 and early 1992 to assess the IDD situation, the impact of the IDDCP on this, and the knowledge and attitudes of the population concerning the nature and causes of IDD. The 30 cluster sample survey method was employed, with children aged 6-11 years and women aged 15-45 years as the target groups. The survey was conducted in the northern districts and the southern border districts. All subjects were examined for goitre and cretinism, and urine and blood samples were collected for urinary iodine and thyroid stimulating hormone estimation respectively. The results of the survey are shown in Table 15.2.

A further aim was to investigate iodine content in salt throughout the country. Certain aspects of salt purchasing, storage and cooking practices needed improvement. However, 96.6% of the 146 salt samples collected from the north, and 95.0% of the 140 salt samples from the south were found to have an acceptable iodine content.

The current iodine status of the population has shown a very encouraging trend towards an iodine sufficient situation, since the control programme began in earnest. Although the prevalence of goitre revealed by this study is considerably lower than in 1983, the goitre prevalence in both children and women is still high.

If this situation improves still further and maintains at that level, the prevalence of goitre and cretinism in all sections of the population can be expected to fall to negligible levels over the next 5 to 10 years.

Democratic People's Republic of (DPR) Korea

The Democratic Peoples' Republic of Korea (DPRK) is geographically prone to iodine deficiency owing to its predominantly mountainous terrain. Based on a small survey conducted in Hyangson in 1991 the National Total goitre rate is estimated to be 14.7 % with females (16 %) more affected than males (13 %). However, a unique traditional practice of distribution and consumption of iodine-rich sea weed, especially to those living in the mountainous areas, has probably helped mitigate the manifestation of IDD. Pregnant and lactating mothers and children in nurseries and kindergartens (recognized as high risk groups) are given sea weed preparations every day. However, it is necessary to carry out a comprehensive survey to establish the status of IDD prevalence in the country.

India

India is the second most populous country in the world with a population of 834 million (1991 census). A high prevalence of goitre and cretinism exists in a broad Himalayan and sub-Himalayan belt. The Himalayan goitre belt involves Jammu and Kashmir, Himachal Pradesh, Punjab, Haryana, Uttar Pradesh, Bihar, West Bengal, Sikkim, Assam, Mizoram, Meghalaya, Tripura, Manipur, Nagaland and Arunachal Pradesh.

In addition to the well known Himalayan endemic belt, iodine deficiency has been reported from many other states in the country. In 1989, the Indian Council of Medical Research carried out a multicentric IDD prevalence study. Nine states outside the traditional goitrebelt were studied for the prevalence of goitre and cretinism. A total of approximately 410,000 individuals were examined and the overall goitre prevalence observed was 21.1 per cent and the overall cretinism prevalence was 0.7 per cent.

Results of sample surveys conducted by different agencies in 239 districts of 25 States and 4 Union Territories of India have shown a high prevalence of IDD. Of the 457 districts in the country, 197 are identified as endemic for IDD. (Fig. 15.2)

A conservative estimate using the epidemiological (Dulberg) model suggests that 150 million are at risk of IDD, 54 million have goitre, 2.2 million suffer from cretinism and an estimated 6.6 million are affected by milder neurological defects attributable to environmental iodine deficiency.

Following the successful trial of iodized salt in the Kangra valley, Himachal Pradesh (Sooch et al 1973), a National Goitre Control Programme was launched by the Government of India in 1962. The objective of the programme was to survey the problem of iodine deficiency in the country, produce and supply iodized salt and then resurvey after five years to assess the impact of the iodized salt programme. Initially 12 salt iodization plants were installed with UNICEF assistance (5 in Rajasthan, 3 in Gujarat and 4 in West Bengal). These plants had an annual production capacity of 376,000 tonnes of iodized salt but actually produced only 120,000 to 150,000 tonnes per year, well below the estimated 1 million tonnes needed annually for the endemic areas alone.

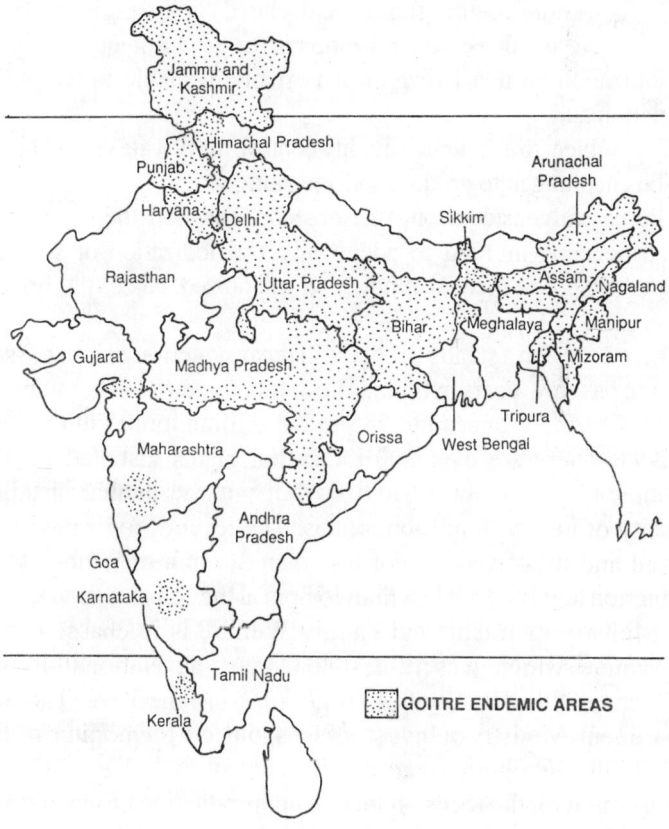

Fig. 15.2 Map of India showing the goitre endemic areas.

As the need for bringing more and more areas under the National Programme was felt, it was realized that the existing arrangements, by which the production and distribution of iodized salt was confined to the public sector alone, were no longer adequate to meet the growing demand. It was also found that supplying only certain pockets of a district or states with iodized salt was administratively difficult. Infiltration of common salt into such 'sealed areas' was frustrating the effectiveness of the programme. The technical goitre control review committee of the Ministry of Health and Family Welfare considered the entire situation at its meeting held in April 1982 and recommended that:

i) the entire country should be declared "goitre prone"

ii) there should be a liberalization in the government's policy on salt iodization so that iodized salt is freely available to the entire population and

iii) subject to a system of quality control, the private sector should also be encouraged to produce iodized salt.

After careful consideration of these recommendations the government took a decision in 1983 to adopt universal iodization of salt and permitted the commercial production of iodized salt in the private sector.

There has been a steady progress in the production of iodized salt over the past few years in India. The annual production has gone up from 0.5 million tonnes in 1985 to 2.8 million tonnes in the year 1992-93. There are over 500 iodization plants installed for the commercial production of iodized salt with an annual installed capacity of nearly 6 million tonnes. The level of iodization was revised and it is fixed at 'not less than 30 ppm of iodine at the production level and not less than 15 ppm at the consumption level'. The Ministry of Health and Family Welfare is in charge of the programme which was re-designated as the National Iodine Deficiency Disorders Control Programme in June 1992. The Salt Department, Ministry of Industry, is responsible for monitoring the production, distribution and quality control of iodized salt. An action plan with the focus on increasing production of iodized salt to meet the goal of USI by 1995; intensification of Programme at national and state level for creating demand for iodized salt and establishing a district level system for monitoring of iodine in salt was developed.

As a result of advocacy, four major salt producing states (Gujrat, Tamil Nadu, Rajasthan and Andhra Pradesh) producing 85% of salt have issued a ban notification against the sale of non-iodized salt. Over 300 manufacturers and traders who together produce 95% of iodized salt participated in the regional orientation and sensitisation workshops on IDD. As a result, iodized salt production increased by 25% - presently estimated to be 3.4 million tons against the total requirement of 5 million tons. The country, however, has installed capacity to iodize the entire edible salt required in the country.

Quality control laboratories under the National Programme have been established by the Salt Department at nine centres to check the quality of salt at the production level. Quality control at the retail level is done by the State Governments through the health directorates. Monitoring at the household level has been introduced recently. In some endemic areas, Non Governmental organizations are also participating in the monitoring activities.

As quality control and effective monitoring is the backbone of the programme, the Government of India with UNICEF assistance, has finalised a project in 1992 for the intensive monitoring of IDD control activities in the 4 endemic States of Assam, Madhya Pradesh, Himachal Pradesh and Uttar Pradesh. The objective of the project is to reduce goitre prevalence in the project area in the age group 10-14 years to less than 5% and to bring down to zero the number of cretins born by the year 2000 A.D. The objective would be achieved by strengthening the monitoring system from production to consumption level to ensure that 100% of the population get only iodized salt in the project area; ensuring dietary consumption of iodized salt and creating awareness about IDD and the need for the consumption of iodized salt by 100% of the population.

The strategy adopted to achieve the goals envisages the establishment of a network of iodine monitoring laboratories for testing the salt at the manufacturing level, at the distribution level and at the consumption level; the testing of urine samples at the district / state level and the monitoring of the thyroid activity of newborns through the screening of cord blood samples in a few of the selected areas. The strategy also envisages the strengthening of training, the establishment of IDD training centres, the formulation of State Information, Education and Communication Plans and the production of educational material for the benefit of the public.

Under the project for 1993-95, nine additional states of east and north-east India, viz. Sikkim, Arunachal Pradesh, Mizoram, Manipur, Meghalaya, Nagaland, Tripura, Bihar and West Bengal are being covered and the possibility of increasing the accessibility of iodized salt or water among the people is being tried out. The co-operation of NGOs in intervention programmes entailing information, education and communication is being sought. 86 more districts in addition to the 20 districts already taken up in 1992 are being covered making a total of 106 districts in 13 states. Thus, virtually the entire IDD endemic area in the Himalayan and sub-Himalayan region is being brought under this project.

Indonesia

Historically, most of the interior regions of Indonesia have been severely iodine deficient. A prevalence rate of over 80 per cent for endemic goitre has been observed in individual villages. Even more important, throughout these regions, the prevalence of endemic cretinism has been found to be more than 10 per cent in villages, and as high as 15 per cent in individual hamlets.

These rates are among the highest reported in the world.

Goitre prevalence surveys were carried out between 1980 and 1982 in 25 of the 27 provinces of Indonesia. The total goitre rate (TGR) was found to be 37.2% and visible goitre rates to be 9.2%. All the provinces had a TGR of >10%. About 30 million people are estimated to live in iodine deficient areas in Indonesia. In 1974, Indonesia initiated a nationwide control programme-the National Goitre Control Programme-consisting of two components: a) iodization of common salt as a permanent measure b) intramuscular injections of iodized oil for the population living in high risk areas, especially where iodized salt would not have easy access.

The salt iodization programme, started with 20 iodization plants supplied by UNICEF and 8 procured by PN Garam, the state-owned company, was charged with the task of iodizing the salt. The total capacity of the 28 plants was 336,000 tonnes per annum against the requirement of 415,000 tonnes of salt for the whole country.

The programme has since been expanded to encompass 183 iodization plants with a combined total capacity of 575,000 tonnes representing the total estimated requirement for the country. To strengthen the programme, the government issued a joint decree of four Ministries (Industry, Health, Trade and Home Affairs), that all salt for human consumption in Indonesia should be iodized to 40 - 50 ppm with potassium iodate. Results of the national monitoring of iodine content in salt at the market level revealed that only 20% of iodized salt met the fortification requirement.

The iodized oil supplementation programme has been operating since 1974. So far 11 million people have received iodized oil injections. Indonesia now has the capacity to produce iodized oil indigenously. Starting from 1993, injected iodized oil supplementation has been replaced by iodized oil through oral administration. The development of this new preparation by Kimia Farma was assisted by earlier investigation in Australia supported by ICCIDD.

At present one laboratory for measuring TSH and urinary iodine exists in Semarang and a second one at NRDC, Bogor is planned. The target of the programme in the Fifth Five-Year Development Plan (1990-1994) is to decrease the total goitre prevalence among school children from the current 32 per cent to 18 per cent and the visible rate from 5 per cent to 4 per cent. With that objective, the salt iodization programme is being strengthened.

Indonesia is part of the international commitment to eliminate IDD. The government has endorsed the recommendations of the 1991 World Health Assembly towards the elimination of IDD by the year 2000 as also the goals of the 1990 World Summit for Children. Furthermore, the Ministry of Health has endorsed the goal of 'elimination of new cretinism by the year 2000'. As already mentioned in Chapter 3, the Indonesia programme has strong support from President Suharto. Assistance with expertise and funding support has been provided through the International Working Group, established by ICCIDD in 1989.

Maldives

It was assumed that IDD is not a public health problem in Maldives. This was probably based on the fact that staple diet of local population consists of sea-fish, a rich source of iodine. However, no systematic surveys were carried out to assess IDD problem.

The Department of Public Health in association with UNICEF undertook a countrywide survey in June-July 1995, to assess the prevalence of IDD and estimate urinary iodine in a sub-sample of the population, The survey adopted the, "EPI-30 cluster" methodology. A total of 30 clusters chosen from a sampling frame of 200 islands. A total of 2834 school children (6 to 12 years) were examined in Maldives. Of these, 725 children had goitre. Thus the total goitre prevalence rate in the surveyed children was 23.6% (Grade 1 = 22.5% and Grade 2 = 1.1%). It is evident that in Maldives IDD is a public health problem The median urinary iodine level was 6.7 µg/dl and 65.5% of children had urinary iodine levels below 10 µg/dl.

Maldives imports its total requirement of salt from India, Sri Lanka, Thailand, Singapore etc. Thus, it is feasible to introduce universal salt iodization in the country.

Mongolia

Mongolia is an agrarian country in Central Asia with a population of 2 million. It is mountainous, high above the sea level and far away from the sea. Studies to determine the degree of iodine deficiency in the environment and its correlation to food and water have been conducted since 1960, leading in 1970 to an appreciation that IDD was a public health problem needing investigation. The studies indicate an overall goitre prevalence usually above 30% with a probable increase in recent years. The most recent survey, conducted in 1989 among school children, indicates a 36 per cent prevalence of goitre. Roughly, 84.8%

of the affected children were aged between 6 and 16 years. The prevalence of endemic goitre among children under 4 years is very low, but rises steeply in the age group of 5-7 years, and increases at a rapid rate with every year from 8-12 years. In general the central and northern parts of Mongolia have a high prevalence of endemic goitre, varying between 30 to 40 per cent. Even animals, sheep and goats in this region have enlarged thyroids. A plan for the prevention and control of IDD in Mongolia is being developed and is expected to be put into operation soon.

Myanmar

Myanmar is bounded by the Himalayas in the north and the Bay of Bengal in the south. With a tropical climate, it has various types of geographical regions - mountainous and hilly areas, plateaus, a central dry zone, a plain and low-lying delta areas. An estimated 14.5 million (36 %) of the 40 million population are at risk of IDD.

The Chin Hills Gazetteer mentioned the high prevalence of goitre and cretinism in certain parts of the country, as early as 1896. Surveys in the northern mountainous areas reported goitre prevalence of 50-90 per cent from the states of Kachin, Chin and Shan. A survey was conducted by the Department of Medical Research in 1981-82 in three townships in the Irrawaddy Division, a delta area, where a goitre prevalence of 40-60 per cent was observed. Another study was conducted by the students of the Institute of Medicine in another 66 townships in Irrawaddy, Magwe, Mandalay, Pegu and Yangon Divisions. A review of the findings of all the surveys up to 1982 by the Department of Medical Research indicates that endemic goitre was prevalent in nearly 50 per cent of the 314 townships in the country. These surveys further reveal that goitre was not confined to the hilly regions, as was thought earlier, but was equally common in the plains and the riverine delta areas of the country. The condition was found in all age groups, but the largest goitres with complications were found in older people. The prevalence was higher among females in all age-groups.

Between 1982 and 1986 another round of goitre surveys was conducted by the Department of Medical Research in 12 townships in 4 divisions and two states. The findings revealed that in half of these townships, the crude goitre rate was more than 10 per cent. Recognizing endemic goitre as a public health problem, a National Goitre Control Committee was established in 1968 under the chairmanship of the Deputy Minister of Health with representatives from the Department of Health and Medical Research, and from Trade and Revenue Corporations. The pilot iodized salt distribution programme was started in two districts of the northern Chin hills, a region previously shown to have goitre. Initially the programme covered about 800,000 people but was later extended to remote endemic areas in Magwe Division, Chin and Shan states. An interim assessment of the programme after 3 years of its operation showed a decline in the prevalence of goitre from 91% to 24.7%.

An important reason for the relative success of the programme was the status of the salt trade in the country, which was state controlled. In 1977, there was a change in trade policy which led to the transfer of salt trade to the private sector and the discontinuation of iodized salt distribution. The production and distribution of iodized salt was stopped in 1980. During the second People's Health Plan (1982-86), preparations were made to revitalize the iodized salt distribution programme. Salt is produced by hundreds of private salt firms on the coast. However all this salt is processed in refineries located around Rangoon. These refineries represent the best point for iodization. Due to recent political and social developments in the country, the establishment of a fully effective National IDD Control Committee was delayed.

The country is to embark on a national salt iodization programme which shall make it mandatory for all human and animal salt to contain iodine as an essential constituent at a prescribed level. The cost of promoting and administering the programme is estimated to be approximately US$ 1 million for a three-year period which is a very small cost for such a major public health intervention. Iodization will add very negligibly (0.20 Kyats/Viss) to the cost of salt which is about 5-8 per cent of the retail price of salt. The programme needs to be supported by promotional measures such as information, education and communication, legislation and enforcement, quality control, monitoring and evaluation and overall administration and co-ordination.

Nepal

Nepal lies in the heart of the Himalayan goitre belt. It is situated between India and the Tibetan plateau of China. It has an area of 147,181 km and has a population of 18.6 million (1991 census). Geographically, Nepal has three distinct regions, i.e., mountainous (>3000 meters), hilly (300 to 3000 meters) and the low flat Terai regions.

In 1965-66 the government carried out a country wide goitre prevalence survey. A total of 5265 persons aged 13 years or more from 19 villages were examined. These 19 villages covered all the three geographical regions of the country. The results showed that 55 percent of the population had goitre and that goitre of high endemicity occurs throughout Nepal including the Terai region.

Subsequently in 1969, very high goitre rates (74 - 100 per cent) were found in school children in Jumla (2,250 meters) and Trisuli (550 meters). This was associated with a wide distribution of cretinism and deaf mutism. Half the population was estimated to be hypothyroid by laboratory indicators. Delange et al (1976) confirmed high rates of goitre (55 per cent) and cretinism (5.1 per cent) in the general population in Trishuli, and also demonstrated a low iodine content in the water, soil and food. In the Kunde region, Ibbertson's group from New Zealand carried out thyroid function studies before and after the administration of iodized oil.

The Government of Nepal has taken two initiatives to deal with the problem. In 1973 a Goitre Control Project was set up and is responsible for the procurement and distribution of iodized salt from India. In 1979 the Goitre and Cretinism Eradication Project was initiated with the responsibility for a mass iodized oil injection campaign primarily in the mountainous and hilly areas of Nepal. The iodized oil injection programme was associated with the Expanded Programme of

Immunization (EPI) of the Ministry of Health with support from UNICEF and WHO. It has covered 40 districts till now, some of which are being covered for the second and third time as well. Each of the remote hilly and mountainous districts is covered again after every five years. So far more than eight million injections have been given. One of the significant achievements of the programme has been that even in the remote mountainous areas, the iodized oil programme has covered more than 85 % of the target population i.e. all people below 45 years of age.

While the iodized oil programme has been a resounding success, the iodized salt programme has been beset by logistic problems. The State Trading Corporation of Nepal was given the responsibility for the implementation of the salt iodization programme. The Goitre Control Project has planned to have six salt iodization plants located along the Indian border to iodize salt imported from India. So far three spray type salt iodization plants have been established. Analysis of salt samples at the household level for iodine content in 1992 showed that 40 % of samples had an iodine content of more than 15 ppm. Ongoing monitoring of iodine in salt is a vital component and is being strengthened. There are major logistic difficulties due to delays in transport, problems with packaging, storage, and delivery to the more remote areas. Presently, there is one urinary iodine monitoring laboratory and four salt iodine monitoring laboratories in Nepal.

The Nutrition Planning Commission of the Government through National Nutrition Co-ordinating Committee since April 1995, is reviewing activities every month. The IDD Plan of Action focussing on issues related to IDD elimination, USI & sustainability has been formulated and a Task Force is appointed to monitor its implementation. A draft plan of action on USI has been developed with special focus on logistical aspects of salt iodination, proper packaging and distribution. The draft legislation on salt iodination has been prepared and will be placed before the Parliament for its approval. Some of the activities identified for priority action are increased levels of iodine in salt to 50 mg/kg, increased availability and accessibility of iodized salt, improved packaging, improved warehouse facilities, provision of iodized oil capsules till 1997 and continuation of transport subsidy till 1997.

Sri Lanka

It is only in recent years that endemic goitre has been recognized as a public health problem in Sri Lanka. The south-east region of the island extending over the hills of the Western Sabarangamuwa, the central and southern Provinces and parts of Uva province are now identified as areas of endemicity. Almost 70 per cent of the total population of 8.5 million inhabit these provinces, and are at risk of iodine deficiency.

A national prevalence survey was undertaken in 1986-87. Seventeen out of 24 districts of Sri Lanka were studied, the remaining 7 deferred because of civil unrest. A random sample of large, medium and small size post-primary schools was selected, containing a total of 59,158 children from 17 districts. The overall goitre prevalence was 18.8 per cent. The prevalence was higher in females (23.2 per cent) than in males (14.0 per cent). These findings clearly show that the goitre prevalence is over 10 per cent in a large part of the country and about 66 per cent of the total population of Sri Lanka live in the goitre endemic area.

An effective national IDD control programme including a comprehensive plan of action with iodized salt has recently been developed. The Emergency (Edible Salt) Regulation No. 1 Act of 1990 stipulates that all salt in the entire country meant for human or animal consumption should be iodized at a prescribed level. Six salt iodization plants have been established at the salt works in Hambantota and Puttalam. In order to achieve the goal of universal iodization, the programme needs strengthening of advocacy, demand generation, and monitoring components.

The Ministry of Health has trained 81 Public Health Inspectors (PHI's) and some of the Divisional Directors of Health Services on IDD and monitoring of iodine content in salt in April-May 1995. A total of 7,000 copies of information booklet on IDD have been distributed to 4,000 Public Health Midwives and health staff in 23 districts for use in interpersonal communication with families and community members. Sarvodaya, an NGO is actively involved in IDD activities. Thus efforts are being made by the different sectors towards achieving USI in Sri Lanka.

Thailand

Initial goitre prevalence surveys done in 1955 and 1957 showed IDD to be a major problem in north east Thailand. The provinces chiefly affected by IDD were : Chiangmai (23.5%), Chiangrai (49.3%), Lampong (41.2%), Prae (39.5 %), Uttaradit (45.4 %). With aid from WHO and UNICEF, the Ministry of Public Health began a pilot salt iodization project in Prae province in 1965. Subsequent surveys among school children in 1968 again showed a high endemicity of IDD in these provinces. An estimated 20 million (39 %) of the 53 million population are at risk of IDD.

Beginning in 1968, the salt iodization pilot project expanded to a national programme. In the seventies, the emphasis was shifted from IDD to other health and nutrition issues. In 1984, however, the IDD control and prevention project was revived with aid from UNICEF and Redd Barna.

A survey conducted in 1987 revealed that endemic goitre was widespread in 8 to 14 provinces in Northern Thailand as well as Loei province in the north-east. The prevalence of goitre in the above provinces had come down to between 10 % to 30 % from the original 20 % to 50 %. The national IDD control project was planned and presented and approved by the cabinet in 1989. The strategy for control includes the supply of iodized drinking water in select provinces, and salt iodization in endemic provinces. Iodized oil capsules are used in remote and highly endemic areas. Eight regional and one central laboratory has been set up to measure the iodine content in urinary and cord blood TSH levels. Five ultrasound machines were purchased to strengthen clinical examinations.

The results of the concerted efforts are reflected in the lowering of goitre prevalence in 1991. The goitre prevalence in the northern provinces have fallen from 19.3 % in 1989 to 15.1 % in 1991 and in the north-east provinces from 30.5 % in 1990 to 16.2 % in 1991.

Innovative strategies to suit the local conditions are being attempted to increase the accessibility of iodized salt. The co-operation of the NGOs is being sought in promoting information, education and communication activities. Recently the Government took a decision to adopt the universal iodization of salt and the salt sector is being motivated and supported to ensure this.

The status of the national programme has been greatly enhanced by the acceptance by HRH Crown Princess Maha Chakri Sirindhon, of the position of Chairperson to Thailand's National Committee for IDD Control.

References

Acharya, S. October, 1991. 'Proceeding of Ending Hidden Hunger–A policy conference on micronutrient malnutrition, Montreal'. Canada.

Bhutan 1992. 'Iodine Deficiency Disorders the Bhutan story'. Directorate of Health Services. Royal Govt. of Bhutan.

Clugston, G.A., E.M. Dulberg, C.S., Pandav, R.L., Tilden, 1987. 'Iodine Deficiency Disorders in South East Asia'. In Hetzel B.S., J.T., Dunn, J.B., Stanbury eds. *The Prevention and Control of Iodine Deficiency Disorders*. Elsevier, p.273-308.

Delange, F., Valix 1976. 'Endemic goitre and Cretinism in Trisuli'. *WHO Preliminary report*.

Dulberg, E.M. 1985. 'A model for predicting the prevalence of developmental iodine deficiency disorder from goiter-a preliminary report'. *IDD Newsletter* 1(1):6.

Pandav, C.S., M.G., Karmarkar, L.M., Nath, 1988. 'National Goitre Control Programme, National Health Programme Series-5'. New Delhi: National Institute of Health and Family Welfare.

Pandav, C.S., R , Mohan, M.G., Karmarkar, P., Subramanian, L.M., Nath, 1989. 'Iodine Deficiency in India'. *The National Medical Journal of India* 2(i) : 18-2.

Sooch, S.S., M.G., Deo, M.G., Karmarkar, N., Kochupillai, K., Ramachandran and V., Ramalingaswami, 1973. *Prevention of endemic goitre with iodized salt. Bull. World Health Organization* 49. 307-12.

Thailand 1992. 'The Control of Iodine Deficiency in Thailand: Past, present and future'. Thailand: Department of Health, Ministry of Public Health.

World Health Organization. 1993. 'Micronutrient Deficiency Information System'. MDIS Working paper # 1.

16

IDD in China

T. Ma and T.Z. Lu

Iodine Deficiency Disorders are a very significant endemic disease in China. Among the 31 provinces, autonomous regions and municipalities, only Shanghai Municipality has no IDD problem; the population at risk of IDD was about 400 million in 1991, representing nearly 40% of the whole population at risk of IDD in the whole world. Endemic areas are not only in remote mountainous regions but also in some flatlands not far away from the sea Fig. 16.1.

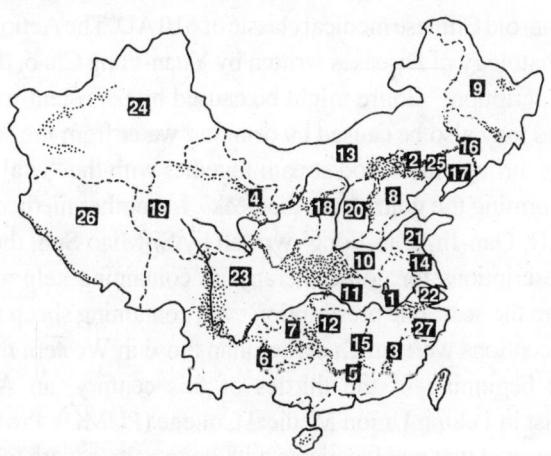

Fig. 16.1 Map of China showing IDD areas. Some of the provinces affected include: 1. Anhui, 2. Beijing, 3. Fujian, 4. Gansu, 5. Guangdong, 6. Guangxi, 7. Guizhou, 8. Hebei, 9. Heilongjiang, 10. Henan, 11. Hubei, 12. Hunan,13. Inner Mongolia, 14. Jiang Su, 15. Jianxi, 16. Jilin, 17. Liaoning,18. Ningxia, 19. Qinghai, 20. Shandong, 21. Shanghai, 22. Shaanxi, 23.Sichuan, 24. Sinjiang. 25. Tiangjin, 26. Tibet, 27. Zhejiang (Source: Micronutrient Deficiency Information System WHO Working paper # 1 1993).

The goitre subjects numbered 34 million prior to prophylaxis, and now there are still as many as 8 million. The typical endemic cretins, mainly neurological and some myxedematous, have been reported to number 230,000. (see further Chapter 1). Obviously, this figure is an underestimate, because the primary health workers are not experienced enough to identify all of them. Besides the typical endemic cretins, in the IDD endemias, the incidence of mild mental retardation is remarkably increased; in some serious endemias, it is as high as 15%. Most of the mild mental retardation in IDD endemias is caused by iodine deficiency, which has been called 'subclinical cretinism'. Some psychologists have reported that the IQ distribution curves of the children in many IDD endemias in China have a generalized tendency to shift to the left by about 10 points. Therefore, if the iodine supply is not sufficient in China, then each year, the Chinese population can be estimated to lose 60 million IQ points, which represents a very serious loss. In ancient Chinese writings long before Christ, such as the 'Mountains and Seas' and also in the 'Huai-Nan-Zi', there were already some records of goitre. In an old Chinese medical classic of 610 AD, The Aetiology and Symptomatology of Diseases written by Yuan-Fong Chao, there was such a description: 'Goitre might be caused by persistent worry and anger; and may also be caused by drinking water from the sand. The sand goes through the blood stream together with the "vital energy" thereby forming the goitre over the neck'. In another medical classic of 682 AD, Qan-Jin-Yao-Fong' written by Si-Miao Sun, there were some prescriptions for goitre therapy all containing kelp and other cures from the seas; one prescription even containing sheep thyroids. Such perceptions were much earlier than those in Western medicine.

In the beginning of the thirties of this century, an American biochemist in Peking Union Medical College (PUMC), Professor W Adolf, reported that many patients with huge goitres were found near the Eastern Qing Tombs outside Beijing. In 1940, another biochemist of PUMC, C Y Zhang first observed the effects of oral iodized vegetable oil on goitrous rats. During World War II, a US Army doctor noticed many patients with goitre in Yunnan Province along the Burma Road. In 1940)2, Dr X Y Yao and Dr T Z Yao of the Ministry of Health of the Republic of China made a goitre survey in 37 counties of Yunnan Province. The table salt produced from the Yi-Ping-Lang salt mine of Yunnan began to be iodized after 1945. This was the first salt iodization programme in China.

In 1950, the second year of the founding of the People's Republic of China, Mr X F Yang, Governor of Hebei Province noticed many mentally retarded people in Qan-Xi County. He sent two of them to the present Teaching Hospital of Tianjin Medical College to be studied upon, when Professor H I Chu (X Y Zhu) was the Director and Drs T Ma and T Z Lu were assistant residents of the Medical Department. However, because endemic cretinism was so different from the sporadic cretinism commonly seen in the urban region, they failed to recognize it. After the establishment of the Endocrine Research Group of Tianjin Medical College in 1959, Drs T Ma and T Z Lu visited a well known village of mentally retarded people in Qan-Xi County, Hebei Province. They believed that the people there were retarded due to iodine deficiency, yet they still considered it to be a localized phenomenon. In 1960, Dr T Ma found that these subjects were prevalent in many goitre endemias in Chengde Prefecture, Hebei Province; and afterwards a large scale study led by Professor H.I. Chu was conducted in Chengde in 1961 which lasted for 5 years. The study revealed that patients suffering from both goitre and cretinism had a low thyroid hormone status and that both goitre and cretinism could be prevented by iodization. Two mothers, with all their previous children being cretins, gave birth to two perfectly normal children after iodine prophylaxis. Subjects with less obvious mental defects (the so called 'subclinical cretin') were first demonstrated during this study. A very important conclusion was arrived at that the mental retardation of the next generation would be a most serious disaster for the community. In 1963 and 1964, two nation-wide symposia were held in Chengde, and after this the new concept of iodine deficiency affecting brain development spread rapidly.

Mao Tse-Tung in his famous poem Farewell to the God of Plague expressed his keen desire to eradicate the endemic diseases from China. For the realization of his hopes, a Central Leading Group for Endemic Diseases Control was set up in 1961 directly under the Central

Committee of the Chinese Communist Party. As it was decided that the chief of the group should be a member of the Political Bureau of the party's Central Committee, it became a leading group with full authority. The Vice-Director of the Chengde Study Group, Mr C Chang was appointed a member of the Central Leading Group.

During the period of the so-called 'Cultural Revolution' most of the public health work was interrupted; and IDD control did not escape from the turmoil. In 1973, however, the Central Leading Group was reconstructed, though its work was still under the influence of the misguided policy prevailing at that time. In early 1950, Dr J B Stanbury pointed out that 'the thyroid hypertrophy is the adaption of the body to iodine deficiency', but some leaders neglected this scientific advice and considered the goitre as a superfluous mass. By their strong desire to cut down the goitre rate more rapidly, they favoured the surgical removal of goitre. In Shaan-Xi Province alone, more than 200,000 goitres were removed surgically within one year, some belonging only to the grade II diffuse type. The injection of tincture of iodine into the goitre was carried out to make it shrink, which was magnified as a new invention at that time. In addition there was a recommendation that a big dose of iodide (1-10 mg/day) could reduce the goitre rate rapidly. Under these circumstances, regular salt iodization programmes were often neglected. As the well known saying of Confucius goes: 'If the term is not correct, then the logic will not be reasonable; if the logic is not reasonable, then the aim cannot be achieved'. For this reason, we support Dr Hetzel using the term 'iodine deficiency disorders' (IDD) instead of endemic goitre and endemic cretinism. In this way, one could consider the various disorders caused by iodine deficiency, including mental retardation, as a whole and avoid the 'goitre fixation', also realizing that iodization programmes should not be neglected.

The 'Cultural Revolution' terminated in 1976; the Central Leading Group was reorganized and a famous Army General D S Li became the chief. The suggestions of the Scientific Advisory Group were re-evaluated and salt iodization again became the sole measure. The Central Leading Group organized a multi-sectoral workshop each year, to be attended by all the vice-governors of the provinces with IDD and all the vice-ministers of related ministries. In addition, a so-called 'Three Ministries and One Co-op' meeting was held regularly each year to co-ordinate the administrative and technical work between the Ministries of Public Health, Light industry and Commerce and the Central Co-operative. In such a way, the salt iodization programme could be carried out readily. The leading groups at the provincial level as well as at the county level were all strengthened at the same time. The up-to-date urinary iodine assessment and radio-immunoassay of thyroid hormones began to be used in monitoring.

Besides Tianjin Medical College in North China, another scientific advisory centre was established in Jiamusi Medical College in north-east China led by Dr J C Li. In 1979, their excellent control work in Jixian Village near Jiamusi, made a great impact in China. (See Chapter 1, Table 1.3) The Guiyang Medical College became the scientific advisory center in south-west China almost at the same time. Guizhou Province is a severely iodine deficient area, but did not have significant IDD earlier, because all the inhabitants were provided with Sichuan well salt which has a high iodine content. In 1955, a railway connecting the province to the sea was built, after which the cheaper sea salt was provided. This had a much lower iodine content. A couple of years later, severe endemic goitre and cretinism suddenly flared up over the whole province like an epidemic. Incidences of cretinism in some severe endemias was more than 5% and affected only the children. Professor H I Chu visited Guizhou Province and organized a large scale study of iodine prophylaxis together with Guiyang Medical College, which lasted five years. By a massive assessment of the thyroid hormone status of the entire population in the endemic area before the iodization, an important conclusion was drawn that even if there were no symptoms or signs present, all the inhabitants in the endemic areas would be suffering from iodine deficiency. Two professors, Dr Z F Shi and Dr G H Zeng of the Guiyang Medical College were appointed Provincial Ministers of Public Health and so Guizhou became a leading IDD control province.

In 1980, the IDD Group of the Institute of Endemic Diseases Control of Xinjiang, led by Drs H M Wang and F F Lin, organized a co-operative IDD control study with Tianjin Medical College in Hetian, Southern Xinjian. Only then the significant IDD problem there was taken more seriously.

In the area of the Dabie Mountain of Anhui Province, there was a claim of a new inherited form of mental retardation related to inbreeding among the local villagers. Some officials believed this and proposed to tackle the problem by massive immigration. Professor H I Chu was very concerned about this suggestion because it could divert attention from the iodization programme. In 1978, he visited the area and demonstrated the very typical endemic cretins to certain local health officers.

Under the leadership of the Central Leading Group, in the decade 1976-1986, the IDD control work advanced successfully. Sixteen provinces attained the Chinese Goal of Control by 1986. Professor H I Chu described the great achievements of China at a regional conference in Japan in 1982. Dr T Ma described the administrative structure, particularly the experience of multi-sectoral leading groups at different levels, at the Sixth Asian Congress of Nutrition in Bangkok in 1983. A representative from south-east Asia said that such an ideal administrative system could hardly imagined in his country.

In 1981, Dr B S Hetzel, from the CSIRO, Division of Human Nutrition in Adelaide, Australia, visited China and initiated discussions with Professor Chu on a proposed China Australia Programme of Technical Co-operation. This programme was finally carried out by Dr C Eastman and Dr G Maberly from the Westmead Hospital, Sydney, with Chinese scientists from Tianjin, Qinghai, Harbin and Guiyang over the period 1986-1991. Thanks to the work of this co-operative programme, supported by the Australian International Development Assistance Bureau (AIDAB), a very severely affected IDD province, Qinghai, reached the Chinese Goal of Control of IDD. Modern monitoring laboratories were set up in 4 provinces.

Southern Xinjiang and Tibet are two significant IDD endemias, but it has been very difficult to carry out the regular iodized salt programmes there. In 1985, the UNICEF Office for China helped Tianjin and Harbin to set up for a proper iodization process in these two regions. Different procedures using oral iodized oil were compared in Xinjiang and the iodized tea brick was shown to be effective in Tibet.

In 1986, Dr X Sun, Director of the Central Leading Group Office attended the inaugural meeting of the ICCIDD in Kathmandu. Chinese scientists have been playing an active role in the work of ICCIDD since its foundation.

Late in 1986, according to the principles of government reform, all administrative work was to be transferred to the specific government organizations. The representatives from all provinces with IDD problems and from all related ministries and almost all members of the Scientific Advisory Group on IDD Control insisted that the organization in charge of IDD control should be one directly under the State Council, otherwise its multi-sectoral function would be lost. Unfortunately, the Minister of Public Health at that time claimed that his Ministry should be the appropriate organization taking this responsibility. Finally a Bureau of Endemic Diseases Control was set up in the Ministry of Public Health; all the experienced IDD control managers of the former Central Leading Group were discharged and the former Scientific Advisory Group was reorganized.

The Director of the Bureau encouraged the dismissal of the provincial leading groups, but this was resisted by the provincial authorities. Finally, although most provincial leading groups were retained, they no longer had the authority they enjoyed before. A new National IDD Control and Research Centre was set up in Harbin on the basis of the centre in Jiamusi Medical College to do the training and monitoring work for the Bureau, but at the same time, the very effective centres in Tianjin and Guiyang gradually collapsed.

The Bureau of Endemic Diseases Control as well as the National Center of IDD Control and Research have made serious efforts to promote IDD Control in China. In order to avoid iodine loss, potassium iodate has been used instead of potassium iodide. A nation wide monitoring system has been set up, although it is still only a preliminary one. A salt iodization regulation was drafted four years ago, but so far has not been approved owing to some controversy between the salt industry and the Health department.

With the reform of the economic system in China, salt production as well as salt purchase is no more monopolized by the government. As a result, the privately produced uniodized salt has begun to flood the market. The former voluntary labour of primary health workers is no more available, so that all the surveys and all the preventive measures require their own budgets. With the exception of potassium iodate, funds for IDD control now all come from the provincial governments. Therefore, the Bureau of Endemic Control has found it very difficult to issue rigorous instructions. In some provinces with financial difficulties, the control work has lacked momentum. The work of the Bureau has been very difficult.

An International Working Group on IDD Control for China (IWGIDD) was organized in 1989 through the help of ICCIDD, with the WHO Representative for China and the UNICEF Programme Officers in Beijing as members, the Executive Director of ICCIDD, Dr. Basil Hetzel as Chairman and the Director of the Bureau of Endemic Diseases Control, Mme Gao Shu-fen as Vice-Chairman. While the function of the Group is to introduce control and monitoring techniques and the experience in advocacy to China, its most important role is to seek financial support from multilateral and bilateral funding agencies. In 1991, after the Ending Hidden Hunger Meeting in Montreal, the IWGIDD proposed a multisectoral meeting in China and tried to set up a supra-ministeric organization again. In early 1992, UNICEF, WHO and UNDP sent a group led by Dr P. Greaves and Dr G. Maberly to draft a 'United Plan of Support' from the UN Agencies with the necessary technology and training to be provided under PAMM in Atlanta, USA.

The International Working Group has given top priority to explaining the significance of IDD control to the Chinese leadership.

A large scale meeting on advocacy was held in Beijing, in the Great Hall of the People (September 22-24, 1993) with the sponsorship of the Chinese Premier Mr Li Peng.

All provincial Governors with their staff attended the meeting in addition to representatives of the international agencies including WHO, UNICEF, UNDP, World Bank and ICCIDD. The meeting was chaired by Madame Peng Pei Yung one of five members of the State Council. The Vice Premier, Mr Zhu Rong Ji made a commitment on behalf of the Chinese Government which was followed by speeches of support from the international agency representatives including UNDP and the World Bank. Mr Zhu subsequently, at a special meeting of the Provincial Governors, assured them that the central government would provide the necessary funding to secure an effective elimination programme by universal access to iodized salt. It is clear that the Chinese government has recognized the major hazard of the effects of iodine deficiency on early brain development in the light of its one child family policy. It is now agreed that the supra-ministerial multi-sectoral organization will be re-established.

At the conclusion of the meeting a plenary session was convened at which the provincial officials endorsed a revised " National Plan of Action". The IDD Advocacy process in China has resulted in the acceptance of the five key principles mentioned below, which have become the foundation for the National Plan of Action.

1. **IDD** include, in addition to goitre and cretinism, a potential diminishment of intellectual capacity of more than 10 IQ points across entire areas affected by only mild iodine deficiency.

2. **IDD** are not restricted to remote or rural areas, but in fact can be found in all geographic areas of the country.

3. **IDD** elimination nation-wide will only be achieved through multi-sectoral co-operation.

4. **IDD** are an issue of national development

5. **IDD** are most cost-effectively eliminated by universal salt iodization

As there are only five years left in the present century, and the IDD problem has been so serious, it is feared that China might remain one of the few countries not able to attain the goal in time. The key to success depends upon two essential factors; first, to mobilize a large number of workers enthusiastic in IDD control, including the salt industry; second, to speak the truth instead of making propaganda, so as not to again produce destructive results as on earlier occasions in Chinese history. The scientific leadership needs to be firm and based only on scientific findings.

The ICCIDD has proclaimed that its mission is to bridge the gap between scientific knowledge and its application at country level in the elimination of IDD. In the course of the history of IDD control in China, the gaps have varied with the times.

Fortunately, there has been an excellent scientific advisory group in China, which has had to evolve with experience. In the sixties, the main problem lay in the fact that cretinism was not considered a result of iodine deficiency. This problem was solved by observation and reference to the scientific literature. Yet the recent inclination to attribute cretinism to heredity is still an evidence of this gap. In the seventies, the main gap existed in the neglect of the wider spectrum of brain damage, with attention focused on goitre. The main gap in the eighties lay in the denial that IDD elimination was a multi-sectoral problem. The present gap is that of the political leaders having overlooked the general deterioration of population quality due to IDD. This has been bridged by IDD control being now given high priority.

The Government of China has a made a stong committment towards the goal of elimination of IDD by the year 2000. The steps taken towards this goal are the establishment of the National Leading and Co-ordination Group for IDD control which is to be supported by a Multisectoral Management Committe, and a National Training and Technical Training and Support Team; the completion of the World Bank loan to support the iodization and the packaging process;ongoing and increasing support from UNDP, UNICEF, UNIDO and WHO; and the push to achieve universal iodization of salt by the end 1996 on an emergency basis.

Reference

'Report of the National Advocacy Meeting to Eliminate Iodine Deficiency Disorders by the year 2000'. China: Beijing. 22-24 September, 1993.

17

IDD in Europe

F. Delange

Epidemiology

Endemic goitre, occasionally complicated by endemic cretinism, has been reported in Europe up to the turn of the twenteth century, especially from remote, isolated, mountainous areas in central parts of the continent including Switzerland, Austria, Northern Italy, Bulgaria and Poland. The problem of IDD has been entirely eradicated in Switzerland thanks to the implementation and monitoring of a program of salt iodization. Probably because of the impact on the medical world of this remarkable program, IDD seem to have been considered no longer as significant public health problems in Europe during the last five decades.

However, reevaluation of the problem in the late 1980s under the sponsorship of the European Thyroid Association clearly indicated that, with the exception of most of the Scandinavian countries, Austria and Switzerland, most of the European countries or at least certain areas of these countries were still affected, especially in the Southern part of the continent. Shortly thereafter, it was shown that differences in the iodine supplies in the adult populations of several countries or areas were accompanied by parallel differences in the iodine content of breast milk and of urine of neonates (Table 17.1). These surveys also revealed a lack of information on IDD in countries of the Eastern part of the continent.

Based on this information and thanks to recent changes in the political situation in Europe, the status of iodine nutrition was reevaluated in all European countries, including in the Eastern part of the continent, at an international workshop entitled 'Iodine Deficiency in Europe: A continuing concern' held in Brussels in

Table 17.1 Comparison of the results obtained in European countries or regions for urinary iodine excretion in adults, for the iodine content of breastmilk and of urine of infants on day 5 of life. The number of determinations are shown in parentheses. Adapted from Delange et al. 1986.

Country or Region	Urinary Excretion of Iodine in Adults (μg/day)	City	Iodine Concentration (μg/dl) Breast milk	Urine infants (Mean ± SEM) day 5 (Median)
The Netherlands	88-140	Rotterdam		16.2 (64)
Finland	238-270	Helsinki		11.2 (39)
Sweden	91-140	Stockholm	9.3 (60)	11.0 (52)
Sicily (non endemic area)	113	Catania		7.1 (14)
Switzerland	126-141	Zurich		6.2 (62)
Spain	89	Madrid	7.7 ± 0.9 (69)	
France	55-126	Paris	8.2 ± 0.5 (68)	
		Lille		5.8 (82)
Belgium	51	Brussels	9.5 ± 0.6 (91)	4.8 (196)
Italy	37	Rome		4.7 (114)
Germany	35	Berlin		2.8 (87)
North	20	Freiburg	2.5 (41)	1.1 (41)
South	16	Iena	1.2 ± 0.1 (55)	0.8 (54)
Sicily (endemic area)	22	San Angelo	2.7 ± 0.3 (59)	

April 1992. During this meeting, one representative from each European country summarized the latest data available in his country on the situation of iodine nutrition, which included the evaluation of iodine intake in all age groups, the epidemiological evaluation of the prevalence of goitre and other thyroid disorders related to iodine deficiency, the impact of iodine nutrition on intellectual development and school performances of children as well as on the results of campaigns of systematic screening for congenital hypothyroidism in the neonates by

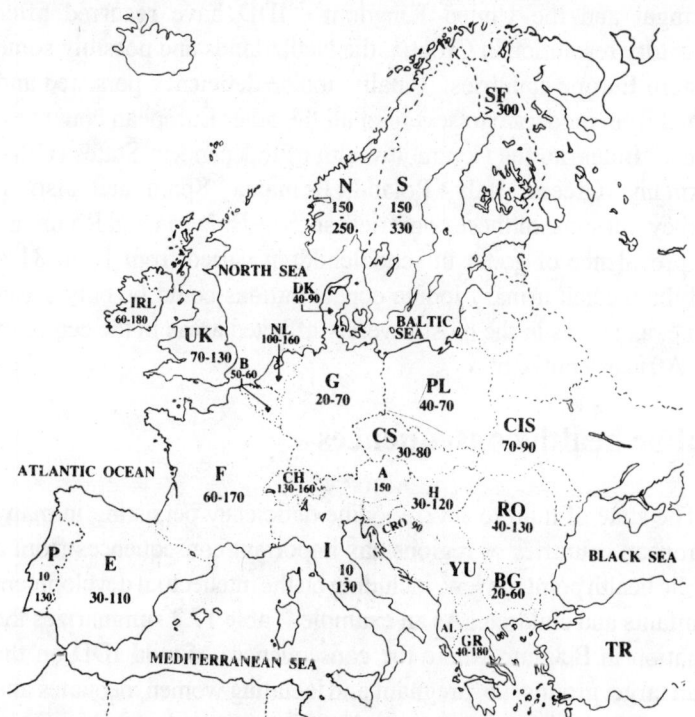

Fig. 17.1 Evaluation of iodine intake in Europe as at 1992 (g/day). Range of the values observed during regional or national surveys. N : Norway, S : Sweden, SF : Finland, DK : Denmark, IRL : Ireland, UK : United Kingdom, B : Belgium, NL : The Netherlands, G : Germany, PL : Poland, CS: Former Czechoslovakia, CIS: The Commenwealth of Independent States, F: France, CH : Switzerland, A : Austria, H : Hungary, Ro : Romania, P : Portugal, E : Spain, I: Italy, CRO : Croatia, Y: Yugoslavia, BG : Bulgaria, GR : Greece, AL : Albania, TR : Turkey. From Delange 1994 (21). With permission.

measurements of serum TSH. Information was also provided on the availability and consumption of iodized salt or on any other prophylactic programme.

Figure 17.1 summarizes the results reported during the workshop on iodine supply in Europe as at 1992. Iodine deficiency was under control in only five countries, namely Austria, Finland, Norway, Sweden and Switzerland. Iodine deficiency was marginal or present mainly in "microfoci" (packets of goitre) in Belgium, the Czech and Slovak Republics, Denmark, France, Hungary, Ireland, Portugal and the United Kingdom. IDD have recurred after transitory resolution in Croatia, the Netherlands and possibly some Eastern Europe countries. Finally, iodine deficiency persisted and varied from moderate to severe in all the other European countries, namely Bulgaria, the Commonwealth of Independent States (CIS), Germany, Greece, Italy, Poland, Romania, Spain and also in Turkey. In some of these countries, such as Bulgaria and Romania, the prevalence of goiter in schoolchildren varied from 16 to 81% and the median urinary iodine concentrations could be only 2 $\mu g/dl$, i.e. as low as in the most severely affected areas in the center of the African continent.

Public health consequences

The state of mild to severe iodine deficiency persisting in many European countries or regions has important consequences from a public health point of view, including on the intellectual development of infants and children. As an example, Table 17.2 summarizes the situation in Belgium where the consequences of mild IDD on the main target groups, i.e. pregnant and lactating women, neonates and young infants, have been extensively investigated.

More generally speaking, the consequences of iodine deficiency in Europe can be summarized as follows:

In adults: the frequency of simple goitre is elevated in many countries and the cost of therapy of thyroid problems resulting from iodine deficiency in the adult population is enormous. For example, the cost for the diagnosis and treatment of goiter due to iodine deficiency in Germany for the year 1986 was estimated at 900 million DM (approximately 700 million US dollars) while prevention by iodized salt would cost only 2-8 US cents per person and per year. Thyroidal uptake of radioiodine varies markedly from one European country to another and is inversely related to the iodine intake. Elevated thyroidal uptake due to iodine deficiency aggravates the risk of thyroid irradiation and development of thyroid cancer in case of a nuclear accident. The best prophylaxis of nuclear hazards in case of radioiodine fallout is to increase the basal intake of iodine of the population.

Thyroid function is usually normal in adults in Europe. In contrast, it is frequently altered in pregnant women. During pregnancy, the gland undergoes stimulatory events due to the synergic effects of three mechanisms : direct stimulation by hCG, stimulation through the usual feedback mechanism via the increase in TBG and the lowering of free hormone concentrations, and finally, the overall enhancing role of limited iodine availability. It has been shown that, at least in conditions of borderline iodine intake as seen in Belgium (50-70 µg/day), pregnancy is accompanied by a progressive decrease of serum free T_4 and consequently by an increase of serum TSH. This state of chronic TSH hyperstimulation results in the development of goiter in about 10 % of the pregnant women and in a progressive increase in the serum concentration of thyroglobulin. Goitre can persist after pregnancy in an important number of women. Pregnancy, especially in conditions of borderline iodine intake, at least partly explains the higher frequency of thyroid problems in women than in men.

The consequences of marginal iodine deficiency during pregnancy in Belgium on the thyroid function of the neonate include even more elevated serum levels of TSH and Tg on cord blood than in the mothers and a slight enlargement of the thyroid gland. The role played by iodine deficiency in these changes is demonstrated by the

Table 17.2 *Functional consequences of mild iodine deficiency in Europe. The case of Belgium. Adapted from Delange 1994.*

Age Groups	Recommended Iodine Intake (µg/day)	Acutal Iodine Intake (µg/day)	Consequences
Adults	150	51 - 60	Elevated thyroidal uptake of radioiodine case of nuclear accident increased risk in
Adolescents	150	30 - 50	'Puberty' simple goitre
Pregnant women	200	< 100 in 90 % of the cases	Increased thyroid stimulation Development of goitre with only partial recovery after pregnancy Prevention of these anomalies by iodine supplementation
Infants-Children	90 -120	< 90 in 80% of the cases (Delange, Wolff, Glinoer and Vertongen, unpublished) deficient in 79% of the cases	Potential risk for brain and intellectual development.
Neonates	90		Elevated serum TSH and Tg at birth (cord blood) Elevated TSH at screening for high recall rate and frequency of 'false positives' Increased risk of transient hypothyroidism in the premature infant

fact that they are prevented by iodine supplementation of the mothers during pregnancy (Table 17.3) and that they do not occur in iodine replete areas in Europe such as some parts of The Netherlands.

In adolescents and children: Euthyroid pubertal goitre is especially frequent in adolescents and occasionally requires substitutive therapy by T_4 or iodide. Iodine metabolism is accelerated during this period of life.

A very important issue is the demonstration that even in Europe today, clinically euthyroid schoolchildren born and living in an iodine deficient environment exhibit subtle or even overt neuro–psychointellectual deficits as compared to controls living in the same ethnic, demographic, nutritional and socio-economic system, except that they are not submitted to iodine deficiency (Table 17.4). These deficits are of the same nature, although less marked, than those found in schoolchildren in areas with severe iodine deficiency and endemic mental retardation. These deficits could result, as demonstrated in severe endemic goitre, from transient thyroid failure occurring during foetal or early postnatal life, i.e. during the critical period of brain development.

In neonates: The most important and frequent alterations of thyroid function due to iodine deficiency in Europe occur in neonates and young infants:

1) The frequency of transient primary hypothyroidism is almost 8 times higher in Europe than in North America. As shown in Figure 17.2, this syndrome is characterized by postnatally acquired severe primary hypothyroidism lasting for a few weeks and requiring substitutive therapy. The risk of transient hypothyroidism in the neonates increases with the degree of prematurity. The specific role played by iodine deficiency in the etiology of this type of hypothyroidism is demonstrated by the disappearance of neonatal transient thyroid failure in Belgian preterms since they were systematically supplemented with 30 µg potassium iodide/day.

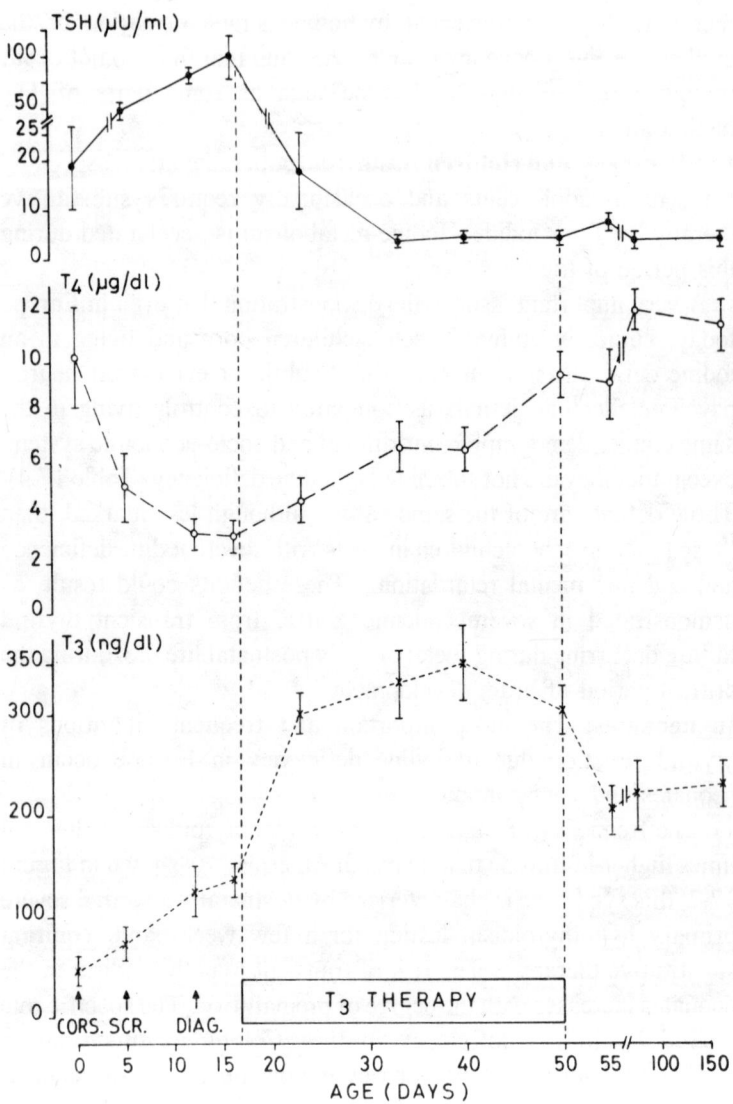

Fig. 17.2 Time course as a function of age of the serum concentrations of TSH, total T_4 and T_3 in 11 infants with postnatally acquired transient primary hypothyroidism. Values recorded as Mean ± SEM. COR S : cord serum; SCR: Screening; DIAG: Diagnosis. From Delange et al. 1984. With permission.

Table 17.3 *Effects on the neonate of iodine supplementation (100 µg iodine per day) during pregnancy in moderately iodine deficient pregnant mothers.*

	Neonates born to	
Variables	Untreated mothers (n = 60)	Iodine supplemented mothers (n = 60)
Urinary iodine (µg/dl)	4.3 ± 0.4	7.7 ± 0.8
Thyroid volume	1.05 ± 0.05	0.76 ± 0.05
Cord serum Tg (ng/dl)	113 ± 9	65 ± 6

Note: Results given as Mean ± SEM. The differences between the two groups are highly significant ($P < 0.0001$). Adapted from Glinoer et al. In press.

2) As shown in Figure 17.3, there is an inverse relationship between the urinary iodine concentration in newborn populations in Europe used as an index of their status of iodine nutrition and the frequency of serum TSH above 50 µU/ml at day 5, at the time of screening for congenital hypothyroidism, i.e. the recall rate under suspicion of congenital hypothyroidism. Consequently, neonatal thyroid screening appears as a particularly sensitive index of the presence and action of goitrogenic substances in the environment and can be used as a monitoring tool in the evaluation of the effects of iodine prophylaxis at a population level.

The reason for the particular sensitivity of the newborn, especially of the preterm infant, to the effects of iodine deficiency appears from the data summarized in Table 17.5. In Toronto, where the iodine intake is elevated, the iodine content of the thyroid in full term infants is 300 µg. In Brussels, with a borderline iodine intake, the iodine content of the thyroid is 82 µg

Table 17.4 *Neuropsychointellectual deficits in infants and schoolchildren in conditions of mild to moderate iodine deficiency in Europe.*

Regions	Tests	Findings	Authors
Spain	Locally adapted Bayley McCarthy	Lower psychomotor and mental development than controls	Bleichrodt et al. 1989
Italy Sicily	Bender-Gestalt	Low perceptual integrative motor ability Neuromuscular and neuro-sensorial abnormamities	Vermigglio et al. 1990
Tuscany	Wechsler Raven	Low verbal IQ, perception, motor and attentive funtions	Fenzil et al. 1990
Tuscany	Wisc Reaction time	Low velocity of motor response to visual stimuli	Vitti et.al. 1992

Table 17.5 *Relationship between the iodine content of urine in adults and neonates used as an index of iodine supply and thyroidal weight, iodine content and estimated turnover rate of thyroidal iodine.*

Cities	Adults	Neonates				
	Urinary excretion of iodine (µg/day)	Iodine concentration in urines		Weight (g)	Thyroids	
		Median (µg/dl)	Values below 5 mg/dl (%)		Iodine content (µg)	Estimated turnover rate [1]
Toronto Canada	600-800	14.8 (81)	11.9	1.00±0.12 (13)	292±47	17
Brussels Belgium	51	4.8 (196) ***	53.2	0.76±0.25 (4)	81±9**	62
Leipzig Germany	16	1.6 (70)***	97.2	3.27±0.39 (10)**	43±6**	125

Note: ([1] Based on a requirement of IT4 of 50 µg/day) in neonates in three areas with markedly different iodine intake. Results given as Mean ±SEM. The number of patients is shown in parentheses. Levels of significance as compared to Toronto ** $p<0.01$, *** $p<0.001$. Adapted from Delange et al. 1993.

Table 17.6 *Overview on legislation for iodized salt in Europe (Survey of 23 countries).*

Prohibited	Denmark
Availability	Nationwide: 17 countries
	In endemic regions only: 5 countries(Bulgaria, Hungary, Portugal, CIS, Romania)
Consumption	Compulsory: 8 countries including Austria and Portugal
	Voluntary: 14 counties including Switzerland
Price versus non iodized salt	Similar: 12 countries
	Higher (+5 to 10%) : 5 countries 9 (Finland, Germany, Greece, Ireland, Spain)
	Lower (-25%) : France Unknown: 4 countries

Note: Adapted from Burgi 1993 and Delange et al. 1993.

and in Leipzig, which used to be severely iodine deficient, the content is only 43 μg. The table also shows that the turnover rate of intrathyroidal iodine is markedly accelerated in iodine deficient neonates. Therefore, thyroid failure is more likely to occur. These neonatal data contrast with adult data which have shown that the iodine stores of the thyroid are not affected by iodine deficiency unless in the case of a severe degree of deficiency.

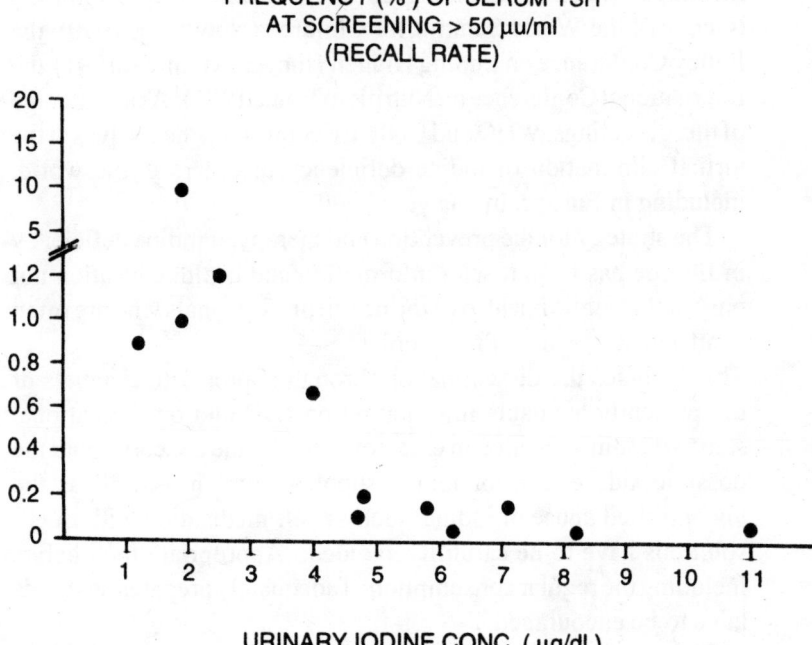

Fig. 17.3 Relationship between the urinary concentration of iodine and the recall rate at the time of screening for congenital hypothyroidism in newborn populations in Europe. From Delange 1994. With permission.

Prevention and therapy of IDD in Europe

It is hard to understand and difficult to admit that iodine deficiency, the most common preventable cause of mental deficiency in the world today, is still so prevalent in Europe. The most probable cause of the phenomenon has been the insufficient awareness until recently of the problem of IDD by the health authorities, including the medical and paramedical world, and by the public.

During the past 10 years, a series of major decision making meetings took place, including the World Health Assembly in 1990 (Geneva), the World Summit for Children (New York 1990), the Policy Conference on Ending Hidden Hunger (Montreal 1991) the International Conference on Nutrition (Rome 1992). As an outcome of these meetings, WHO and UNICEF committed themselves at the virtual elimination of iodine deficiency disorders in the world, including in Europe, by the year 2000.

The strategy for the prevention and therapy of iodine deficiency in Europe has to start with information and health education not only of the public but also of the health professionals who are often insufficiently aware of the problem.

This includes the dissemination through appropriate channels of the presently available information on IDD and on the national status of iodine nutrition in each country. Undue concern about the possible side effects of iodine supplementation as well as the uncontrolled abuse of iodine, such as self medication with Lugol solutions have to be carefully avoided. Appropriate food habits including the regular consumption of adequately prepared seafoods have to be encouraged.

The major measure, however, for the prevention of iodine deficiency in Europe, is the systematic introduction and control of iodine supplementation through programs of Universal Salt Iodization (USI), i.e. the fortification of all salt for human and animal consumption.

In 1992, iodized salt was available in most European countries, usually nationwide, with the exception of Denmark where it was prohibited (Table 17.6). It was compulsory in 8 countries. The price was most usually barely higher than non iodized salt; it was even lower in France. In spite of this apparently satisfying situation and with the remarkable exceptions of Switzerland, Austria, Sweden and Finland, national programs of salt iodization were not sufficiently operational and efficient in Europe. This partial failure could result from the fact that many of the iodized salt samples were grossly inadequate with respect to their iodine content, at least when available at the level of the consumer. It also could result from a gross overestimation of household salt consumption: the actual ingestion of salt, measured by the lilium marker technique, was only 15% of the total salt intake. Therefore, iodized salt should be made available not only for household but also for industrial food production, including cheese and bread, as well as for animal consumption.

Of course, in the context of USI programs particular attention must be paid to the usual recommendation to limit as much as possible the daily intake of salt for medical reasons. The level of iodization of salt has to be adapted in order to meet permanently the appropriate daily requirements of iodine. For example, in Switzerland, because of the progressive decline in salt intake, the iodine intake slightly decreased in the early eighties. The level of salt iodization was therefore increased from 7.5 to 15 ppm. This resulted in an increase of iodine intake from a borderline value of 90 µg/day to a perfectly adequate value of 150 µg/day. Interestingly enough, this change was not accompanied by any significant increase in the incidence of iodine induced hyperthyroidism but rather, by a steadily decline in the incidence of both toxic nodular goitre and Graves disease. It thus appears that the many European countries which are actually in a state of moderate iodine deficiency could make the transition to iodine sufficiency not only with no ill effects, but with the unexpected large benefit of a marked decrease of the incidence of thyrotoxicosis in addition to the disappearance of euthyroid goitre.

From 1992 onwards, and especially following the endorsement by WHO Euro of the recommendations resulting from the Brussels meeting to appoint national iodine committees in all countries and to generalize the use of iodized salt, quite significant progress has been achieved in many countries. National programs have been organised which could result, as for example in Poland, in an exhaustive revaluation of the situation and in practical measures aiming at the implementation of USI. At the initiative of UNICEF Europe, co-operation took place between the salt industry (European

Salt Producers Association, ESPA) UNICEF, WHO and ICCIDD in order to implement and control USI on a European basis. The European Union was officially approached in order to generate European rules for the level of iodization of salt.

Presently ongoing reevaluation of the status of iodine nutrition in 11 European countries by means of standardized measurements of thyroid volume and urinary iodine in school children (ThyroMobil project, unpublished) indicated that substantial progress towards the control of iodine deficiency occurred in some European countries or regions such as Southern Germany, the Czech and Slovak Republics. In others, however, such as Belgium, the situation of borderline iodine deficiency has not improved yet.

As long as USI is not systematically implemented in Europe, special attention has to be devoted to the protecton of the two main target groups, i.e. pregnant and lactating mothers and young infants. If iodine deficient, these age groups should be supplemented with physiological quantities of iodine, for example by including iodine in the polyvitamins administered to these two age groups. Moreover, the iodine content of formula milk should be increased in Europe above the classical recommendation of 5 µg/dl. The present recommendation, endorsed by WHO Euro and by ICCIDD, is 10 µg/dl milk for fullterms and 20 µg/dl for preterms.

In addition, in some European areas affected in the past by overt endemic cretinism, the iodine deficiency was and remains extremely severe, with impairment of neonatal thyroid function and, consequently, with potentially harmful consequences for brain development. In such situations, emergency and transient more drastic measures can be justified from a public health point of view, such as the oral administration of iodized oil.

It is now demonstrated that in many industrialized countries such as the United States, Great Britain and Northern European countries, the main source of dietary iodine is neither salt nor seafoods but dairy milk. This results either from the use of iodiphors in the industrial processing of milk or from iodine supplemented diets for the animals, or from both. European rules for monitoring the iodine content of milk and a precise evaluation of the possible role of milk as a substrate for iodine supplementation in Europe are desirable.

Iodinated water has proved to be efficient in the control of iodine deficiency in developing countries in situations where the access to water is well localized, for example by wells, an where most of the water is used for human and animal consumption. these conditions are probably rarely met in European countries.

Finally, it is conceivable that in exceptional circumstances where iodide or iodate are not accepted as sources of iodine for salt iodization for philosophical reasons, the use of natural seaweeds as a source of iodine could be considered.

In summary, iodine deficiency still affected some 150 million people in Europe in 1992 and 97 million had a goitre. Substantial but insufficient progress has been achieved during the last few years. More precise evaluation of some national situations, dissemination of information, health education, universal salt iodization and adequate monitoring are the priorities in order to reach the goal of elimination of IDD in Europe by the year 2000.

References

B.L., Baltisberger, C.E., Minder and H., Burgi. 1995. 'Decrease of incidence of toxic nodular goitre in a region of Switzerland after full correction of mild iodine deficiency'. *Eur. J. Endocrinol.* 132, 546-9.

Berghout, A., E, Endert., A, Ross., H.V., Hogerzell, N.J. Smits, and W.M., Wiersinga. 1994. 'Thyroid function and thyroid size in normal pregnant women living in an iodine replete area'. *Clin. Endocrinol.* 41:375-9.

Bleichrodt, N., F., Escobar del Rey, G., Morreale de Escobar, I., Garcia and C., Rudio. 1989. 'Iodine deficiency. Implications for mental and psychomotor development in children'. In DeLong, G.R., J. Robbins and P.G., Condliffe eds. *Iodine and the brain.* New York, Plenum Press publ. pp. 269-287.

Burgi, H., Z., Supersaxo and B., Selz. 1990. 'Iodine Deficiency diseases in Switzerland one hundred years after Theodor Kocher's survey: A historical review with some new goitre prevalence data'. *Acta Endocrinol.* (Kbh) 123:577-90.

Burgi, H. 1993. 'Iodization of salt and food, technical and legal aspects'. In Delange, F., J.T., Dunn and D. Glinoer eds. *Iodine deficiency in Europe. A continuing concern*. New York, Plenum Pres Publ. pp. 261-268.

Burrow, G.N. and J.H., Dussault. 1980. *Neonatal Thyroid Screening*. New York, Raven press publ. pp. 1-322.

Delange, F., P., Bourdoux, M., Laurence, L., Peneva, P., Walfish, H., Willgerodt. 1993. 'Neonatal thyroid function in iodine deficiency'. In Delange, F., J.T., Dunn and D. Glinoer eds. *Iodine deficiency in Europe. A continuing concern*. New York, Plenum Press publ. pp. 199-209.

Delange, F., J.T., Dunn and D., Glinoer. 1993. 'Iodine deficiency in Europe'. *A continuing concern*. New York: Plenum Press publ. pp. 1-491.

Delange, F., P., Heidemann, P., Bourdoux, A., Larsson, R., Vigneri, M., Klett, C., Beckers and P., Stubbe. 1986. 'Regional variations of iodine nutrition and thyroid function during the neonatal period in Europe'. *Biol. Neonate*. 49:322-330.

Delange, F., F.B., Iteke and A.M., Ermans. 1982. 'Nutritional factors involved in the goitrogenic action of cassava'. Ottawa: International Development Research Centre publ. pp. 1-100.

Delange, F. 1990. 'Iodine nutrition and risk of thyroid irradiation from nuclear accidents'. In Rubery, E. and E., Smales eds. *Iodine prophylaxis following nuclear accidents*. Pergamon Press Publ. pp.45-53.

Delange, F. 1991. 'Endemic cretinism'. In Braverman, L.E. and R.D., Utiger eds.*The Thyroid. A fundamental and clinical text*. Philadelphia, J.B. Lippincott publ., pp. 942-955.

Delange, F., J., Dodion, R., Wolter, P., Bourdoux, A., Dalhem, D., Glinoer and A.M., Ermans. 1978. 'Transient hypothyroidism in the new born infant'. *J. Pediatr*. 92 : 974-976.

Delange, F., A., Dalhem, P., Bourdoux, R., Lagasse, D., Glinoer, D.A., Fisher, P.G., Walfish and A.M., Ermans. 1984. 'Increased risk of primary hypothyroidism in preterm infants'. *J. Pediatr*. 105 : 462-469.

Delange, F. 1994. 'The disorders induced by iodine deficiency'. *Thyroid* 4:107-128.

Delange, F., P., Bourdoux and A.M., Ermans. 1985. 'Neonatal thyroid screening used as an index of an extrathyroidal supply of iodine'. In Hall, R and J. Kobberling eds. *Thyroid disorders associated with iodine deficiency and excess*. New York, Raven Press publ. pp. 273-282.

Delange, F and H., Burgi. 1989. 'Iodine Deficiency Disorders in Europe'. *Bull. WHO*. 67:317-326.

Delange, F. 1994. 'Iodne deficiency in Europe'. *Thyroid International* 3 : 1-20.

Delange, F. 1993. 'Requirements of iodine in humans'. In Delange, F., J.T., Dunn and D., Glinsoer eds. *Iodine deficiency in Europe. A continuing concern*. New York Plenum Press publ. pp. 5-16.

Dunn, J.T. 1993. 'Sources of dietary iodine in industrialized countries'. In Delange, F., J.T., Dunn and D., Glinoer eds. *Iodine deficiency in Europe. A continuing concern*. New York, Plenum Press Publ. pp. 17-24.

Ermans, A.M. 1993. 'Dietary iodine supply and radioiodine uptake: the case for generalized iodine prophylaxis'. In Delange, F., J.T., Dunn, and D. Glinoer, eds. *Iodine deficiency in Europe. A continuing concern*. New York, Plenum Press Publ. pp. 237-242.

Fenzi, G.F., L.F., Giusti, F., Aghini-Lombardi, L., Bartalena, C., Marcocci, F., Santini, S., Bargagna, D., Brizzolara, G., Ferretti, G., Falciglia, M., Monteleone, M., Marcheschi and A., Pinchera. 1990. 'Neuropsychological assessment in schoolchildren from an area of moderate iodine deficiency'. *J. Endocrinol. Invest* 13 : 427-431.

Fisch, A., E., Pichard, T., Prazuck, R., Sebbag, G., Torres, G., Gernez and M., Gentilini. 1993. 'A new approach to combatting iodine deficiency in developing countries : the controlled release of iodine in water by a silicone elastomer'. *Am. J. Publ. Health* 83 :540-545.

Glinoer, D., P., De Nayer, P., Bourdoux, M., Lemone, C., Robyn, A., Van Steirteghem, J., Kinthaert, and D., Lejeune. 1990. 'Regulation of maternal thyroid during pregnancy'. *J. Clin. Endocrinol. Metab*. 71:276-287.

Glinoer, D., P., De Nayer, F., Delange, V., Toppet, M., Spehl, J.P., Grun, J., Kinthaert and B., Lejeune. 'A randomized trial for the treatment of excessive thyroidal stimulation in pregnancy : maternal and neonatal effects'. *J. Clin. Endocrinol. Metab*. In Press.

Gutekunst, R and Scriba, P.C. 1989. 'Goiter and iodine deficiency in Europe'. *The European Thyroid Association report as updated in 1988.* J. Endocrinol. Invest. 12:209-220.

Koutras, D.A. 1980. 'Europe and the Middle East'. In Stanbury, J.B. and B.S. Hetzel eds. *Endemic goitre and endemic cretinism.* New York: John Wiley publ. pp. 79-100.

Konig, M.P. 1968. 'Die Kongenitale Hypothyreose und der Endemische Kretinismus'. Berlin: Springer Verlag publ. pp.1-175.

Langer, P. 1980. 'Eastern and Southeastern Europe'. In Stanbury, J.B. and B.S. Hetzel eds. *Endemic goitre and endemic cretinism.* New York: John Wiley publ. pp.141-44.

Malvaux, P. 1985. 'Thyroid function during the neonatal period, infancy and childhood'. In Delange, F., D.A., Fisher and P., Malvaux eds. *Pediatric Thyroidology.* Basel, S. Karger publ. pp. 33-43.

Mannar V.M.G. 1994. 'The iodization of salt for the elimination of iodine deficiency disorders'. In Hetzel, B.S and C.S. Pandav eds. *SOS for a billion. The conquest of iodine deficiency disorders.* Delhi: Oxford University Press publ. pp. 89-107.

Nordenberg, D., K., Sullivan, G., Maberly, V., Wiley, B., Wilcken, F., Bamforth, M., Jenkins, H., Hannon and B., Adam. 1993. 'Congenital hypothyroid screening programs and the sensitive thyrotropin assay : strategies for the surveillance of iodine deficiency disorders'. In Delange, F., J.T., Dunn and D. Glinoer eds. *Iodine deficiency in Europe.* A continuing concern. New York, Plenum Press publ. pp. 211-218.

Pfannenstiel, P. 1989. 'The costs of continuing iodine deficiency in the Federal republic of Germany'. *IDD Newsletter vol. 5* No.1:7-8.

Szybinsky, Z. 1993. 'Investigations on iodine deficiency and model of iodine prophylaxis in Poland, Nationwide programme'. *Polish J. Endocrinol.* vo;.44, pp. 1-399.

Thilly, C.H., J.B., Vanderpas, N., Bebe, K., Ntambue, B., Contempre, B., Swennen, R., Moreno Reyes, P., Bourdoux and F., Delange. 1992. 'Iodine deficiency, other trace elements and goitrogenic factors in the etiopathogeny of iodine deficiency disorders (IDD)'. *Biol. trace elem. Research.* 32:229-243.

Vermiglio, F., M., Sidoti, M.D., Finocchiaro, S., Battiato, V.P., Lo Presti, S., Benvenga and F., Trimarchi. 1990. 'Defective neuromotor and cognitive ability in iodine-deficient schoolchildren of an endemic goiter region in Sicily'. *J. Clin. Endocrinol. Metab.* 70 : 379-384.

Vitti, P., F., Aghini Lombardi, L., Antonangeli, T., Rago, L., Chiovato, A., Pinchera, M., Marcheschi, S., Bargagna, B., Bertuccelli, G., Ferretti and B., Sbrana. 1992. 'Mild iodine deficiency in fetal/neonatal life and neuropsychological performances'. *Acta Medica Australia* 19 : 57-59.

18

IDD in Latin America

E.A. Pretell and J.T. Dunn

The history of iodine deficiency disorders in Latin America is long and varied. Pre-Colombian statues in the Andean regions and in Mexico show that endemic goitre existed there long before the Conquistadors arrived. Many early accounts by explorers describe the frequent occurrence of goitre. For example, the western part of what is now Argentina had particularly severe endemic goitre, and the city of San Miguel de Tucuman was moved in the 1680s, 120 years after its founding along the Puente Jeijo River, allegedly because 'its population was becoming idiotic'. The French physician, Boussingault, also reported one of the first uses of iodized salt in what is now Colombia. The severity of iodine deficiency followed geologic patterns similar to those elsewhere in the world. The worse endemias were in isolated mountain communities. Central Mexico and the Andean regions were the most afflicted, but many other parts of the hemisphere were also severely involved, and virtually no country in mainland Latin America was free of iodine deficiency (Fig. 18.1).

Modern surveys for goitre within individual countries began in the 1930s. Almost all had at least some regions where the goitre prevalence was more than 50% and several countries such as Peru, Bolivia, Ecuador, Mexico and Guatemala, had iodine deficiency in most of their geographical area. During the 1950s and 1960s, virtually every country passed a law mandating iodized salt. Some programmes of prophylaxis with iodized salt were transiently successful, but most were not. Those that were successful initially later relapsed. For example, Guatemala in 1952 had a goitre prevalence of 38% nationwide, reaching 74% in some areas. A highly effective salt iodization programme reduced the prevalence to 5.2% by 1965 and

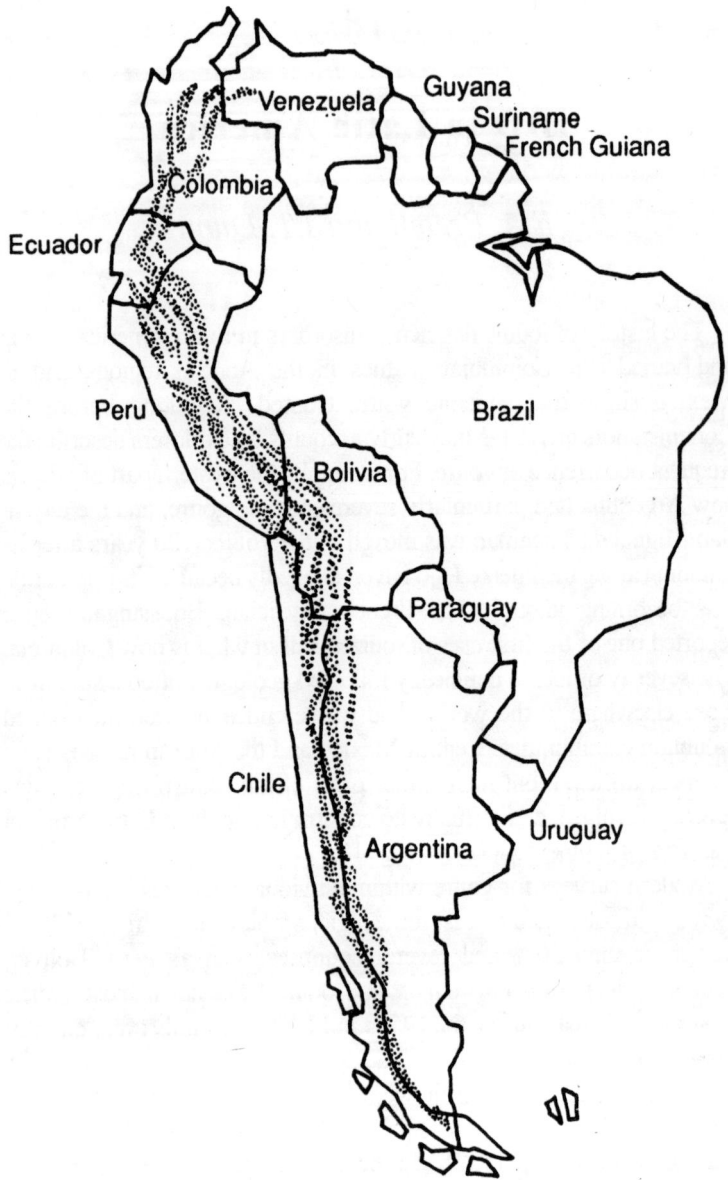

Fig. 18.1 Map of South America showing the Andes Mountains. (Courtesy: Dr M Gueri, PAHO).

endemic goitre was no longer considered a significant health problem. However, effective monitoring of salt iodization deteriorated, controls were not enforced, and as a result the goitre prevalence returned to 21% by 1989. Colombia experienced a similar recrudescence of IDD after a temporarily successful salt iodization programme.

Why did these programmes fail? Several common problems emerge. First, laws were not enforced and did not fix responsibility for absorbing the cost of salt iodization. Iodine itself is not expensive nor is the process of adding it to the salt, but other costs associated with packaging, distribution, and the upgrading of outdated technology inevitably add to the price of salt. Governments are often unable or unwilling to subsidize these costs, producers resent being asked to shoulder this responsibility, and consumers naturally resist price increases. No Latin American country addressed these issues satisfactorily. Secondly, monitoring was either absent or inadequate. Thus, after initial enthusiasm on the part of the government and producers for regular checks on iodine levels in salt, interest waned, monitoring lapsed, and the iodine content of randomly selected salt samples was either absent or greatly diminished. Thirdly, the importance of iodine deficiency and its correction was not adequately communicated to the concerned sectors-different branches of the government, the health establishment, industry, and most importantly, the consumers.

This general failure in Latin America provides a valuable lesson as efforts for iodine prophylaxis are renewed in this region or initiated in countries elsewhere in the world. Despite the 30 year existence of laws mandating iodized salt, only a few countries are now nearing iodine sufficiency, and their successes stem mainly from very recent efforts.

We can divide Latin American countries into three groups based on current IDD status. The first consists of countries with effective IDD control programmes that are moving steadily towards successful elimination; examples of these are Bolivia, Peru, Ecuador, Panama, and Guatemala. A second category includes countries where IDD is known to exist that are now developing renewed interest in control programmes; examples are Mexico and Paraguay. A third category, comprising the rest, includes countries where IDD was known to exist in the past but with inadequate recent information. We will focus particularly on three countries from the first group, because these countries offer valuable experience regarding the possible problems and successes that may help other countries throughout the world as they develop their own IDD control programmes.

Bolivia, Ecuador, and Peru share the rugged mountainous terrain of the Andes and eastern jungles as dominant features of their geography. In the early 1980's, goitre prevalence of these regions were 71% for Bolivia, 80% for Ecuador and 36% for Peru. The strategy for prophylaxis in each has been based on iodized salt, but its implementation needed to be adapted to the unique features of each country. Varying degrees of other supplements have been necessary until the iodized salt programmes were successful. All three countries have indigenous salt supplies. In addition to the sea salt of Peru and Ecuador, all three countries have scattered inland salt deposits.

In Bolivia, the fact that many small producers were located throughout the country created enormous logistic difficulties in trying to introduce iodization into salt production and distribution. One large modern salt producer offered highly refined salt that could be easily iodized, but at a price much higher than the going rate for the crude locally produced salt widely available and almost universally preferred for human consumption. With assistance from outside donors, the government developed a semi-autonomous corporation (EMCOSAL) that built salt iodization plants to be used and operated by co-operatives of local small salt producers. Bolivia has a strong history of co-operatives in many other activities, and this programme was enthusiastically accepted by the salt producers and the communities. EMCOSAL trained the producers to operate the iodization plants, and supervised packaging, marketing, and distribution. Currently 37 iodization plants produce enough iodized salt to cover the country's entire population. Salt for animals is also being iodized. EMCOSAL is becoming progressively self-supporting and the supply of iodized salt is reaching all parts of the country. In 1989, it was recognized that about 1.5 million people, mostly in remote rural areas, would not receive iodized salt for a few years, so a massive programme using iodized oil as a temporary measure was carried out over several months in that year. In addition to the vigorous introduction of iodized salt, the Bolivia programme gave intense attention to programme support measures. Education for the consumer was a key component, and the country was blanketed with pamphlets, radio spots, and presentations at community meetings and fairs. Education also took place at the level of the government ministries involved, including health, industry and communication.

Factors relevant to IDD and its control were different in Ecuador and needed different approaches. Most of its salt comes from the sea and producers are concentrated in a small coastal area. About half the country's population lives along the coast, and is iodine sufficient; the remainder lives in the mountains and jungles, where there is severe iodine deficiency. An Ecuadorean/Belgian co-operative programme targeted 10 Andean provinces for IDD elimination, relying almost exclusively on iodized salt. It began with rapid but careful surveys of villages, including a thorough analysis of salt use. It enforced the existing laws and relied on meticulous monitoring at the factory and consumer level to ensure that the salt was adequately iodized. Simultaneously, it devoted major efforts to education at all levels-government, salt producers, and the general population in the affected areas. Currently, the production of iodized salt is sufficient to cover 100% of the population. The adequacy of salt iodization is monitored at the plant and in the communities, and any lapses are automatically reported by means of a sophisticated monitoring system so that prompt action can follow. As in Bolivia, key factors for the success of the programme so far are: (1) making the use of iodized salt practical, cost acceptable, and attractive to the consumers; (2) careful and aggressive monitoring; and (3) intense education.

About 11 million, or half of Peru's population, live in the sierra and jungle regions where iodine deficiency is severe. Salt production and distribution was in the hands of a state monopoly until 1990. However, this monopoly was dissolved, and the number of plants producing iodized salt abruptly increased from 3 to 38. Only 6 of the 38 are well equipped and 3 of them cover about 95% of the country's salt production. Currently 80% of the salt in the four major plants is satisfactorily iodized with adequate quality control, but only 40% of that in the smaller plants, and 88% of the salt targeted for human consumption is now iodized. Progress in the programme was hampered by changes in the country's political system and by the radical shifts in the salt trade. As in Bolivia, it was recognised that certain high risk areas would not receive iodized salt soon enough, and a massive programme of administering iodized oil was carried out, with over two million doses given. The programme continues to provide iodized salt to all communities in the mountains and jungles. Education is a corner stone of the programme. and includes informational messages at all levels, especially targeted to government, health workers, and affected communities. Despite significant obstacles in the past ten years substantial progress has been made and it should be possible to achieve elimination.

As these examples already show, the approach to IDD control has varied widely among different countries in the region, reflecting the diversity of their cultural, political, and geographical situations. Brazil, by way of further example, has had significant IDD in its vast inland area, particularly in the extreme west. Salt iodization has been the chosen prophylactic measure, and the government met the increased cost associated with iodization by purchasing iodine and donating it to the salt manufacturers. The government analyses salt samples on a routine basis, and good quality control has recently been achieved, but biological monitoring is also needed. Mexico had a highly successful programme in the 1960's that subsequently became complacent and no longer monitored the iodine content of salt effectively. Predictably, manifestations of iodine deficiency reappeared in some of the areas that had previously had severe IDD, particularly in the country's centre. The government has now woken up to this situation, and renewed efforts with iodized salt are being made.

These examples give us an idea of IDD and current efforts at its correction in Latin America. The problems are similar to those elsewhere in the world; (1) the government and people have not been sufficiently aware of IDD and the ease of its solution; (2) the issue of an increased cost associated with iodization and the problem of who will pay for it has not been addressed; and (3) monitoring has not been satisfactory or maintained.

Several lessons can be learned from identifying these problems. To have sustained success, a programme must motivate the entire country, particularly the government and the consumer, and make them understand the importance of attaining an adequate level of iodine intake. Iodized salt must be available at an acceptable cost to all consumers. The government must adopt sustainable procedures for the quality control of salt iodization and for the biological monitoring of its effects. As described above, Latin America has had nominal salt iodization programmes long enough to provide excellent examples of how they can fail. These lessons should have a sobering effect as other countries initiate salt iodization programmes or as they become complacent once they achieve apparent initial success.

In summary, Latin America has had salt iodization programmes for at least 30 years, and most of them have been unsuccessful until recently. They will continue to fail unless a way is found to make them sustainable. Other public health problems such as smallpox have been eradicated because the vector no longer exists. Iodine deficiency is different, and its consequences will recur whenever the means for its correction are withdrawn. In the case of salt iodization, this means that effective long-range monitoring is essential for a successful and sustainable programme. While the progress currently being made in Ecuador, Peru, Bolivia, and other countries is exciting, its ultimate success will be measured by long-term results, not so much in the year 2000, but in 2010 and beyond. Future generations have problems enough without adding to them the need for rediscovering prophylaxis.

Latin America Promotes Universal Iodization for IDD Elimination

In Quito, Ecuador, April 9-11, 1994, representatives of countries, international organizations, and various sectors relevant to IDD, particularly the salt industry, learned how each group could contribute towards IDD elimination, and pledged to work together in the region to achieve universal salt iodization and IDD elimination.

The program included presentations from the President of Ecuador, the Minister of Health, the Executive Director of UNICEF, the personal representative of the Director of Pan American Health Organization (PAHO) and the Executive Director of ICCIDD.

Additionally, the meeting heard from representatives of the salt industry, social communicators, economists, and educators. Special topics included regional overview of IDD, experiences in Bolivia, Ecuador, Guatemala, Mexico and Peru, a discussion of the role of different sectors in IDD elimination, and a symposium on strategies for supporting program against IDD.

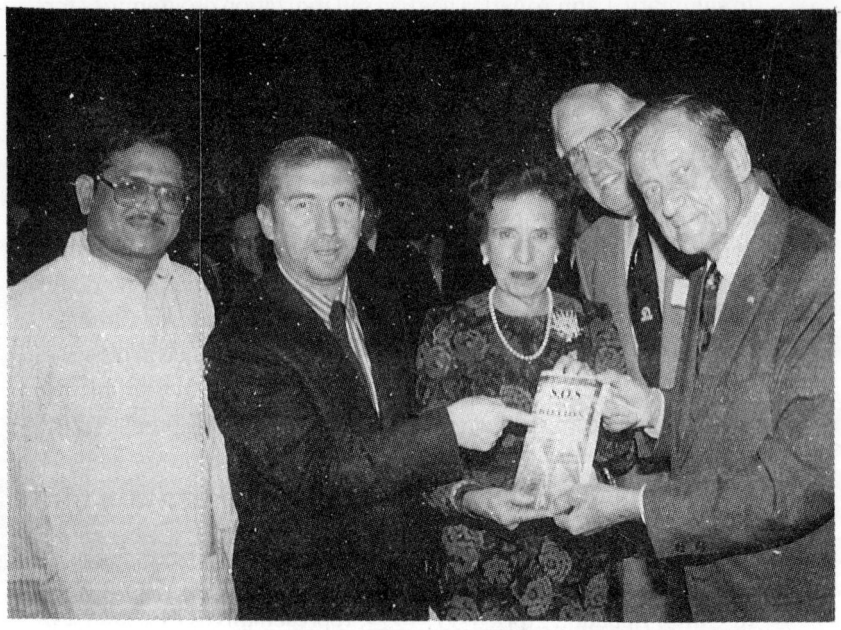

Fig. 18.2 Photograph showing the release of the first edition of the book – *'S.O.S for a Billion - The conquest of Iodine Deficiency Disorders'*.
From Left to Right: Chandrakant S. Pandav (Regional Co-ordinator for S.E. Asia, ICCIDD); Dr. Patricio Abad-Herrera (Minister of Public Health, Ecuador); First Lady of Ecuador, Josefina de Duran Ballen; Basil S.Hetzel (Chairman, ICCIDD); Mr. James P. Grant (Executive Director UNICEF)

In a special poster session, 18 countries presented up-to-date summarises of their IDD status and corrective measures against it. Another session, organized by ICCIDD, demonstrated approaches and techniques in IDD control.

On this occasion the Executive Director of UNICEF Mr. James P. Grant launched the first edition of this book *S.O.S FOR A BILLION : The conquest of Iodine Deficiency Disorder*. Mr James P. Grant in his speech on the launching of the book said ' This book could not have been more timely, it should be a vital handbook for everyone who is engaged in the global efforts to eliminate IDD over the next few years - not just for doctors, public health officials and University lectures, but for government planners and administrators, for food industry executives, for salt manufacturers and distributors, for educators and teachers and for interested and concerned people everywhere.'

The meeting concluded with a 'Declaration of Quito' that reaffirmed the commitment of IDD elimination and universal salt iodization in the Americas.

Quito Declaration on Universal Salt Iodozation

The countries participating in the Regional meeting on Universal Salt Iodization Towards the Elimination of Iodine Deficiency Disorders in the Americas, held in Quito, Ecuador, from 9 April to 11 April, 1994 recognizing that:

— A large proportion of the people living in the region are at risk of IDD, due to inadequate amounts of iodine in soil, water and food;

— Iodine deficiency impairs the development of children, and is the single largest cause of mental retardation;

— Many countries in the region have already successfully tackled the problem of iodine deficiency through fortifying all edible salt with iodine, and that this has proven to be the most practical and low-cost approach to eliminate IDD; and

— In the few countries in the region where salt iodization has been introduced but not sustained, an increase in IDD has been recorded.

We therefore declare:

1. That all people in the Region have a right to receive adequate amounts of iodine and that our Governments have an obligation to ensure compliance with this human right;
2. That the most efficient way of ensuring adequate levels of intake is to iodize all salt consumed by people and animals, including salt used in the manufacture of processed food;
3. That, by continuing to work with salt producers, distributors, exporters, importers, and consumers, our Governments will establish legal, technical, and administrative provisions, as well as other measures needed to ensure that all salt for consumption is adequately iodized; our Governments will also implement adequate information strategies for awareness-raising and participation in using iodized salt through relevant ministries (health, education, economy) and other public and private institutions involved in this problem, such as municipalities, research centers, community organizations, nongovernmental organizations, social welfare entities and external co–operation agencies;
4. That the iodization of all salt for human and animal consumption should be maintained and that all the countries of the region will develop and support mechanisms, its sustainability and compliance with the goal of universal iodization of salt by 1995 in order to guarantee that new cases of iodine deficiency disorders will not appear and that they be virtually eliminated in the Americas; and
5. That all alimentary salt traded between countries in our region should be adequately iodized.

Overview of Countries Situation Following the Quito Meeting

Following the Quito Meeting, all the countries in the Region have re-enforced their activities to reach the main goal of universal salt iodization of the edible salt by the end of 1995.

With the exception of two countries, in all the others the production volume of iodized salt is practically covering the human potential demand. The country with the lowest production is Uruguay, because up to now the iodized salt consumption was mandatory only in those areas previously recognized as endemic. However, a new legislation towards the universal salt iodization is to be approved.

The legislation concerning the level of iodization of the salt has been corrected in the three countries (Venezuela, Brazil an Paraguay) where used to be very low.

Monitoring of iodized salt is being carried out in practically all the countries. The minimum required level of iodization (>20 ppm) at retail level in more than 70% of samples has been already met in 7 out of 12 countries where data has been available. Assessment of iodized salt consumption by the population is carried out by means of surveys among school children and/or the use of kits, which have proven to be a very easy and convenient tool. Peru is producing kits at a reasonable low price.

Urinary iodine excretion analysis as an indicator of the impact of intervention and of the IDD situation is being implemented in many countries. Peru and Bolivia are the ones using it more extensively. ICCIDD is helping in the implementation of laboratory facilities for this purpose.

Governmental support and IEC have significantly increased in the majority of countries.

It is exciting to say that the goal of virtual elimination of IDD is already reached in three countries, Costa Rica, Ecuador and Bolivia, and that there are other countries working hard towards it.

19

IDD in the Middle East

K. Bagchi and A. Verster

Endemic goitre, as a clinical condition, has been known in this part of the world for decades. In fact, Pakistan, one of the countries in this region, has the distinction of being mentioned in international medical literature as a country where, in a particular region, almost everyone had enlargement of the thyroid gland. McCarrison in 1908 published a famous paper in the Lancet focussing attention on the alarming prevalence of goitre and cretinism in the Chitral and Gilgit districts of Pakistan, (McCarrison 1908).

Today, 13 out of 22 countries in the Eastern Mediterranean Region of the World Health Organization have reported the prevalence of iodine deficiency disorders (IDD) which includes most of the Middle Eastern countries (Fig. 19.1). Roughly 93 million people are affected by various types and degrees of iodine deficiency in this region. In fact, iodine deficiency disorders are now considered as a priority public health problem in many countries, and an increasing number of countries are in the process of adopting control measures.

It is of interest that a mild thyroid enlargement in plump or obese women is not at all obvious in many cases, as it gives a fullness of the neck which is clearly compatible with moderate obesity, a very common feature of most Arab women and a condition actually favoured by men in many Arab countries.

The Regional Strategy which was formulated in 1989 and adopted by the Regional Working Group on IDD, was presented to the Intercountry Workshop on Iodine Deficiency Disorders (IDD) Control, held, 5-9 August 1990 at Teheran, Islamic Republic of Iran. A technical paper, presented to the 37th session of the Regional Committee Meeting in Damascus, Syria, assisted greatly in sensitizing the Member States, who unanimously adopted Resolution EM/RC37/R.9.

In November 1991 a Tri-Regional Traveling Seminar in India and Nepal exposed participants from 22 countries in three WHO regions (from Morocco to China) to the practical aspects of salt iodization and iodized oil supplementation. Participants included IDD programme managers, salt engineers, representatives of the salt industry and several agencies.

In December 1992, an Intercountry Training Workshop was held in Damascus, Syria to expose Managers of IDD laboratories to techniques used in IDD Control. Laboratory managers and programme managers from 14 countries received practical instruction in various laboratory methods, as well as in ultrasonography for determination of thyroid volume and palpation for goitre in field conditions.

The WHO office of the Eastern Mediterranean Region provided consultancy services to Egypt, Lebanon, Libya, Sudan, UAE and Yemen.

So far, Egypt, Islamic Republic of Iran, Syria, Saudi Arabia and Algeria have carried out a national IDD prevalence survey. Six countries are now producing iodized salt, while five more have some iodized salt production capacity or are in the process of establishing this. Six countries use iodized oil, either as an interim measure or in hyper-endemic areas.

Geography of Iodine Deficiency Disorders in the Middle East

The endemic areas in most countries of the region are the usual mountainous regions, as in the Hindukush mountain range in Pakistan, which itself is the extension of the Himalayan range. Coming westward, the same Hindukush range continues into Afghanistan. As in the entire sub-Himalayan region of India, the continuing mountainous areas in Pakistan and Afghanistan are highly endemic. Iran has two mountain ranges-one in the north and the other in the middle-spreading from east to west, and here again, the endemic foci of iodine deficiency are situated in these ranges. The same pattern of endemic foci in the mountainous regions is also seen in Sudan, Iraq, Somalia, Lebanon, Tunisia and Morocco.

In several countries there is an additional feature of iodine deficiency endemicity in desert areas. There are reports of significant prevalence of endemic goitre in the oases of Egypt (New Valley) and Libya (Fezzan Province) where the soil, with almost no vegetation, and the well water, are almost devoid of iodine. Rainfall is insignificant in these desert areas thus depriving these oases from receiving any iodine from the rain water.

Increased Political Commitment in Middle Eastern Countries

Earlier regional action to control "endemic goitre" was the effort by the Eastern Mediterranean Regional Committee of WHO to motivate Member States, affected by iodine deficiency, to mount control programmes against endemic goitre in the biennium 1978-1979 as WHO Collaborative Programmes. However, the Member States at that time gave a low priority to 'goitre control' in view of pressing needs for other health programmes, and thus WHO resources were diverted for other programmes.

IDD is now recognized as much more than endemic goitre, as described in Chapter 1. IDD stands for a number of health disorders and crippling conditions spread over the entire span of human life. The tragic fact that iodine deficiency can be an important cause of stillbirth, abortion and infant mortality and varying degrees of mental defect is being increasingly now fully grasped by many senior health administrators and decision makers. Creating an awareness among them about the wide-ranging health disorders caused by iodine deficiency and the fact that it is an important public health problem needing immediate action has now been given top priority by the WHO Regional Office for the Eastern Mediterranean. Due to this joint effort by WHO (EMRO) & ICCIDD, many senior health administrators and decision makers have become more aware of the effects of IDD.

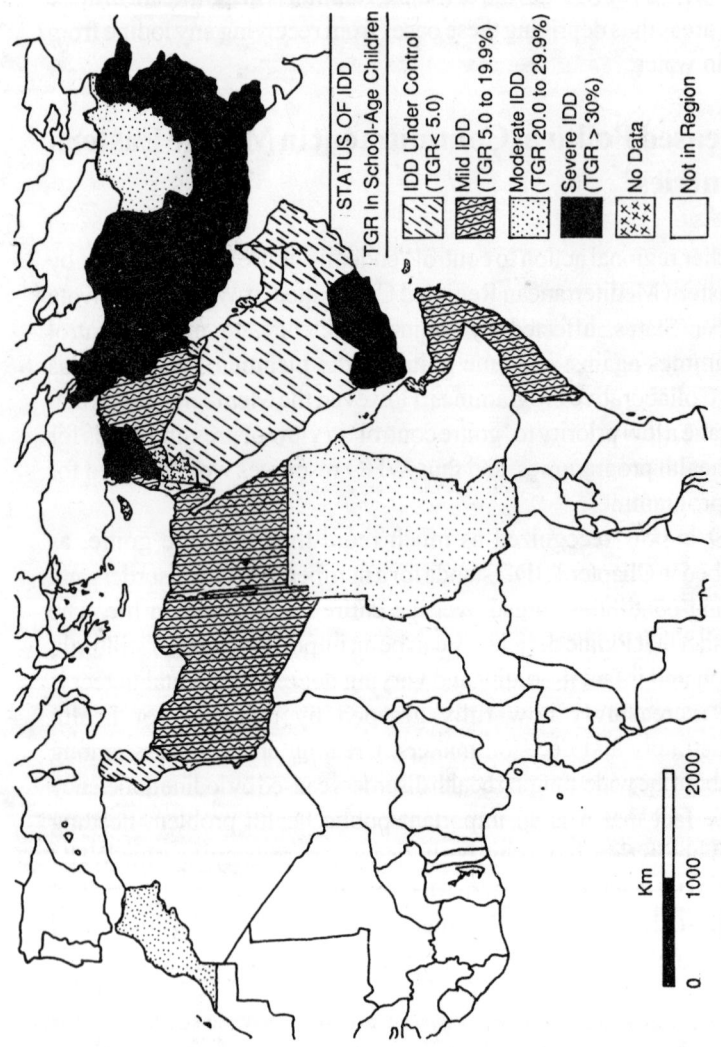

Fig. 19.1 Map showing extent of IDD in Middle Eastern countries within the Eastern Mediterranean Region, World Health Organization. (From Micronutrient Deficiency Information System, World Health Organization, 1993).

Action by World Health Organization Regional Office

An exhaustive review of IDD was made by the Regional Office and published in the September 1987 issue of the Eastern Mediterranean Health Services Journal. This was widely circulated among health policy and decision makers. For the first time, this review brought to the attention of the health administrators the fact that at least 10 countries in this region have a high to alarming prevalence of IDD in some regions, while at the same time not a single country had a control programme in operation.

The review was based on published and unpublished records of surveys, the latter taken mostly from assignment reports of WHO consultants assigned to countries. It specifically emphasized the fact that the absence of data from any given country does not imply that the country has no iodine deficiency problem. In fact, the geological character of the countries in the region indicated that many more countries must have this problem which could only be revealed if a careful survey is done in more remote areas.

The WHO Regional Office pursued this advocacy measure by taking two further steps - the first one by convening a consultation of experts from several countries of this region, including members of the ICCIDD, in order to collect more recent information about the prevalence, details of ongoing national control measures, with an exchange of experiences about their implementation. This led to the formation of an IDD Working Group as in other regions to develop guidelines that would assist countries to define the extent and magnitude of the IDD problem and put into operation national control programmes. The outcome of this Working Group was the publication in 1990 of a booklet reporting the development of a strategy for IDD control in the region. This publication in English and Arabic has been widely disseminated, and has been reprinted several times in order to meet the continuous demands from the countries. This publication describes in easy language the wide spectrum of human health disorders due to iodine deficiency and draws attention to the fact that endemic goitre manifested by a swelling of the thyroid gland is just one visible manifestation of iodine deficiency and that there are much more serious and non-visible manifestations of iodine deficiency (varying degrees of mental defect) which are not even known to many health workers. It has now been revised to respond to the new global goals for virtual elimination of IDD.

The renewed interest generated among the countries of this region in the control of iodine deficiency through these measures prompted the WHO Regional Office to select the topic of control of iodine deficiency disorders for technical discussion in the 37th session of the Eastern Mediterranean Regional Committee in October 1990 in which Health Ministers and Senior Health Administrators of the 22 countries from this WHO Region participated. This form of advocacy at the highest level of the health sector paved the way for government commitment and support for the control of iodine deficiency disorders in several countries. Today, the Regional Office of WHO for Eastern Mediterranean, in collaboration with the International Council for Control of Iodine Deficiency Disorders (ICCIDD) and UNICEF is assisting increasing number of countries in undertaking measures for the elimination of this scourge. A meeting on programme management was organized in 1990, a tri-regional seminar on practical issues of salt iodization and iodized oil distribution was held in 1991 and a training course on IDD laboratory techniques followed in 1992. A regional joint WHO/UNICEF/ICCIDD meeting held in Alexandria (April 1993), reviewed the progress, discussed the communication strategies and provided a forum where programme managers and IDD experts could exchange experiences.

National Programmes for the Elimination of Iodine Deficiency Disorders

All countries in this Region are motivated and committed to the elimination of iodine deficiency disorders, and have taken administrative steps towards this objective in which there are two major segments:

— an intersectoral committee supervising the implementation of the control programme in which the health sector, the salt industry and the information dissemination sector are major partners;

— a focal point or technical unit in the Health Ministry responsible for the control of iodine deficiency disorders.

These two administrative steps, taken by the countries embarking upon IDD elimination programmes deserve special attention. In recent years a number of evaluations of national programmes revealed that, in many cases, the failure or faltering of these programmes was due to the entire responsibility of its implementation being entrusted solely to the Health Ministry and to the lack of full involvement by other equally important sectors, as for example the salt industry. The countries of this region are now taking steps to overcome these administrative flaws.

Another noteworthy step taken by several countries (notably Egypt, Iran and Syria) is to conduct a comprehensive survey to assess the extent and magnitude of the problem utilizing clinical and laboratory methods. For the first time in this region, the prevalence of neonatal hypothyroidism is being assessed. Such surveys will yield valuable information on the basis of which effective elimination programmes can be developed.

In the recent WHO/UNICEF/ICCIDD Regional Meeting it was found that five countries have carried out national surveys, several more are preparing to do so, while others have in the past carried out ad-hoc surveys which indicated problems. Six countries produced iodized salt, and six countries are providing iodized oil to target populations with severe IDD. Several workshops on laboratory methods have been organized by WHO with ICCIDD support. Special attention was given to communication aspects at the Regional Meeting.

Looking back over the past decade one can conclude that though IDD elimination efforts have started relatively late in the countries of this region and the momentum of countries adopting such programmes is slow, steady progress is now being made with the help of lessons learnt from other countries and regions. The recent major international fora - The World Summit for Children (1990) and the International Conference on Nutrition (1992) are also making a significant impact at the country level in this region.

References

McCarrison, R. 1908. 'Observations on endemic cretinism in the Chitral and Gilgit Valley'. *Lancet* 2:1275-80.

WHO 1993. 'Global prevalence of iodine deficiency disorders' MDIS Working Paper 1.

PART IV

Sustaining Elimination of Iodine Deficiency Disorders

PART IV

Sustaining Elimination of Iodine Deficiency Disorders

20

Monitoring and Verification of Progress Towards the Elimination of IDD by the Year 2000 and Beyond

J.T. Dunn, C.S. Pandav and B.S. Hetzel

In 1990, at the World Summit for Children, most of the world's nations pledged the 'virtual elimination' of iodine deficiency disorders by the year 2000.' As described in earlier chapters vigorous efforts to achieve this goal are underway, and the progress is heartening. At the same time, we need to look not only to the year 2000, but also to the decades beyond. Thus, the goal needs to be extended and restated as 'the sustainable elimination of IDD by the year 2000.'

This insistence on sustainability is not a trivial concern. The spectacular success in eradicating smallpox is frequently taken as a model for the IDD elimination campaign but these two public health menaces represent fundamentally different problems. A virus caused smallpox and once the virus was killed the possibility of the recurrence of the disease ended. Iodine deficiency, on the other hand, is not caused by a single etiologic vector but is a condition similar to poverty, crime, and hunger, and can only be controlled, not eradicated. Thus, to have sustainable elimination of iodine deficiency, a country must have a programme that will endure long beyond the initial achievement of iodine sufficiency.

Several historical examples justify this concern for sustainability. Some were described in the chapter on Latin America, where a long experience with iodine prophylaxis programmes has provided enough time to document their frequent failure. For example, initially successful efforts in Guatemala, Colombia, and Thailand later lapsed, in each instance because of complacence, lack of vigilance and monitoring. In the current rush towards achieving the virtual elimination of IDD by the year 2000, we must keep the added requirement of sustainability firmly in view. Otherwise, the effort will consume an enormous expenditure of resources and time, to achieve only a temporary reprieve from the ravages of iodine deficiency.

In relation to sustainability two key issues deserve consideration.
1) what criteria can a country use to verify that it has achieved virtual elimination of IDD, and
2) how can a country ensure that this elimination, once achieved, will be sustained?

To address these questions, several international groups are collectively considering criteria for assessing the progress towards IDD elimination. The following guidelines have been proposed by ICCIDD, in consultation with many experts from countries and international agencies.

Proposed Guidelines for Tracking Progress Towards Elimination

A. A country with universal neonatal screening, preferably by TSH in a sufficiently sensitive assay, may be declared free of iodine deficiency if fewer than 0.3% of neonates need to be recalled for suspicion of congenital hypothyroidism. It is not necessary that any other criterion be established.

B. For countries where there is no universal screening of newborns at least two of the following three criteria should be met to establish that sustainable elimination of iodine deficiency is being achieved.

1. **All salt for human and animal consumption** in all regions where IDD is known or suspected, should be iodized at a reasonable level (usually 30-100ppm) at the factory, so

that representative salt samples obtained regularly from retail outlets, or preferably from homes, have an iodine content at or above a level of 20ppm in all regions.
2. **Samples of urine** obtained on a regular basis in a statistically valid mode should have a median iodine content of 10 µg/dl or more in all regions of the country.
3. In regions where IDD is known or suspected, the **prevalence of total goitre**(i.e., grades 1 and 2, palpable plus visible) in representative surveys of children of school age (eg, 8-10 years old) should be less than 5% as ascertained by competent observers and preferably confirmed by ultrasonography.

In addition to meeting two of the above three criteria, **sustainability** must be established according to the following guidelines, as applicable.
1. **A National IDD Commission** should be in operation with a responsibility for the continuous monitoring of the status of iodine deficiency and of the iodine content of salt, according to established criteria, including mandatory public reporting of IDD status at regular specified intervals (e.g. every three to five years) by designated units (e.g. the programme, the Ministry of Health) that are technically competent and adequately financed.
2. **The government, the private sector, and consumers** should have a high awareness of iodine deficiency and be committed to its sustained elimination.
3. **The salt industry** should have the commitment, technical resources, and responsibility (frequently mandated by legislation) to sustain effective iodization of salt, including its production, distribution, and financing including the consumer.
4. **The supply of iodine for salt iodization** is assured either through private purchase by the salt manufacturers or through the government the availability of foreign exchange.

5. The availability, realtive cost, and **perceived health benefits** of iodized salt should make consumers prefer it to the uniodized product.
6. The IDD programme should have ready access to local or regional facilities to **measure iodine levels** in salt and to a central laboratory competent to measure urinary iodine or neonatal blood TSH concentrations, or both, at affordable rates.

These guidelines are built on the results of a 1992 joint WHO/UNICEF/ICCIDD consultation 'Indicators for assessing IDD and their control through salt iodization' which has been mentioned in Chapters 2 and 4. They are internationally wide-ranging enough to cover highly industrialized countries as well as the least developed. For example, neither the United States nor Japan has a compulsory salt iodization programme, but universal neonatal screening for hypothyroidism shows that both can meet the criteria satisfactorily. Most of the less developed countries do not have universal neonatal screening, and many do not use iodized salt. For them, a survey of urinary iodine levels and goitre prevalence should be undertaken, although occasionally existing data on normal subjects, obtained as a part of the general health assessment, are enough to indicate iodine sufficiency. These guidelines will help chart a country's progress towards IDD elimination, but they need the oversight of appropriate national and international experts to see that they are applied intelligently and responsibly. We propose that oversight committees be set up to provide this guidance, both within individual countries and globally.

In reviewing why programmes succeed or fail, the three key factors are **awareness, monitoring, and responsibility.** With regard to the first, we have advanced a long way since the IDD control programme of a generation ago, when a government simply passed a law mandating salt iodization but failed to involve the relevant parties, particularly the salt industry, the affected communities, and the health, education, agriculture, and commercial sectors. For a successful programme, each of these groups must consider itself as a stakeholder in the effort, and that viewpoint will motivate the group to work on the programme's behalf. Obtaining the collaboration of all relevant sectors requires continuing and extensive education, and this activity must be a major priority for the programmes.

The second factor, **monitoring,** is equally essential. The programme must include mandatory periodic assessment of results and their public reporting, on a regular schedule that continues well beyond the year 2000 AD. The key indicators for monitoring are iodized salt distribution, urinary iodine levels, thyroid size and neonatal TSH screening. The optimal use of these indicators, singly or in combination, will vary depending on the individual features of a particular country, but designing a cost effective monitoring programme is usually a straightforward procedure that any country with appropriate advice and resources can achieve.

The third key element in sustaining a programme is a clearly assigned **responsibility for its maintenance.** Some government institution or its designate should play this role. Usually this is the nutrition division of the Ministry of Health, but other components of the government are also essential, particularly those dealing with salt, commerce, transportation and education. As pointed out in earlier chapters a national commission, with representation from several sectors, both government and private, is essential, so that they are fully involved in the elimination of iodine deficiency. Consumers should be included. Such a committee should meet on a scheduled basis and be required to report on progress regularly. The programme's suspension should depend not on specific persons but on institutions, to provide permanent accountability for its results.

In addition to these key programme elements, other broader socio-economic factors play a pivotal role in determining the ultimate success of an IDD programme. Iodine deficiency rarely exists as an isolated entity, but instead is part of more chronic nutrition, health, economic and social problems. Attention to these problems will contribute to a 'silent prophylaxis', in which progress in the socio-economic sphere indirectly improves iodine deficiency. Better education allows people to understand the importance of iodine prophylaxis and creates a demand of this intervention. Better general health improves education potential and also enhances the body's ability to utilize iodine effectively; for example, prevention of diarrhoeal diseases helps iodine absorption, and improved general nutrition enhances the thyroid's ability to make and utilize thyroid hormones. Better transportation networks give greater diversity of food sources, making iodine-rich foods more available as well as enhancing the distribution of iodized salt. Many other examples could be cited. The goal of correcting iodine deficiency is closely entwined with that of socio-economic advancement, and progress towards either goal helps the other.

Recommendations for achieving sustainability follow naturally from the above discussion.

First, each country must educate all relevant sectors to be aware of the magnitude of IDD and its correction. This is done through intense and continued efforts.

Second, each country must set up a sound monitoring programme both for the quality control of iodized salt and for monitoring the effects of iodine deficiency in humans.

Third, the programme must assign responsibility for its suspensions and maintenance, including mandatory periodic reporting, to make sure that problems do not recur as has happened in the past. Only by meeting these conditions can sustainability be achieved, and any programme that omits them is shortchanging its target population, its workers, and its donors.

So far we have described the necessary monitoring process at country level required to ensure sustainability.

Beyond this is the need for independent verification. As already mentioned (Chapter 2) the ICCIDD has proposed to WHO and UNICEF that a Global Verification Commission be established to provide an independent verification of progress at country level towards the goal of elimination. This verification process would be available to countries on request. Monitoring data would be submitted by them and assessments could be made by the Global Verification Commission through a Regional Committee including the ICCIDD Regional Co-ordinator and representatives of WHO and UNICEF.

The independent verification of progress towards the goal of elimination is all-important to the sustainable achievement of the goal. National governments will have the opportunity to satisfy themselves about the status of their elimination programme. The UN agencies including donors will also have the opportunity of independent verification by appropriate monitoring data.

A verification mechanism will need to be in place for the forseeable future in order to safeguard elimination of the mental defect consequent on iodine deficiency. An adequate dietary iodine intake is just as important as clean water.

As we have seen the knowledge required for the elimination of IDD is available. The solution is practicable and sustainable.

Let the global partnership go forward with great determination towards achieving the sustainable elimination of an ancient scourge of mankind. Subsequent generations will always be in debt to our present generation even though they will not know it.

Reference

WHO/UNICEF/ICCIDD November, 1992. 'Indicators for assessing Iodine Deficiency Disorders and their control through salt iodization'. *Report of a Joint Consultation* 3-5. WHO, Geneva. Document WHO/NUT/94.6.

PART V

Statement on Safety of Iodized Salt and Iodized Oil

21

STATEMENT ON SAFETY OF IODIZED SALT AND IODIZED OIL

Iodine and Health
Eliminating Iodine Deficiency Disorders Safely through Salt Iodization

A statement by the World Health Organization

A deficiency of iodine, which is among the body's essential trace elements, is both easy and inexpensive to prevent. Iodine deficiency nevertheless continues to be a significant public health problem in many countries. Iodine deficiency not only causes goitre; it may also result in irrereversible brain damage in the foetus and infant, and retarded psychomotor development in the child. Iodine deficiency is the most common cause of **preventable** mental retardation. It also affects reproductive functions and impedes children's learning ability. The cumulative consequences in iodine-deficient populations spell diminished performance for the entire economy of affected nations.

Iodine deficiency disorders (IDD) are currently a significant public health problem in 118 countries. An estimated 1571 million people world wide live in iodine-deficient enviornments and are thus at risk of IDD; 20 million of these are believed to be significantly mentally handicapped as a result. A large proportion of the severly deficient are women in their reproductive years whose babies are at high risk of irreversible mental retardation unless they recieve adequate amounts of iodine.

In the last 50 years, many countries in the Americas, Asia, Europe and Oceania have successfully eliminated IDD, or made substantial progress in their control, largely as a result of salt iodization with potassium iodide or pottassium iodate and through dietary diversification. For example, in Switzerland, where salt iodization began in 1922, cretinism has been eliminated and goitre has disappeared, while there has been negligible evidence of any adverse effects from iodine intake.

Universal salt iodization[a] has been endorsed in numerous international forums[b] by heads of state, senior government officials, and representatives of international intergovernmental and nongovernmental organizations. Nevertheless, WHO countinues to receive queries from national health authorities and other seeking reassurance about the safety of providing iodized salt to non-deficient populations. As with all preventive public health measures, the decision to ensure universal salt iodization will be made by weighing the potential risk of excess intake for the few against the well-documented risk of mental and physiological impairment for the many if a deficiency is uncorrected.

In response to concerns expressed and to facilitate decision-making in countries, this statement summarizes the cumulative scientific and epidemiological evidence in this regard.

Physiological need for iodine

Based on studies of balance and excretion over a 24 hour period, a safe daily intake of iodine has been estimated to be between a minimum of 50 µg and a maximum of at least 1000 µg. A generally

---

[a] Universal salt iodization is defined as fortification of salt for human and animal consumption.

[b] The most important of these are the World Health Assembly, in resolutions WHA 39.31 (1986) and wha 43.2 (1990), the World Summit for children (New York, 1990), the Policy Conference on Ending Hidden Hunger (Montreal, 1991), and the International Conference on Nutrition (Rome 1992).

accepted desirable adult intake is 100-300 µg/day. At all intake levels, a proportionate amount of iodine is excreted in the urine, which is the biochemical basis for assessing iodine status.

Usual food sources of iodine

Sea fish, other sea food, and seaweed are rich sources of iodine suitable for human consumption. Iodine is also found in vegetables grown in soils containing adequate amounts of this trace element, and in milk products, eggs, poultry and meat from animals whose diet contained sufficient iodine.

Usual salt intakes

Average daily salt intakes vary from country to country. Usually, consumption levels are within the 5-15 g/day range for children and adults. No increase in salt consumption is called for. Rather, the recommended level of salt iodization should be adjusted to provide approximately 150 µg of iodine/day actually consumed, taking into account usual climatic factors like heat and humidity, which can affect retention of this element. The recommended quantities of iodate to be added to salt under different conditions are provided in Table 21.1. Although potassium iodide was first used in salt iodization, the use of iodate is now recommended since it is more stable than iodide under varying climatic conditions. Because iodate, on ingestion, is very rapidly reduced to iodide, its use in iodinated salt is equivalent to iodide.

Adverse effects associated with high nutritional intakes of iodine

Since iodine, when ingested in large amounts, is easily excreted through the kidneys into the urine, iodine intakes even at very high levels (milligram amounts) can be consumed safely. However,

Table 21.1 ICCIDD-UNICEF-WHO recommended levels of iodine in salt

Examples of desirable average levels at various points in the salt distribution chain, depending on climate, salt intake, and conditions affecting packaging and distribution

Parts of iodine per million parts of salt, i.e. micrograms per gram, milligrams per kilogram or grams per tonne

Climate and daily salt cosumption (g/person)	Requirement at factory outside the country		Requirement at factory inside the country		Requirement at retail site (shop/market)		Requirement at household level
	Bull (sack)	Retail pack (<2kg)	Bulk (sack)	Retail Pack (<2kg)	Bulk (sack)	Retail Pack (<2kg)	
			Packing				
Warm moist							
5g	100	80	90	70	80	60	50
10g	50	40	45	35	40	30	25
Warm dry or cool moist							
5g	90	70	80	60	70	50	45
10g	45	35	40	30	35	25	22.5
Cool dry							
5g	80	60	70	50	60	45	40
10g	40	30	35	25	30	22.5	20

Source: Adapted from World Summit for Children - mid-decade goal; iodine deficiency disorders. Geneva, 1994. UNICEF-WHO Joint Committe on Health Policy, document JCHPSS/94/2.7 and reference 5.

N.B. 168.6 mg of KIO$_3$ contains 100mg of iodine.

N.B. These are indicative initial levels, which should be adjusted in the light of urinary measurement.

the following adverse affects, though rare, have been reported.
Allergic reactions to iodine in food. Skin rashes and acne have occasionally been attributed to iodized salt. Such reports are extremely rare, however, and thus these conditions are unlikely to occur following satl iodization. For example, among 20,000 children in the USA suffering from allergy during the period 1935-1974, not a single case was reported of allergic hypersensitivity to iodine in food. Following publication in *Annals of Allergy* of a request for notification of allergy to iodine, not a single report was recorded between 1974 and 1980.
High intskes of dietary iodine and thyroid diseases. Through adaptive mechanisms, normal people exposed to excess iodine remain euthyroid and free of goitre. In certain susceptible individuals, iodide goitre and Hashimoto thyroiditis with hypothyroidism have been observed after iodine intakes of 500-3000 µg/day. The prevalence of susceptible individuals in different countries is not fully known. It has been suggested that high nutritional intake of iodine substantiated by urinary iodine of 1000-10,000 µg/litre-as observed in one country in up to 2% of the population-could have an adverse effect in susceptible individuals and in patients with pre-existing abnormalities of the thyroid gland. In this small proportion of the population, chronic excess intake might contribute to the development of Hashimoto thyroiditis, iodide and colloid goitre, and thyroid carcinoma. However, the incidence of follicular thyroid cancer, a more severe form of cancer, is lower in iodine sufficient than in iodine deficient areas. There is little indication that iodine in the amounts noted influences the development of any of these thyroid diseases.
In Japan, where dietary iodine takes are high, it has been shown that:

- normal people who are not iodine-deficient can maintain normal thyroid function states even at intakes of several milligrams of dietary iodine/day;
- the incidence of non-toxic diffuse goitre and toxic nodular goitre is markedly decreased by high dietary iodine intake;

- the incidence of Graves disease and Hashimoto disease does not appear to be affected by high intakes of dietary iodine.

However, high intakes of dietary iodine may induce hypothyroidism in auto-immune thyroid diseases and may inhibit the effects of thionamide drugs.

There are well-documented reports of iodine induced hyperthyroidism (Jod-Basedow phenomenon) where iodine, sometimes in normal quantities, was introduced among iodine-deficient populations. Administration of ordinary amounts of iodine has also been reported to induce hyperthyroidism in people with nodular thyroids, and in other individuals who have no apparent underlying thyroid disease. However, these are transient phenomena, which cease after correction of iodine deficiency; they do not occur in populations with sufficient (i.e. normal) iodine intake.

Current estimates of daily intakes in Canada and the USA are substaintially above physiological need–in the range of 460 µg/day among 9-16 year old children, to greater than 1 mg among as many as 10-20% of adults. With a level of iodization that provides these populations approximately 260 µg/day of iodine from salt, it is thus apparent that much of the intake comes from non-salt sources (see below. A survey conducted in 1968-1970 in ten states (USA) showed that where total goitre prevalence was greater than 3.5%, the percentage of individuals with high iodine-excretion values, i.e. more than 800 µg/litre, was 16% compared with 6% in states with lower total goitre prevalence.

Other sources of iodine

In industrialized countries there are many adventitious sources of iodine which increase daily intake levels far above the physiological amount provided through iodized salt, for example:

- poultry and eggs from animals that consume fish flour as part of their feed and iodoform in water that is used as a disinfectant;

- cow's milk and dairy products from animals fed seaweed, producing an iodine content of milk as high as 694 µg/litre, or that come into contact with iodiphors used to clean milking apparatus or as teat dips and udder washes;
- bread and baked goods through the iodates used as oxidants in dough conditioners and cleaning agents for bakery equipment (reports of the iodine content of bread in the USA range from 0 to 268 µg/slice);
- the iodine-containing colouring agents added to some drugs (including many multivitamins, minerals, and antacids as a coating or colouring agent), beverages, foods (including some brands of dry cereal that contain as much as 850 µg of iodine per 20 µg of product) and cosmetics.

Iodine availability

The iodine content of food actually consumed is not necessarily equivalent to that of raw food since some iodine is lost during cooking. For example, losses of about 20% occur in the iodine content of fish by frying or grilling and as much as 58% by boiling. Iodine consumed in food is generally well absorbed, with the possible exception of people suffering from protein-energy malnutrition, which is of particular concern in high-prevalence, endemic-goitre areas of developing countries.

The uptake of radioactive iodine by an individual thyroid is dependent on the amount of stable, i.e. non-radioactive, iodine in the diet. This is the basis for using radioactive iodine to evaluate thyroid function. Studies from Chernobyl following the nuclear reactor accident in 1986 indicate high thyroid cancer rates, especially among young children. It is postulated that the thyroids of children in this iodine-deficient area experienced an unusual uptake of radioactive iodine released into the atmosphere following the accident. It has been estimated that, in general, iodine prophylaxis, e.g. use of iodized salt, should reduce by twofold to threefold the risk of thyroid irradiation resulting from a nuclear accident.

Conclusion

Issues relating to the safety of universal salt iodization have been carefully examined by WHO and by joint FAO/WHO, ICCIDD/UNICEF/WHO and WHO/FAO/IAEA expert groups in the process of preparing recommendations. All concerned agree that universal salt iodization is the principal public health measure for eliminating IDD.

Daily iodine intakes of up to 1 mg, i.e. 1000 µg, appear to be entirely safe. Iodization of salt at a level that assures an intake of 150-300 µg/day thus keeps intakes well within a safe daily range for all populations, irrespective of their iodine status. Daily consumption of 10 g of salt containing 50 parts per million of iodine would add a maximum of only 500 µg of iodine. Thus the likelihood of exceeding an iodine intake of 1 mg/day from iodized salt is quite small.

In susceptible individuals a minority of adults, usually over 45 years of age, who may or may not have nodular goitres-transient side-effects have been reported at usual intakes exceeding 500-3000 µg/day. The benefits to be derived from universal salt iodization by the more than 1500 million people estimated to be at risk or deficient, and the absence of significant adverse effects among others in the same areas who are not iodine-deficient, far outweigh any risk of excess intake for a small minority.

References

Barsano, C.P. 1981. 'Environmental factors altering thyroid function and their assessment'. Environmental Health Perpectives. 38:71-82.

Dunn, J.T., H.E., Crutchfield, R., Gutekunst, A., Dunn, 1993. 'Mthods for measuring iodine in urine'. ICCIDD/UNICEF/WHO.

Rubery, E.L., E., Samles. 1990. eds. *Iodine prophylaxis following nuclear accidents*. Proceedings of a joint WHO/CEE workshop. July, 1988. New York, Pergamon Press.

Stanbury, J.B., B.S., Hetzel, 1980. 'Endemic goitre and endemic cretinism'. *Iodine nutrition in health and disease.* New York, John Wiley & Sons, Inc.

Trace elements in human nutrition and health. Geneva, World Health Organization (in preparation).

Trowbridge, F.L., D.A., Hand, M.Z., Nichaman. 1975. 'Findings relating to goitre and iodine in the ten-state nutrition survey'. *American Journal of Clinical Nutrition.* 28:712-16.

World Health Organization. 1993. 'Micronutrient Deficiency Information System. MDIS Working paper # 1.

World Health Organization, 1991. Evaluation of certain food additives and contaminants. Thirty-seventh report of a joint FAO/WHO Expert Committee on Food Additives, Geneva. 49 (WHO Technical Report Series No. 806).

WHO/UNICEF/ICCIDD November, 1992. 'Indicators for Assessing Iodine Deficiency Disorders and their Control through Salt Iodization'. Report of a Joint Consultation. 3-5. WHO, Geneva. Document WHO/NUT/94.6.

Iodized Oil in Pregnancy

A statement by the International Council for Control of Iodine Deficiency Disorders

Iodised salt is the preferred means for correcting iodine deficiency, but occasionally other measures are needed, for example, in areas where iodine deficiency is extremely severe and successful implementation of iodized salt is delayed. In such circumstances, iodized vegetable oil is the usual alternative. Iodized oil administration can be implemented quickly. A single dose can provide iodine sufficiency for at least six months to a year when given orally and for one to three years intramuscularly. The value of iodized oil in iodine prophylaxis is clearly established and many millions of doses have been given over more than three decades. The disadvantage of iodized oil are that each target subject must be contacted directly, the cost is greater than that of iodized salt, complete coverage may be difficult, and iodine levels in the blood are not constant. In selecting targets within the community, the first priorities are women of childbearing age, to protect their unborn or unconceived children, and young children.

In pregnancy, the foetus is exposed to most substances administered to its mother. Therefore, sound medical practice demands scrutiny of all such substances carefully, and it is reasonable to ask whether administration of iodized oil has any adverse effects on the foetus. ICCIDD considered this issue in 1992 at the request of UNICEF, and gave the opinion then that pregnant women should be included in programs of iodized oil administration. Because of lingering questions, WHO in 1994 convened a small group of expects, many from ICCIDD, to render a formal recommendation. The group included Dr. Moulay Benmiloud, Dr. Francois Delange, Dr. Constance Pittman, Dr. Summer Yaffe, and Dr. Claude Thilly, as well as WHO secretariat. Their conclusion, now being finalized and published, is that pregnant women may safely receive iodized oil to combat moderate or severe iodine deficiency. The WHO report also presents the recommendations for dose and frequency that originated from an ICCIDD/WHO/UNICEF consultation in Geneva in 1992.

> ## ICCIDD Statement on the Safety of Iodized Oil During Pregnancy
>
> "Iodized salt is the recommended means for iodine supplementation to correct iodine deficiency. For those areas of moderate or severe iodine deficiency that will not be effectively covered by iodized salt within an acceptable period of time, iodized oil is the preferred interim measure. Because damage to the developing brain is the most severe consequence of iodine deficiency, women of childbearing age and children are the first priorities for receiving iodized oil. Extensive scientific experience has clearly established the beneficial effects of maternal iodized oil for the foetus, while failing to show adverse effects. Therefore, ICCIDD recommends that pregnant women should be included in programmes where iodized oil administration is appropriate."

Dr. Delange prepared a background review of published scientific evidence on the use of iodized oil during pregnancy as an appendix to the WHO report. He carefully examined one study from an area with severe iodine deficiency in which iodized oil has been administered to a group that included pregnant women. Of 154 neonates whose mothers had received an intramuscular injection of iodized oil containing 480 mg of iodine a mean 3.5 weeks before delivery, the cord blood of 10% had elevated TSH and low T_4 levels, suggesting neonatal hypothyroidism. However, as Dr. Delange points out, the same incidence of neonatal hypothyroidism (7.5-13.3%), was reported in the same region without any iodized oil, and in addition, there was no biochemical evidence in the cited study that these mothers actually received iodine. Thus, that report did not make a convincing case for an adverse effect of iodized oil during pregnancy. In contrast to that one study, numerous reports, particularly from New Guinea, Algeria, Peru, Zaire, and Malawi, have provided overwhelming evidence that the progeny of mothers who received iodized oil during pregnancy in severely iodine deficient areas fare much better than those of mothers who remained iodine deficientThe benefits include increased birth weight, better neonatal survival, and more normal physical and mental development.

During its Dhaka meeeting in April 1995, the ICCIDD Board once again reviewed the existing evidence on this issue. It reached a consensus and unanimously passed a resolution endorsing the use of iodized oil during pregnancy in areas of moderate to severe iodine deficiency (see statement in accompanying box).

Iodine Induced Thyrotoxicosis

A statement by the International Council for Control of Iodine Deficiency Disorders

Introduction

Iodine Induced Thyrotoxicosis **(IIT)** also called Iodine Induced Hyperthyroidism or "JODBASEDOW" is one of the Iodine Deficiency Disorders **(IDD)**.

It has been reported in Europe and Latin America in the 1960's and 1970's following the introduction of iodized salt. The epidemiology was documented in Tasmania, Australia, following the introduction of iodized bread in 1966 and the addition of iodophors to milk by the dairy industry. Milk iodine has also been a major factor more recently in Europe.

The condition is recognized to be an inevitable consequence of increase in intake of iodine from any source into an iodine deficient population. It continues to be a significant problem in Europe. Its occurrence depends on the existence of an older age group (over 40) that has been deficient since birth.

It can be totally prevented in the next and subsequent generations by correction of iodine deficiency.

In view of the enormous benefits consequent on the correction of iodine deficiency in the whole population it is not regarded as a contraindication to iodine supplementation programmes.

These benefits include: improvement in child survival, child learning, women's health, economic productivity and quality of life.

Description

The condition occurs in older goitrous subjects with thyroid nodules due to longstanding iodine deficiency. Many of these nodules are autonomous, or independent of usual physiologic controls, and have responded to iodine deficiency by enhancing their uptake and utilization of iodine. When presented with a significant increase in iodine intake, these nodules may produce too much thyroid hormone, making the subject hyperthyroid or 'thyrotoxic'. The clinical features vary among individuals, but in older subjects the most common and serious manifestations are rapid heart beat, nervousness, weakness, heat intolerance, and weight loss. Frequently IIT is mild and follows a self-limited course, but in some cases it is more severe and sustained and can sometimes be lethal. The usual treatments - antithyroid drugs (such as methimazole, propylthiouracil, and carbimazole), radioactive iodine, or surgery are highly effective. The greatest threat is delay in diagnosis and treatment.

The incidence of IIT in a population is difficult to establish and relates to case finding, severity of iodine deficiency, and degree and duration of effective iodine supplementation. In some studies the incidence of thyrotoxicosis has doubled over several years following introduction of iodine into iodine-deficient population, but the incidence then characteristically decreases to a level below that existing before correction of iodine deficiency.

Strategy for approching IIT

When IIT is recognised in a community, we recommend the following:
1. To the extent practical, advice older subjects, particularly those with nodular goitres, to reduce their salt intake.
2. Examine the iodine levels in salt and urine to ensure they do not exceed those prescribed in the country's IDD elimination program, and correct production practices that might lead to excess iodine in salt or other factors that may cause excess iodine intake in older age groups.
3. Alert the medical community to proper awareness, diagnosis, and treatment of IIT and provide necessary resources for medical care.

4. Document the number of cases and clinical details in order to assess the magnitude of the problem and then to design appropriate measures for responding.

5. Implement effective biological monitoring systems, as have already been recommended by ICCIDD and others as an essential component of IDD elimination programs.

6. Reassure health officials and the community that IIT is transient and treatable, and that its consequences are far outweighed by the benefits of iodized salt for the development of children.

7. Over the longer range, depending on the number and severity of cases and the actual content of iodine in the salt, consider lowering the required amounts of iodine added to salt.

Conclusions

Some iodine induced thyrotoxicosts can be anticipated as iodine deficiency is corrected worldwide. Prompt diagnosis and treatment of individual cases are the best approaches to IIT. While IIT is significant, correcting the other iodine deficiency disorders, particularly those affecting the mental and physical development of children, is much more important for the health of the community. Therefore, concern about the development of IIT should not be used as an argument to delay, compromise, or stop a program of iodized salt.

PART VI

New Alliances and Progress Towards Elimination of IDD

PART-I

22

IDD in Livestock - Ecology and Economics

C.S. Pandav and M.G. Venkatesh Mannar

Introduction

Although manifestations of Iodine Deficiency Disorders (IDD) have been recognized since ancient times in human beings, IDD in animals has only recently received attention. Most of our knowledge of the effects of iodine deficiency comes from medical research using experimental animals in order to understand the role of iodine in development, homeostasis, and reproduction. Livestock health and productivity, however, are also affected by environmental iodine deficiency, much the same way as with humans.

It is generally believed that those geographical locations where IDD is more pronounced in human beings are likely to be the same as for animals (such as sheep, goats, cows, buffalo, pigs, and chickens) due to the ecology of iodine. A lack of iodine in the diet of farm animals has been shown to substantially reduce the yield of eggs, milk, meat, agricultural draught power, and dung for cooking fuel and maintaining soil fertility. This is especially relevant to rural people given the intimate interrelationship in the health of both humans and animals (see Figure 22.1-newspaper article). An examination of the whole ecology of iodine deficiency is therefore, necessary to ensure the health of both human and animal populations through appropriate interventions. Figure 22.2 serves as a model for this discussion of the effects of iodine deficiency in the food chain starting at the source and moving upwards in an ecological fashion. Measuring iodine deficiency and the effects of iodine supplementation are subsequently discussed.

HEALTHFILE

People keep as well as the animals they live with

By Kalpana Jain

Thirty-five-year-old Hardevi went to a primary health care centre with her three children suffering from pneumonia. The doctor on duty asked her to immediately admit the children to the centre. Hardevi was asked to stay back and help take care of the children as staff was scarce.

Hardevi, despite the serious condition of her children, said she could not do so. Back in her village, some five km from this centre, her buffalo was also lying ill. And she couldn't risk the death of the buffalo for the lives of her other three children, her husband and his parents depended on the survival of the animal.

The doctor pleaded with the woman. He explained that if she took them away they would all die. Hardevi did not relent. She took the children back. One by one her three children -- two-year-old Satpal, four year-old Hira and six-year-old Dayal died. The buffalo survived.

This incident occurred sometime back at the primary health care centre at Ballabgarh run by the All India Institute of Medical Sciences. But more shocking is the fact that this is not an isolated case. "Such incidents are common, " says associate professor of pediatrics N.K. Arora explaining that the health of the entire food chain is vital. Health of soil, plants and animals is what contributes to the overall health and growth of a child, he says.

The economic consequences of diseases of livestock are important while considering public health measures, especially for the rural areas where dependence for livelihood is entirely on livestock. The yield from this livestock affects others who are not directly dependant on livestock for economic sustenance. It affects health depending on the nutrients given to the livestock through plants and other fodder. To achieve this complete food chain the health of soil and plants has also to be ensured.

"The economic consequences of livestock ailments are acute. And it is important to look after the health of livestock if the health of human beings is to be taken care of," says Dr C.S. Pandav, who for the first time brought medical scientists handling issues of health of human beings and veterinary scientists together.

The two-day meeting was held at Pantnagar's Agricultural University. Participants included experts from the National Institute of Nutrition, paediatricians, medical scientists from the All India Institute of Medical Sciences, agriculture scientists, soil scientists, and entomologists.

These scientists are approaching health in its totality which means healthy soil, plants and animals. The soil where plants grow should have adequate amounts of all nutrients.

Animals, who are also feeding on the same plants that are deficient in micronutrients suffer in several ways. The effect of iodine deficiency in farm animals has been studied extensively. The rate of miscarriage is high, says Dr Pandav. No abortions occurred in goats when their intake of iodine was increased ten times. The rate of miscarriage in these goats was as high as 47 per cent.

It was found that iodine deficiency leads to several other disorders. The calves may be born blind, hariless, or extremely weak. The rate of conception goes down and there is infertility as well. The yield of milk and wool is also reduced substantially.

In those parts where iodine deficiency disorders are common amongst human beings, they are known to affect animals as well. But in places where iodised salt is available for human beings, uniodised salt is kept for giving to livestock, adds Dr Pandava, the regional coordinator for iodine disorder control for south- east Asia.

Experts feel that with this step scientists are moving ahead of superspecialisation. They are now connecting disciplines and completing a chain to arrive at better solutions to health care.

Fig. 22.1 Newspaper article.

PEOPLE	**Humans** ↑	health and socioeconomic impact
EFFECT ON ANIMALS	**Livestock**	clinical and reproductive disorders, decreased productivity
LOW AVAILABILITY OF IODINE	**Plants**	iodine-poor feeds and fodders, goitrogens
	Water, Soil	environmental iodine deficiency

Fig. 22.1 A hierarchial food chain where iodine deficiency is attenuated at each trophic level with consequences.

Iodine Ecology - a Review

The iodine cycle in nature affects the distribution of this element in soil, plants, and animals within a system (see chapter 2 for a review of the ecology of iodine). Iodide ions (IO_3^-) found in soil and sea water are easily oxidized when exposed to sunlight into volatile molecular iodine (I^-) which escapes to the atmosphere and returns to the soil by rain. The rate of replenishment, however, is slow, resulting in an indefinately low iodine soil content that is compounded by soil erosion and repeated flooding. Consequently, iodine has over time become irregularily distributed over the earth's surface resulting in acute deficiencies in mountainous regions (ie. the Swiss Alps, the Himalayas) and flooded riverines (ie. the Great Lakes, the Indo-Gangetic Plain). Today, the problem is aggravated by accelerated deforestation and agricultural soil erosion and overgrazing where iodine is leached from the soil.

Thus, iodine deficiency results from geological rather than social and economic conditions. IDD in animals may also be more severe due to a relatively closed foodchain, where as humans have an access to consume a variety of foods imported from non-deficient areas.

Availibility of Iodine

An understanding of the causes of IDD livestock first requires an examination into the 'environment' which precipitates the disease. This approach emphasizes an understanding of the root etiology of IDD in livestock and it's prevention, as opposed to a purely medical approach.

The amount of iodine available to animals from vegetation is generally affected by three factors:

1) Iodine content of water, soil, and plants
2) Presence of Goitrogens (anitmetabolites)
3) Parasitic Infection

1) Iodine Content of Water, Soil, and Plants

Unlike other nutrients, such as iron, calcium, or the vitamins, iodine does not naturally occur in specific foods; rather, it is present in the soil and imbibed through foods grown on that soil. As a result, animal and human populations which are totally dependent on food grown in such soils are unable to obtain the physiological amount of iodine that they need and deficiency symptoms appear.

The iodine contents of water, soils, feeds, and fodders in different countries are the main determinants of iodine deficiency in all livestock species (Table 22.1); however, no real consensus has been established on any threshold values of iodine as research is scant on this subject. For sake of comparison, the concentration of iodine in sea water is 50 µg/L; in rain water, 1.8 - 8.5 µg/L; in water of severely iodine deficient areas, 0.1 - 2 µg/L; in mildly deficient area, 9 µg/L; in plants grown in iodine deficient areas, 10 µg/kg (dry matter); and in plants grown in iodine sufficient areas, 10,000 µg/kg (dry matter).

Table 22.1 *Iodine contents of soil, drinking water, feeds, and fodders in different countries (Kapoor and Rao)*

Country	Soil	Water	Feeds	Fodder
USSR	2.59 (1.5 - 4.00)	2.80 (2.30 - 0.58)	171 (9.8 - 660)	0.150 (0.02)
New Zealand	1.5	_	_	<0.1
Ireland	2.92 - 30.15	_	_	0.08-0.42
Germany	-	1.3	-	-

The abundance of iodine and other trace elements in soil and plant systems is a complex problem influenced by various factors: soil type and pH, local geology, type of fertilizers used, source of irrigation, average annual precipitation, crop species and rotation pattern, stage of plant maturity, and climatic factors.

Availaibility of herbage iodine, for example, is affected by atmospheric temperature and season. The probable reason suggested is that at low temperautres, root nodule activity is reduced which affects the mobilization of iodine and plant growth. The ripening and flowering of a plant species in a higher ambient temperature may also decrease iodine content. Soil iodine content is also affected by type and pH of a soil. The iodine content of Tarai soil is lower than expected because of it's basicity. At higher pH's values, iodine is presumably displaced from clay surfaces by hydroxlions (OH^-); and with increased acidity of clay suspensions, there is a progressive increase in iodine absorption. Another factor affecting the iodine content of plants is the introduction of high grain yielding dwarf varieties of certain cereals and mechanical harvesting. Fodder crops and straw production have declined as a result, accentuating the gap between demand for and availability of conventional feeds and fodders for livestock for trace minerals, including iodine. Table 22.2 lists the iodine content on a dry matter (DM) basis of several varieties of animal feeds and fodders. Cereal, oil cakes, and wheat bran are poor natural sources of iodine as compared to straws and green fodders which contain low to marginally adequete levels of iodine. Fresh feeds and fodders have a higher iodine content before being dried. Cereals, which form the bulk of the daily diet of humans, are poor sources of iodine. Wheat has been shown, however, to contain relatively more iodine than rice. Fruits and vegetables grown in iodine deficient areas are poor sources, although roots and tubers contain more iodine in such areas. Pulses are the best source of iodine and meat has the highest amount of all foods.

Table 22.2 *Iodine content of different feeds and fodders*

Feed / Fodder	Iodine Content (μg/kg - DM basis)
Cereals (maize, wheat, barley)	115 - 192
Oil cakes (deoiled G.N.C., Mustard, mahua)	185 - 263
Bran, wheat and rice (deoiled)	95 - 287
Green fodders (maize, barja, berseem, oat, subabul)	216 - 574
Green fodders (beet leaves and brassicas)	73 - 196
Legumes and graminae	49 - 66
Ensiled wilted red clover	163
Sugar beet tops	63
Straw (wheat, rice)	293 - 309

2. Goitrogens

Goitrogens are chemical substances found in certain plants that interfere with normal iodine metabolism and can precipitate IDD despite an otherwise adequete iodine intake. They are a secondary factor to dietary iodine deficiency, which is more common, and also because goitrogens are easily counteracted with sufficient dietary iodine supplementation. Three general categories of goitrogens exist for the purpose of animals: i) cyanogenic glucosides, ii) mimosine, and iii) other iodine antagonists.

i) Cyanogenic glucosides

A number of cruciferous plants (e.g. rape seed, mustard seed, and kale) are valuable sources of protein and various amino acids. Although the protein quality of these plants is quite good, they are goitrogenic in nature. The goitrogenic substances in these plants are glucosinalates, which are capable of producing thiocyanate in the rumen of cows.

Thiocynates and sulfocyanates are formed during the process of detoxification of cyanide in the liver and these substances restrict the uptake of iodine by thyroid, probably by inhibiting the metabolic activity of the thyroid epithelium and thus thyroxine (T_4) production. A continued intake of a low level of cyanogenic glucosides is commonly associated with a high incidence of goitrous offspring. These goitrogenic substances may appear in an animal's milk and also provide a toxic hazard to both animals and humans.

Members of the brassica family (ie. cabbage, turnip, kale, soybean, linseed, pea, ground nut, and white clover) and cruciferous crops can promote goitre development as they contain moderate to high levels of glucosides. Linseed meal, for example, contains the glucoside linamarin, which is thought to be the agent producing goitre in new born lambs from ewes fed with the meal during pregnancy. Mustard meal contains sinigrin, which is metabolized into allothiocyanate, another cyanogentic glucosside goitrogen. Rapeseed meal contains the glucosinalate progoitrin which in pigs is metabolized into goitrin causing thyroid disorders, even when it comprimises as little as 2% of rations. Some other pasture and fodder plants, such as subterrane an clover and rye grass are known to have a moderate content of cyanogenetic glucosides. These goitrogenic substances may appear in an animal's milk and provide a toxic hazard to both animals and man.

Thiocyanate production, however, can depend on the variety and maturity of a plant, as with kale, where small young leaves of certain varieties produce five times as much thiocyanate in the rumen as compared to large fully formed leaves. Kale in a lamb's diet has been shown to reduce milk yield, increase neonatal mortality and infertility due to suppressed estrus illustrating the some of the consequences of goitrogens on livestock.

ii) Mimosine

Mimosine is a toxic amino acid commonly found in the feed/fodder species subabul (Leucaena leucocephala). Subabul fed to female adult goats adversely affects fertility, neonatal survival, and congential goitre in kids born.

iii) Other iodine antagonists

Inorganic elements, such as: excess Arsenic, Iron, Calcium, or perchlorates, low amounts of Copper, Molybdenum, or Sellenium, and excess nitrogen (in the form of nitrates, urasil, and thiourea) have been shown to aggravate iodine deficiency in livestock.

Common crop and pasture plants and numerous weeds may accumulate toxic levels of nitrates. In ruminants, nitrate is readily reduced to nitrite which is absorbed and causes toxicosis. Chronic nitrate toxicity causes goitre, infertility, etc. Abnormal accumulation of nitrate in plants can be provoked by excessive nitrogen fertilization.

A high dietary intake of calcium decreases intestinal absorption of iodine. In some areas, heavy application of lime on pastures is followed by the development of goitre in lambs. This factor may also be important in areas where drinking water is heavily mineralized (hard water).

Gross bacterial contamination of drinking water and feedstuffs by sewage can also precipitate goitre in livestock. Records exist of severe outbreaks of goitrous calves grazing on pastures heavily dressed with crude sewage and sludge as fertilizer.

3) Parasitic infection

Hypothyroidism in animals may also be aggravated by parasitic infection. Histopathological evidence has demonstrated sclerotic lesions in the thyroid glands of cows due to Onchocerea infection.

The effect of intestinal worms in decreasing iron intake in humans is perhaps analogous to iodine uptake in parasitized animals.

Effects on Animals

Most of our knowledge on the effects of iodine deficiency in humans comes from medical research using experimental animals such as rats, monkeys, marmosets, etc. All of these studies have been conducted in order to understand the role of iodine and the consequences of its deficiency so as to take the necessary corrective measures in humans. A body of literature has, however, emerged over the years on the specific effects of IDD in livestock given their importance as a valuable source of animal protein (in the form of milk, eggs, and some meat) and in the livelihood of rural people. It is generally believed that geographical locations where iodine deficiency is more pronounced in human beings are likely to be the same as for animals. Based on this assumption, about 100 million animals (cattle, buffalo, goat and sheep) are in the IDD risk zone of the Himalayan and the Sub-Himalayan region of Asia.

Iodine deficiency occurs in many species of animals and manifests itself differently in different animals; productivity, however, is inevitably reduced in all animals. Decreased resistance to stress and disturbed energy metabolism is commonly known. The major clinical manifestations in animals is neonatal mortality and visible or palpable enlargement of the thyroid gland in some animals. Colloid goitre is less common in animals, however, and probably represents an evolutionary stage after primary hyperplasia. For example, obvious enlargement of the thyroid gland is more often seen in adult sheep than in adult cattle. Clinically detectable enlargement of the thyroid gland through inspection and palpation is more common in goats, sheep, and young cattle than in other animals. Goitre, therefore, should not be considered as the only criteria for iodine deficiency in animals as it's manifestation is species dependant. The importance of subclinical iodine deficiency - the death of a newborn without goitre - is more important.

Reproductive failure is the oustanding manifestation of iodine deficiency in farm animals. Irregular or suppressed estrus causing infertility has been reported in animals in iodine deficient areas. Development of the fetus is retarded or arrested at some stage during gestation resulting in early death or resorption, abortion, or stillbirth, the birth of a weak, "hairless" offspring associated with prolonged gestation, or parturition and the retention of the placental membrane. The danger increases in cases of multiple births. The main point is that iodine deficiency, and not simply goitre, also influences the iodine status of offspring.

Cattle

Alimentary tract motility has been shown to be reduced in hypothyroid ruminants as well as monogastric animals. Dairy cattle fed insufficient iodine are less able to resist stress and may even have a higher incidence of ketosis. Failure to express estrus in dairy cows and loss of libido and deterioration of semen quality in bulls affect the fertility of a herd. Iodine deficient calves may be born blind, hairless, weak, or even dead, depending on the severity of the deficiency. Morbidity is high, especially after birth. Goitre is often observed in newborn calves even when there are no clinical symptoms in the herd, although they may also be afflicted. If affected calves are not assisted for a few days to suck because of weakness, they may die. Endometritis, ovarian cysts, and a host

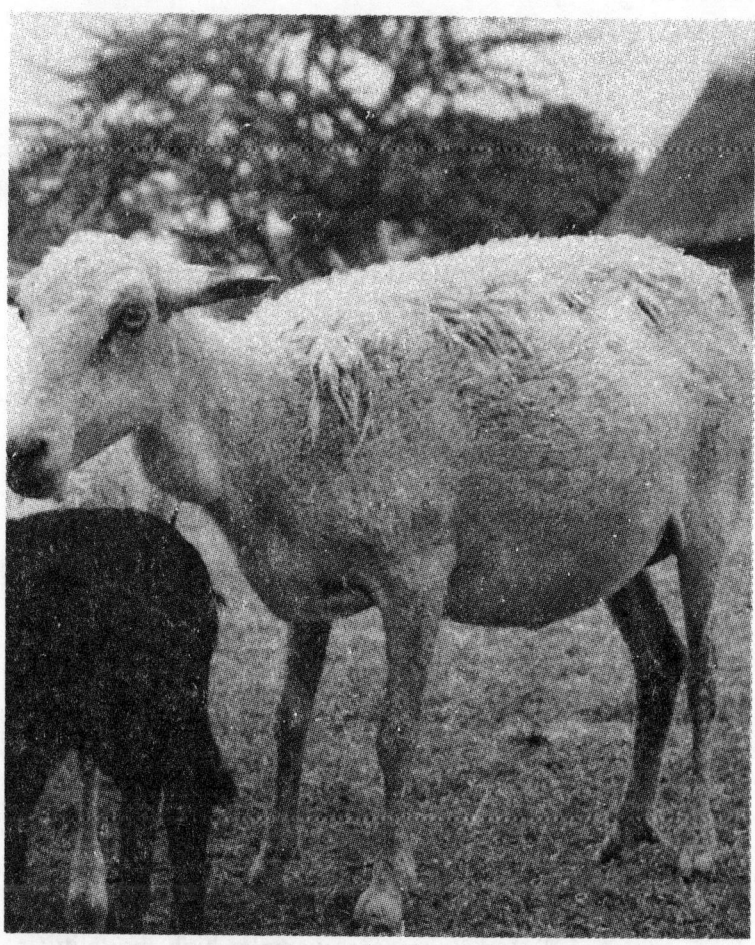

Fig. 22.2 Sheep with goitre in a region of iodine deficiency. (Photo E. Cabezas - Reproduced with permission from -Salt Iodization for the Elimination of Iodine Deficiency by M.G.Venkatesh Mannar and John T. Dunn a ICCIDD/MI/UNICEF/WHO Joint publication, 1995).

of other repoductive disorders and infections have also been shown to accompany impaired thyroid function in cattle.

Horses

Pregnant mares may not show external signs of iodine deficiency but may produce a stillborn foal or one showing extreme weakness at birth. Foals born alive with a well developed goitre usually die or remain weak for the duration of their life. Foals show a normal hair coat and little thyroid enlargement but are very weak at birth. In most cases, they are unable to stand without support and many are too weak to suck. Excessive flexion of the lower forelegs and extension of lower parts of the hindlegs has also been observed in affected foals. Defective ossification has also been reported, the manifestation being the collapse of the central and the third tarsal bones leading to lameness and deformity of the hock. Thoroughbreds and light horses are more susceptible to IDD than draft animals.

Sheep

The symptoms of iodine deficiency in mature sheep are goitre, reduced yield of wool, reduced conception rate, or lambs born weak, dead, or without wool. Severe iodine deficiency in pregnant ewes causes reduction in the brain and body weight of the foetus from 70 days gestation to parturition. Prolonged gestation has also been reported in ewes. New born lambs manifest weakness, extensive hairlessness, and palpable, if not visible, enlargement of thyroid glands. Animal productivity has been reported to be impaired even in conditions of marginal iodine deficiency that does not cause clinical goitre; for example, high mortality in lambs from ewes showing minimal thyroid enlargement in Tasmania has been observed. Adult sheep in iodine deficient areas may show a high incidence of thyroid enlargement although they are clinically normal in other respects.

Goats

Goats present a similar clinical picture to sheep, except that all abnormalities are more severe. Thyroid glands of goats/kids palpated may be graded as palpable and plum size (+), easily palpable and lemon size (++), and duck egg size, hanging and visible from a distance (+++). The incidence in kids is higher than in adults and the degree of enlargement is more in kids than in their dams. Goats

Table 22.3 *The influence of iodine supply on the reproduction of goats*

Description	Iodine Content in Fodder (mg/kg dry weight)	
	0.04 (n=19)	0.40 (n=18)
Success of conception (%)	79	83
Success of first insemination (%)	27	73
Abortion rate (%) of gravid goats	47	0
Length of gravidity (days)	158	152
Kids per gravid goat	1.4	1.7
Kids carried to term per gravid goat	0.9	1.7

which survive the initial danger period after birth may recover, except for partial persistence of the goitre. The thyroid gland may pulsate with the normal arterial pulse and may extend down a greater part of the neck and cause some local edema. Auscultation and palpation of the jugular furrow may reveal the presence of the murmur and thrill (the 'thyroid thrill') due to the increased arterial blood supply of the glands. Early studies on the thyroid glands of goats were the first to demonstrate increased levels of T_3 hormone in response to iodine deficiency, reflecting the compensatory me chanism of the thyroid gland to iodine deficiency. The abortion rate in iodine deficient goats is 46% as compared to 0% in iodine sufficient goats. More kids are born to iodine sufficient goats and the probability of survival of kids born to iodine sufficient goats is twice than those that are born to iodine deficient goats.

Pigs

Symptoms of iodine deficiency in piglets born to iodine deficient sows have thickened skin, puffy necks, hairlessness, and bloated appearance. Some piglets are born dead while those that are born alive are weak and usually die within a few hours. Survivors are lethergic, do not grow well, have a waddling gait, and leg weakness of ligaments and joints. Thyroid enlargement may be present, but is never sufficiently large enough to cause visible swelling.

Poultry

Poultry appear to be able to withstand a considerable degree of iodine deficiency without marked loss of production or hatchability of eggs. On an iodine deficient diet for 35 weeks, hens did not show any effect on hatchability or embryo weight. After a period of two years, however, a decrease in hatchability, prolongation of hatching time, reduced egg production, and retarded embryo development were observed. Thyroid enlargement in the embryos is also observed. Iodine deficiency in breeding hens results in an enlarged thyroid and in some cases lower body weight in growing chicks.

Productivity

Milk production is positively correlated with iodine intake for many animals. Long term deficiencies may result in decreased milk yields that are important to offspring health as well as for human consumption. Approximately 10% of dietary iodine goes into milk depending on the level of production. Increase in milk iodine content due to increased dietary iodine has been reported. Iodine supplementation has generally been shown to increase milk yield from 4% to 15%. Some reports also suggest that iodine supplementation not only influences milk yield but also it's composition. A decrease in volatile fatty acids in the rumen and an increase in milk fat, protein, casein, lactose, calcium, and phosphorus is observed with iodine supplementation.

Increase in milk iodine can also be affected by factors other than dietary iodine supplementation. Dutch workers have reported that iodine concentration of summer milk is low (ie. 9.7 µg/L) as compared to winter milk (21.1 µg/L). Increase milk iodine can occur with the use of iodophor teat dips used as a disinfectant where a good amount of iodine is believed to be absorbed through the skin of the teats; iodine concentration can rise to 113-346 µg/L with the use of a teat dip as compared to 13-23 µg/L without. Milk iodine concentration also decreases as lactation progresses, falling during the first few days after parturition, climbing to a higher level for the first three months of lactation, and then gradually decreasing with time, concurrent with a reduction in total milk yields.

Measuring Iodine Deficiency

Measuring the degree of biochemical iodine deficiency in livestock species is useful in determining the severity of the disease and what supplementation or therapy interventions are needed. Various chemical methods developed from time to time for the estimation of microquantities of iodine have their merits and demerits. They can be broadly classified into three categories:

    1. Methods for the estimation of relatively larger amounts of iodine (e.g. in iodized salts, mineral blocks, and mineral mixtures). The methods in the first category are comparatively simpler and with the current availability of spot testing kits, approximate concentration can be obtained in a given sample.

    2. Methods for the estimation of small amounts of iodine (e.g. in blood, milk, urine and water). The estimation of iodine in

blood, milk, urine and water is complex, however, a simplified procedure has been developed, particularly for urine, providing a very useful tool in determining the present status of iodine intake given that about 90% of ingested iodine is excreted through urine. This procedure however, requires some sophisticated equipment which restricts its large scale application in the field.

3. Methods for the estimation of very small amounts of iodine (e.g. in feeds and plant materials). Plants and feed material require the most difficult and complicated methods of estimation as they contain very small amounts of iodine (0.01 to 0.20 ppm). Methods generally involve fixation of plant iodine and oxidation and reduction processes requiring extra pure chemicals and well-equipped laboratory facilities.

Iodine deficiency can be clinically diagnosed if the thyroid gland is palpable or visible in the animal species. Thyroid histology, iodine levels in urine and milk, serum precipitable iodine, and protein-bound iodine are the subclinical indicators of iodine status. In the last three decades, radioimmuno assays of triiodithyroinine and thyroxine have provided precise indications of iodine deficiency in various species where these assays measure the uptake of iodine by the thyroid gland. Iodine concentration of milk has been closely linked with dietary iodine intake and so it has been suggested as an indicator of goitre status in a given area. Thyroid size, iodine levels in urine, milk, serum precipitable iodine, protein bound iodine, and levels of thyroxine, and triiodothyronine are all useful indices of iodine status. High levels of protein bound iodine (PBI) with a normal diet suggest adequate iodine intake. The normal range of plasma inorganic iodine in animals is 0.08 to 0.60 µg/L. Values below 0.08 µg/L are generally considered as iodine deficient status. Levels above 1 µg/L are harmful to animals.

Requirements of Iodine

The minimum dietary iodine requirements of farm animals is difficult to express with accuracy as the requirements for growth may not be identical with those for reproduction and lactation. The normal recommended dietary intake of iodine is considered to be 0.1 - 0.3 mg/kg DM of feed. The minimum requirement of iodine in dairy animals has been reported to be around 0.6 ppm of dry matter feed. Other estimates suggest that dietary concentrations of iodine should be 0.8 ppm for pregnant and lactating animals and 0.12 ppm for non-pregnant and non-lactating animals when no goitrogens are fed; additional supplementation of 1.2 ppm of iodine is recommended with feed containing goitrogenic substances. Iodine should be at least double the requirement if the diet on DM basis contains 25% of a strongly goitrogenic feed such as soyabean. For example, it has been reported that the iodine requirements of lambs can be met by a supplemented diet containing 0.18 - 0.27 ppm of iodine when kale, ryegrass, and clover were the main dietary consituents.

Iodine Supplementation

The choice of control measures in animals is largely dependant on the severity of the problem and the economic stakes involved. Supplemental iodine may be incorporated into salt, mineral mixtures, or concentrate feeds of animals. Iodine has been found to be most efficiently delivered, however, through salt for many reasons.

Iodized Salt

Salt is a natural carrier for trace minerals since all animals need salt. Requirement of sodium is 53 to 64 mg/kg of body weight, which would be provided by 0.3% of salt in the dry matter of the ration. A continuously low salt intake affects the health of animals through loss of appetite and weight. Feed utilization decreases and more feed per unit of gain is required. Salt iodised with either iodide or iodate can be made available to livestock, however, iodate is less soluble and more stable than iodide and so is preferred in humid tropical conditions. Potassium iodide, sodium iodide, or calcium iodide are some other possible iodine supplementation compounds. It has been suggested, however, that potassium iodide given alone is unsuitable, but when mixed with calcium stearate (8% stearate in potassium iodide), it can be added to salt at the rate of 200 mg/kg of salt.

Farmers can supply trace mineralized salt in a mineral block or box with free access, although this can lead to overconsumption of salt.

Table 22.4 *Daily iodine requirements and average daily salt consumption of several common livestock species and suggested salt iodization levels*

Class of Animal	Iodine Requirement Total Diet (ppm)	Maximum Dietary Tolerance Levels (ppm)	Salt Consumption (Maximum) (grams)	Iodine Content Required in Salt (ppm)
Swine	0.14	400	4.1	28
Beef Cattle	0.2-2.0	50	10	40-400
Dairy Cattle	0.25-0.50	50	24.3	50-100
Horses	0.1	5	10.9	20
Sheep	0.1-0.8	50	4.1	20-160
Goats	0.15-0.80	50	4-8	30-240
Poultry	0.3-0.4	300	0.21	20-160

For grazing animals in inaccessible parts of the world, iodised salt blocks are air dropped. EIDD is an organic iodide used at relatively high dosages for treatment of foot rot, lumpy jaw, and other conditions and so the use of iodine in farming practices is aleady quite familiar. In the developed countries, there are a range of trace mineralized salts that cater to each variety of livestock and poultry, typically at a concentration of 70-80 ppm of iodine. Organised livestock rearing is a growing industry, but is still limited in some countries which can limit the potential for large scale interventions. In many countries, it is very difficult to have separate grades of iodised salt for animals and so a separate monitoring of iodine intake of animals is necessary to determine if additional supplements are required. The normal iodine concentration in salt for human consumption is in the range of 30-100 mg/kg (parts per million:ppm). Such iodised salt can be easily administered to animals either orally or mixed with animal feeds, fodder, and concentrates for regular prophylactic use in endemic areas or as specific therapy when required. Table 4 summarizes the daily iodine requirements of several common livestock species and suggests iodization levels based also on their average daily consumption of salt.

Other Methods of Iodine Supplementation

As with humans, many iodine-containing compounds (elemental iodine, iodides, iodates, organic iodine preparations, seaweed meal, thyroid gland meal etc.) have been used in livestock to prevent and treat iodine deficiency. Vehicles of iodine include: common salt, vegetable oils, water, feed, soil, plants and even some specifically designed porous vessels and intraluminal devices. The modes of administration include oral (water, capsules, drops) and intramuscular oil injection, directly or with different carriers. The choice of method may depend on the objectives (prophylaxis or therapy), targeted livestock species, scale of operation and economic considerations.

In certain situations, the use of iodised salt in drinking water may also prove useful. The appropriate amounts of potassium iodide or potassium iodate can be added to water containers, drinking water wells, or water pipelines. Although water iodisation has been tried in the range of 50 to 500 ug/L, a dose of less than 120 ug/L has been found to be ideal from the point of view of odour. The use of porous polymer vessels containing iodine in community water supplies could be conveniently utilized for animal systems with appropriate adjustments made in dosage. In some countries, chemical iodine is already used to purify water and reduce bacterial pollution, which certainly benefits iodine deficient human and animal populations in the area. Lugol's solution (Potassium iodide) containing 6 mg of iodine per drop has been widely used as a disinfectant for wounds and for oral prophylaxis of iodine deficiency in human beings. Such supplementation has been adapted for correction of iodine deficiency in livestock, as with pregnant goats which was found to be effective in preventing IDD in offspring.

Iodine in the form of tablets or drops has been used in some countries to correct iodine deficiency in human. Tablets containing 100-500 ug of potassium iodide are available for daily consumption (as in Germany). Direct use of oral potassium iodate in pregnant ewes has been reported by Rodel (1971) and in lambs by McCauley et al (1973). Direct use of potassium iodide in poultry feed at the rate of 5000 ppm has been reported by Roland et al (1977) for IDD therapy investigations.

Certain seaweeds, such as sargasso and Laminaria japonica tresch, etc. and thyroid glands of animals have been known to be effective in controlling IDD since ancient times. In more recent times, powders and extracts of these iodine-rich sources have been used for medicinal purposes. These natural sources could be used to fortify the animal diet. The use of seaweed meal containing 1 to 10% iodine has been reported to be useful in poultry production.

Injectable iodine is another form of iodine supplementation for livestock. One of the most widely used prophylactics is Lipoidal which contains 480 mg of iodine conveniently bound to 1 mL of poppy seed oil. One main advantage in the use of iodised oil preparations is that they can be administered weekly, monthly, or even yearly. Intramuscular injection treatment with potassium iodide in aqueous solutions was found to be effective in increasing protein bound iodine (PBI), weight gain, and reduction of thryoid size in cattle.

The use of an intraluminal device in sheep has been reported to be successful in a goitre prone area of Northern Tasmania. Pregnant ewes were treated with an intraluminal device designed to release a regular quantity of iodine into the rumen.

Iodine Toxicity

In humans, it has been reported that an intake of 2000 μg of iodine/day is potentially harmful. In all cases, however, there is no risk of toxicity to any class of animal, even with salt containing high levels of iodine of 200 ppm.

Dairy cattle require a minimum level of 0.60 ppm of iodine in their diet and a maximum level of 50 ppm which is almost 100 times the minimum requirement. Iodine toxicity, however, may appear in dairy cattle at an intake of 50 ppm of iodine in calves weighing 80-112 kg. The main symptoms of excess iodine intake in cattle have been shown to be: anorexia, severe pityriasis, restlessness, hyperthermia, and bronchopneumonia. In contrast, milking cows showed no symptoms of toxicity at dietary iodine intakes of 50 ppm through various sources (ie. NaI, KI), although extremely high iodine levels become present in the serum, milk, urine and faeces.

Pigs are much more tolerant to excess iodine than cattle, however, symptoms of toxicity at 400 and 800 ppm level of potassium iodate have been observed.

Potassium iodide doses in lambs exceeding the range from 94 to 785 mg per day per lamb caused lambs to be lethargic, consume less feed, and gain less weight than lambs given smaller doses.

An early study by Malan et al (1932) reported the detrimental effects of iodine on reproduction when 0.02 g of potassium iodide was given as a daily supplement to merino ewes for 16 months.

In this context, there is a much greater danger of iodine deficiency than iodine toxicity affecting livestock.

These minimum requirements can be achieved by ensuring that feed contains 1% of iodised salt (iodised at a level of 0.01%) and if concentrates and forage are fed proportionately.

Human Health and Socioeconomic Impacts of IDD in Animals

From the point of view of human self-interest, it is important to prevent IDD in livestock if good yield of milk, eggs, wool, and meat are to be ensured.

Using the most conservative estimates, the cost-benefit ratio of IDD elimination programmes is 1:3. If benefits related to education and livestock populations are included, the ratio would be 1:8 or even more.

Another study showed that the cost of trace minerals was 4.7 US cents per pig but returned $ 1.64 US (a cost benefit ratio of 1:35).

A study in Colombia indicated a return of 15.6 Pesos for each Peso invested in mineral supplements for animals compared to common salt supplements only.

Reports from Montana, USA indicate that before iodine feeding was practised there, goitre had caused an annual loss of thousands of pigs. Records from other areas show serious losses in the sheep and cattle industries prior to the discovery of the lack of iodine as the causative factor. The cost of iodisation is low: normally in the range 2-7 US cents per kilogram which is less than 5% of the retail price of salt in most countries.

If salt for human consumption is only iodised, then there exists a situation in the market where non-iodised salt, which is cheaper than iodised salt, is available for animal consumption. This leads people to purchase the cheaper, non-iodised salt, especially when farmers buy one type of salt from the market for both their livestock and their family.

The availability of two types of salt also poses a major problem to law enforcing agencies as they cannot take legal action against those selling non-iodised salt since it is intended for animal consumption.

Legislation conversing the iodisation of salt for human use should be extended to include all salt for livestock consumption. This will have the double benefit of ensuring that animals receive iodine supplementation and also that there is only one variety of salt in the market (iodised salt).

The majority of livestock, however, is owned by landless, marginal and small scale farmers who are categorized as the poorest of the poor in society. The livestock sector provides valuable animal protein for the human diet in the form of milk, meat, eggs and chicken. It also provides draught power for agricultural operations and rural transportation and dung for maintaining soil fertility and for energy for cooking in rural homes. Wool, hair, hides, skins and bones are some of the by-products from animal enterprise which are used as raw materials for garments, carpets, shoes, and the mineral industry, all of which help in earning valuable foreign exchange. Livestock generate employment for the rural population, particularly for women.

In view of the importance of livestock in the economy, it is necessary to tackle the situation of iodine deficiency in livestock with the same determination as with humans. Research between investigators in the medical and veterinary sciences is currently being united in an effort to collaborate on efforts to eliminate iodine deficiency disorders in both humans and livestock.

References

Bell, T. Donald. 1960. 'Sodium chloride in Animal Nutrition'. In Kaufmann, D.W. ed. *Sodium Chloride*. New York: Reinhold Publishing Corporation.

Conrad, J.H., M.P., Plumbee, W.M., Beeson. Aug. 1959. 'Trace mineral additions to corn soybean meal rations for growing-finishing pigs'. *Purdue Agr. Exp. Sta. mimeo*. AS-264.

Cunha, T.J. 1987. 'Salt Trace Minerals for Livestock, Poultry and Other Animals'. *The Salt Institute: Alexandria*. USA: Virginia.

Groppel, B., M., Anke, E., Scholz, B., Kohler, 1986. 'The influence of different iodine supply on reproduction and the intrathyroidal iodine content of goats and sheep'.

Healy, W.B., G., Croucheley, R.L., Gillett, P.C., Rankin, H., Watis, 1972. 'Ingested soil and iodine deficiency in lambs'. *New Zealand Journal of Agricultural Research*.

Heinrich, H., G., Wenk. 1989b. 'Iodine content of feeds and water used for cattle, sheep and pigs in the Erfurt area'. In *6th International Trace Element Symposium*. 3: 749-55.

Hetzel, B.S., G.F., Maberly. 1986. 'Ioine in Trace Elements'. In: *Human and Animal Nutrition*. Vol.2. New York: Academic Press. pp. 139-208.

March, B.E., R.E., Austic, L.S., Jensen, D., Polin, J.L., Sell, P.E., Waibel P.W., Waldroup. 1984. 'Nutrition Requirements of Poultry'. Washington: NAS-NRC. D.C.

McDowell, L.R. April, 1992. 'Minerals in Animals and Human Nutrition'. Academic Press.

McGrath, D., G.A., Fleming, 1988. 'Iodine levels in Irish soil and grasses'. *Irish Journal of Agricultural Research*. 27: 75-81.

Salakhutdinov, K.G. 1985. 'Iodine Deficiency in Farm Animals'. USSR: Kazanskii Veterinarnyt Institut: Kazan. pp. 96-99.

The major portion of this chapter is based on A Multidisciplinary Report on the Proceedings of: Technical Review Meeting on Iodine Deficiency Disorders in Livestock Populations Held at: G.B. Pant University for Agriculture and Technology, Pantnagar, Dist. Nainital, Uttar Pradesh (India) 27 - 28th January 1995, key references are listed below. Authors would like to thank Mr. Rashid Ahmed for editorial assistance.

23

Partnership to End Hidden Hunger Collaboration of Stakeholders in Sustaining the Elimination of Iodine Deficiency Disorders

C.S. Pandav, David P. Haxton and Hema Viswanathan

Introduction

In response to the need of accelerating progress towards eliminating IDD as a public health problem in the South Asian region, a conference between all those different people working on the problem, the 'stakeholders', was held in Dhaka, Bangladesh from 9th April to 12th, 1995. A multisectoral group of over 80 participants from Bangladesh, Bhutan, India, Nepal, Pakistan, Sri Lanka, and 16 other nations represented the interests of IDD experts, NGOs, salt industries, government, salt regulators, policy makers, communicators, educators, and health care providers in achieving the following conference objectives:

1. To renew commitment to the World Summit goal of IDD elimination by 2000.
2. To forge alliances between all stakeholders involved in IDD elimination.
3. To facilitate the development of strategies for sustaining elimination of IDD and foster combined synergistic efforts towards this end.

'We are committed to the elmination of iodine deficiency disorders by the years 2000. To achieve that goal, we have taken all possible measures. The Iodine Deficiency Prevention Act has been strengthened. At the same time, import of noniodized salt in the country has been banned. Iodization machines have been installed free of cost in all salt mills. We hope, by the end of the year, we will be able to ensure supply of iodized salt for all. I want to assure you that your recommendations will receive our close attention and we will do whatever necessary to eliminate the scourge of iodine deficiency disorders. I wish the conference all success. Thank you all'.

- Excerpt from a speech made by the Honorable Begum Khaleda Zia, Prime Minister of Bangladesh, at the Partnership to End Hidden Hunger Conference on 11th April 1995

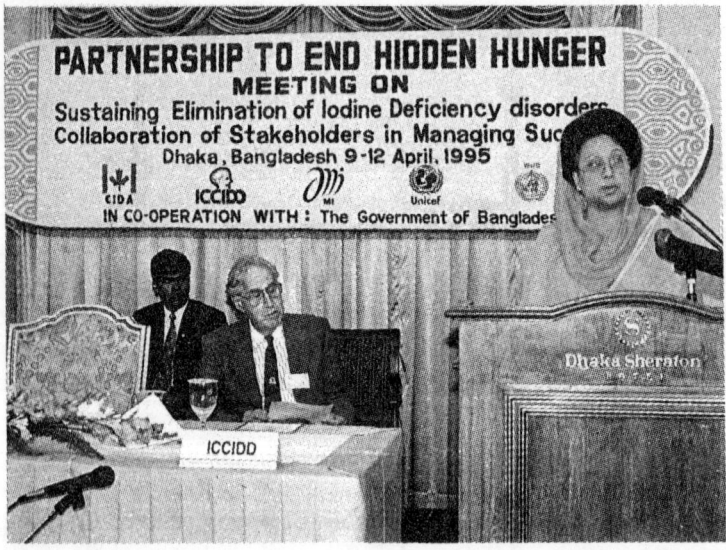

Fig. 23.1 The Prime Minister of Bangladesh Honouarable Begum Khaleda Zia addressing the 'Partnership to End Hidden Hunger' Conference on April 11th, 1995.

Salt iodization has proven to be the cheapest and most effective method of eliminating IDD in South Asia, where over 50% of the world's population is at risk of stillbirths, stunted growth, neurological debilities, goitre, lower IQ scores, decreased energy metabolism, and many other manifestations of dietary iodine deficiency. Despite the sense of a technical solution, the implementation of salt iodization has been slow, difficult and frustrating. Once IDD is eliminated, however, there is the further challenge of sustaining its elimination. It was with this goal in mind that CIDA, ICCIDD, UNICEF, WHO, and the Government of Bangladesh organized this first-ever conference.

Guided by an innovative 'Future Search' conference methodology, participants worked in small groups on a series of five creative and intensive tasks over three days:

1. A review and analysis of the past of IDD elimination
2. The construction of a composite picture of everything that is happening in the present, that is external, and that will have a impact on the future regarding IDD
3. The development of one or more future scenarios for the elimination of IDD five to twenty years into the future
4. The discovery of common ground amongst the scenarios
5. The construction of action plans for both the short and long term for sustaining the elimination of IDD

Outcomes of the conference stressed the importance of transposing IDD from a medical problem into a socioeconomic issue by soliciting the help of different concerned, but 'new', groups. Compliance with production of adequately iodized and packaged salt, an efficient and non-competitive distribution and market system for only iodized salt for human and animal consumption, education of communities on the consequences of IDD and the benefits of iodized salt through various media (including schools, mass media, and rural IEC activities), private sector and government collaborations on food fortification, and periodic salt-iodine monitoring and IDD health surveys are some of the ways of helping ensure a sustained effort to eliminate IDD through out the region and future.

The process emphasized dialogue between the various stakeholders and cumulated with each South Asian country delegation drawing on these multidisciplinary insights to develop specific strategies within and outside their country.

With the discovery of new strategies through 'future searching' and alliance-building between all IDD stakeholders, namely, Government, Salt Regulators, Policy Makers, IDD Experts, Salt Industry, Communicators, Educators, Non-Governmental Organizations (NGOs) the Partnership to End Hidden Hunger conference aimed to build and maintain a network of collaborators in the South Asian region working towards eliminating IDD by 2000.

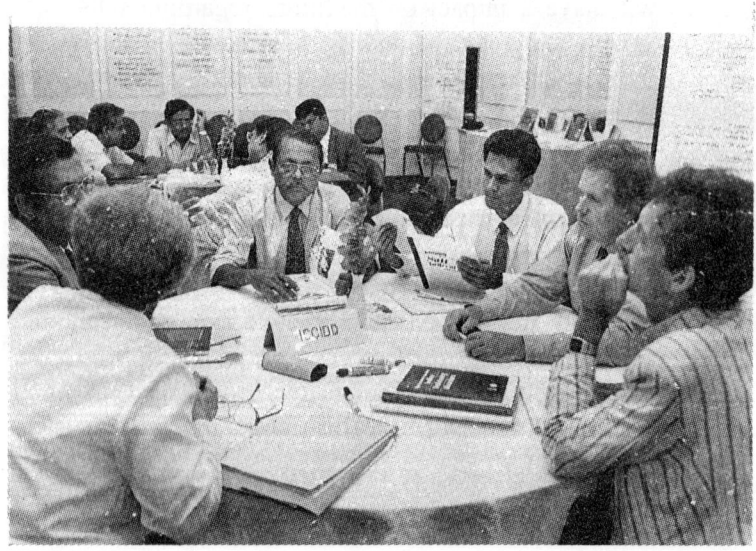

Fig. 23.2 Partnership to End Hidden Hunger Conference (Participants).

Future Search: Conference Methodology

The Future Search methodology is a form of strategic, long term planning that involves the participation of a whole organizational system or community, such as all those that have a role in seeing IDD eliminated in the South Asian region. Assembled in one place at one time, key representatives of various groups come together to design a preferred future and to discover common ground. The process is one that seeks to honor diversity and deal with complexity and ambiguity. Everybody works as peers, confronting the past, the present, and the future in dialogue with each other. Participants explore the whole system, its history, ideals, constraints, opportunities, and trends within and outside the system. Freed from the pressure to solve intractable problems, the methodology seeks to establish common ground that none knew existed. The most radical aspect of this type of conference is the treatment of conflict. Group dynamics are structured so as to encourage participants to find common ground and thus plan for a shared future, while still dealing directly and intensely with the issues. Other types of conferences usually involve speeches, presentations, and formal papers: not this one.

The Future Search Conference was designed around four basic principles:

- getting the whole system under one roof
- developing desired future scenarios, rather than problem solving
- working together on a series of structural tasks
- working as peers and equals in small, self-managed groups

The conference involved more than 80 participants who came together for 3 days with the goal of developing a consensus on the desired future for eliminating IDD in South Asia. Although facilitated by two consultants to the system, the work of the conference was self-managed by the participants. Five tasks were completed by the participants working in small groups of about 8 people each. Each group represented a mix of stakeholders and countries at various times. Each of the five took about 3 hours and are as follows:

1. A review and analysis of the past of IDD elimination
2. The construction of a composite picture of everything that is happening in the present, that is external and that will have a impact on the future regarding IDD
3. The development of one or more future scenarios for the elimination of IDD five to twenty years into the future.
4. The discovery of common ground amongst the scenarios
5. The construction of action plans for both the short and long term for sustaining the elimination of IDD

The Past: Creating a Common Database

After introductions and a preliminary overview of the conference, participants were given the task of developing a shared database of critical issues and events that had shaped the past and form the backdrop for the present stage of IDD in South Asia. This was done by asking participants to list key events on three large 'timelines' which had been posted on the walls of the meeting room. The first timeline focused on global society or world wide events, the second line centre on the efforts to eliminate IDD, and the third line was for the personal history of the participants.

The next step was to analyze the data on the timeline. Participants were asked to identify patterns and connections between the three timelines to see the relationship between global events, the effort to eliminate IDD, and the participants' own lives.

Derived from the exercise was the insight that the effort to eliminate IDD has evolved from a local problem into an international issue. Recently, elimination efforts have gained support from the growing recognition of human rights and the rights of children, the creation of national policies on salt iodization, and increased recognition of IDD as a serious and widespread problem.

IDD was also perceived to have evolved from a medical problem into a political problem. Although a technical solution to IDD has been known for more than seventy years, the elimination of IDD has been far slower than anticipated partly because it is not a political priority and partly because it is essentially a problem of the poor. There is cautious optimism about the possibility of eliminating IDD given continued scientific advances in evaluation and intervention measures and the potential for mass communication.

Commitment to IDD elimination was found to have increased over the year with the awareness of the relationship between iodine deficiency and brain development. Opposition to iodization from some groups and individuals, however, has also increased; their fears and misunderstandings are communicated by word of mouth and through the media.

The Present: Mindmap, Prouds and Sorries, and an Assessment

i) Mindmap

The next task was to develop a shared understanding of the present environment in which the campaign to eliminate IDD exits. As participants brainstormed together on the question 'What are the most important forces and trends that have an impact on efforts to eliminate IDD?', the conference managers drew a 'mindmap' on the wall. A mindmap is a diagrammatic listing of all influential trends and forces with suggestions of some key relationships between these trends. The resulting mindmap demonstrates graphically the complexity of the problem and the interrelationships of issues to a far grater extent than would a conventional outline. Participants were then asked to mark those trends which seemed most critical to them and which deserved significant attention in the future. A short list of the most important items was created.

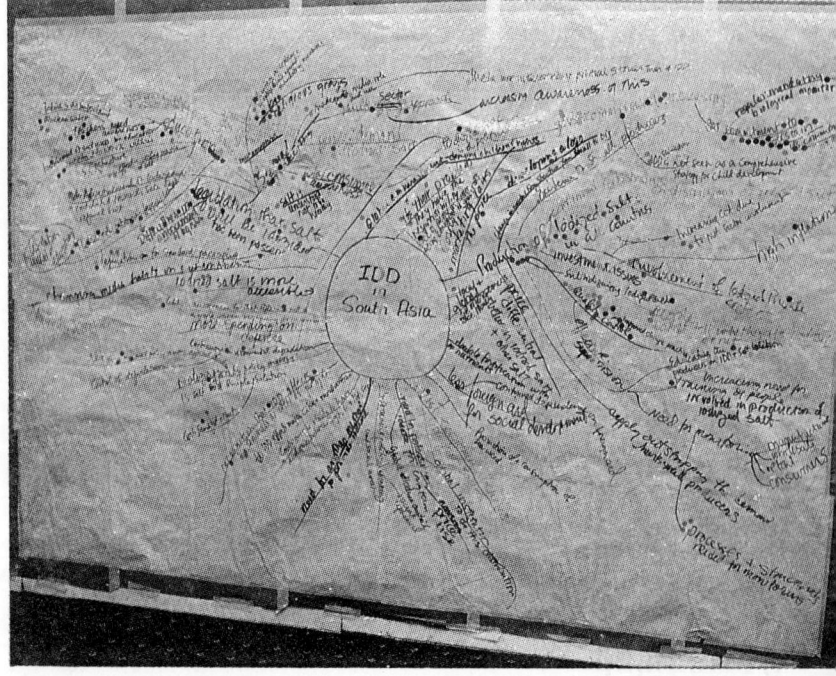

Fig. 23.3 The Mindmap.

ii) 'Prouds' and 'Sorries'

Meeting as country groups, participants were asked to list those efforts and achievements in eliminating IDD in their country about which they felt happiest (the 'prouds'). Things that had been done (or not done) in their country which they regretted were also listed (the 'sorries') For example, the Sri Lankan group was 'proud' of recent salt iodization legislation which took effect in January 1995, their technical expertise in salt iodization, and their ongoing national education programs on IDD. They 'felt sorry' that social marketing efforts had not reached many of the target groups, that there were inadequate buffer stocks of common salt for iodization, and that in many cases, salt manufacturers still do not comply with legislation.

Participants from Nepal were 'proud' of the political commitment at the highest level to eliminate IDD, their special IDD programs, data they have collected on IDD, and the fact that they have a single salt supplier. They 'felt sorry' that the delivery of salt is hampered by the landscape of Nepal, that salt is not indigenously produced, that the country is landlocked, and that salt iodization legislation in Nepal is inadequate.

The Indian delegation was 'proud' of the government's commitment to eliminate IDD, their technical expertise, and the database on IDD which exists in India. They 'felt sorry' that global methods for monitoring salt iodization have not yet been adopted, that salt is not packaged in small packets, and that some professional antagonism exists among those working on the issue of IDD.

Participants from Bhutan were 'proud' of the dramatic reduction in the prevalence of goitre and cretinism in their country, the effective regulatory measures that have been enacted, and the fact that iodized salt is available even in the most remote areas. They "felt sorry" about their late start in instituting a program to eliminate IDD.

The Bangladesh participants were 'proud' of the ordinance on universal salt iodization, the low-cost testing kits available for home and factory, and that salt iodizing machinery is produced locally and has been supplied to all 265 salt producers. They 'felt sorry' about the lack of monitoring of salt iodization, the lack of awareness about IDD, the lack of buffer stock, and the faulty import policy regarding salt.

Participants from Pakistan were 'proud' of their success in transforming the salt industry through private investments, the high level of political commitment in Pakistan, and their innovative ways of engaging private and public sector cooperation. They 'felt sorry' about the failure to respond quickly to misinformation about iodized salt that has been communicated, the lack of federal legislation, and that supply and demand are not well coordinated.

CIDA was "proud" of their growing budget and 'sorry' that CIDA staff see nutrition as welfare. WHO was 'proud' of their increased productivity and their role in facilitating national plans of action; they were 'sorry' to see their budgets decreasing. The group from UNICEF was 'proud' of the mid-decade goal of Universal Salt Iodization and that their involvement in IDD has not been marginalized. They regretted the misdirected emphasis on iodized oil capsules. Kiwanis was 'proud' of their decision to adopt the IDD project and 'felt sorry' about the time it has taken to get proper management underway. The participants for Myanmar were 'proud' of the involvement of private salt plants in iodization, the formation of multisectoral coordination in a target division, and the fact that health staff have been trained about IDD in 10 out of 14 divisions (states); they felt sorry that legislators have not been enlisted.

iii) Assessing Present and Desired Activities

The third step in the exploration of the present situation was for each stakeholder group to identify what they were presently doing to eliminate IDD and what they wished they were doing. Notes from the stakeholder groups follow.

Policymakers

This stakeholder group would like to see all government make a commitment to sustaining the elimination of IDD. They want budgets provided and resources allocated so that progress can be monitored. They would like to see national policies on nutrition, enforcement of existing laws, and a regional policy regarding the export and import of salt across national borders.

Government

In some or all of the participant countries, government officials are currently using the media to inform people about IDD, conducting workshops, advocating the elimination of IDD, distributing testing kits, using a logo for iodized salt, and enacting legislation. They would like to involve more religious leaders, social workers, and NGOs. They want iodized salt to be compulsory for both animal and human consumption. They would like to see iodized salt packaged in small bags and financial and technological help provided to all salt producers. They expressed a desire to assist with the development of effective monitoring systems.

Salt Industry

Although manufacturing practices (such as testing, record keeping, and storage) currently exist in many cases, this group of participants reported that they would like to see far more quality control and improvement in raw salt production techniques. They would like a better buffer stock of common salt to ensure supply, more efficient technology and more technology transfer.

NGOs

Presently, some NGOs are involved in activities such as sponsoring discussions, pushing for legislature, promoting awareness, promoting quality control, and distributing packets of iodized salt. This is not typical of all NGOs, however, and efforts are in adequate. Participants from the NGOs wished that there was agreement among them about the most important course of action to adopt. Fundamentally, they expressed the need to come to an agreement that they can do something about eliminating IDD.

Educators

Educators reported that they want to see awareness of IDD built into the curricula of schools at all levels, including activity-based use of iodized salt kits. They also believe that there is a need to educate and gain the commitment and cooperation of planners, producers, traders, consumers, and other groups.

The Future: Creating Scenarios

At this point, participants were given the task of coming to a consensus within their groups on the best pathway from the present situation to the goal of having sustained the elimination of IDD till the year 2010. After agreeing on the best path, they enacted for the entire conference their group vision of what the future will be like once IDD is eliminated and how the elimination of IDD will be achieved. Costumes, music, a bit of acting talent, and a lot of participant energy and enthusiasm made the eight scenarios thought provoking, spirited, and sometimes hilarious.

Visualizing the future and the steps towards it is one of the best ways of gaining confidence in one's abilities - much like how an athlete prepares for the Olympics by training her body and mind towards winning.

Common Ground and Promising Ideas

The next task was to determine what ideas were common to most or all of the stakeholder groups. Each group came up with a list of elements that had appeared in several of the scenarios on which they agreed and for which they would be willing to work. First two groups, then four groups, and then finally the entire conference came together and gradually developed a list of elements upon which everyone agreed. This list became 'Common Ground'. Other ideas that not everyone in the room could support were placed on the 'Promising Ideas' list.

Common Ground

- Demand quality iodized salt at production, retail, and consumer level.
- Improve quality control and management practices.
- Ensure that clean, iodized, packaged salt becomes the norm.
- Issue guidelines for proper storage of salt at the household level.
- Education involving teachers.
- Develop curricula about IDD for schools, including the use of test kits.
- Make test kits available and be sure testing is continued.
- Integrate IDD monitoring into other social monitoring programmes.
- Iodize all salt including that for animal consumption.
- License a logo to be used for the quality control of iodized salt.
- Establish standards for salt and communicate them to peer groups, families, schools, and health sectors.
- Enforce more existing laws about iodizing salt.
- Enact and strictly enforce needed legislation.
- Create an alliance between the private sector, governments, and NGOs to work on this issue.
- Develop a multisectoral approach to eliminating IDD.
- Obtain commitment to eliminating IDD at the highest political level exerting pressure.
- Establish global cooperation and international solidarity on IDD elimination and develop shared objectives.

Promising Ideas

- Work for acceptance of quality control concept by all salt producers.
- Assist with the transfer of technology among salt industries.
- Develop ways to provide assistance to small scale producers.- Improve the salt distribution/transport system.
- Develop efficient and cost-effective distribution systems for salt.
- Improve technology for storage of iodized salt.
- Develop policies to set the price of salt.
- Create a stable price for iodized salt.
- Communicate success stories about the 'elimination of hidden hunger'.
- Advocate IDD elimination referring to the UNs 'Rights for Children.'
- Clarify the message about why iodization is necessary.
- Develop appropriate safety messages on the use of iodized salt.
- Ensure that messages about iodization are specific and brief.
- Be certain that each slogan has only one message.
- Hold press conferences to sustain awareness.
- Involve religious leaders to promote iodized salt.
- Enlist popular personalities as IDD ambassadors.
- Acquire free time of TV and radio for coverage of IDD.
- Institute and IDD week or day.
- Use folk songs, puppet shows, theater, etc., for the promotion of iodized salt.
- Disseminate sub-district data on IDD control.
- Share information about progress broadly.
- Use modern technology to communicate about IDD, i.e. the Internet.
- Monitor a sample of school children for IDD (for every five years) using a clinical and biochemical monitoring system.
- Continuously monitor all government, school and households.

- Empower international body to monitor standards.
- Include IDD as part of a large nutrition and social contract.
- Utilize hand-held ultrasound for diagnosing goitre.
- Consider whether ICCIDD is redundant.
- Fortify salt with iron.

Action Planning

The third day of the conference was devoted to action planning. Participants worked in three configurations. First, they worked in stakeholder groups brainstorming possible collaboration across country boundaries. The next step was to work in their organization delegations and to begin the process of formulating specific strategies for their country organizations. Finally, a representative from each group discussed what needs to be done on a regional basis and how that can happen.

The plans that emerged must be seen as the first step of the action process. The notes from the various country and agency delegations are stated in this report but it is important to be aware that these are only preliminary plans. What is most critical is what happens after the conference.

Bangladesh

The delegation from Bangladesh recommended that their country:

i) Take a multisectoral approach to awareness building and monitoring of iodized salt.
ii) Strictly enforce laws regarding production and marketing of iodized salt.
iii) Increase the quality control of marketed salt.
iv) Use both traditional and non-traditional methods to communicate the IDD message.
v) Include materials on IDD and its causes in school curricula.

They suggested that their focus for the next six months be on:
- Assuring that all the salt factories produce iodize salt.
- Strengthening IEC activates using posters, handbills, flyers, etc.
- Developing networks among relevant partners on strategies to build awareness, monitor iodized salt, and provide information on IDD.

During the following eighteen months they hope to:

- Produce IDD films, T.V. spots, etc.
- Strengthen IDD surveillance as an element of the regular disease surveillance system.
- Establish a quality control system and monitor iodized salt at all levels.
- Include IDD and iodine related information in school curriculum as part of other health related issues.

They see barriers to the implementation of these plans coming from:
- Superstition and misconception
- Misinformation or lack of information
- Social and official inertia or sluggishness in accepting new ideas
- Other competing priorities
- 'Profit' motive of business groups

Bhutan

The group from Bhutan sees a four prong strategy as the best path for their country:

i) Universal salt iodization
ii) Education
iii) Monitoring
iv) Quality Control

In the coming months, they will inform the government of the need for:

- A nationwide assessment (two years) of IDD
- A revitalization of information/communication activities (two years)
- Inclusion of IDD in school curricula (two years)
- A review of IDD control programmes with ICCIDD (six months)
- A meeting of the stakeholders with UNICEF Bhutan to followup on this meeting.

India

The delegation from India will focus their efforts in six areas:

i) Assuring universal availability of standard powdered iodized salt in consumer packs.
ii) Enacting a comprehensive uniform law to prevent manufacture, sale, and use of non-iodized salt and supporting its strict enforcement.
iii) Increasing quality control.
iv) Taking a multisectoral approach to social marketing and increasing consumer awareness of IDD.
v) Monitoring progress through the examination of routine health statistics and administration of special surveys.
vi) Supporting compilation of statistics on the production, sale, and consumption of iodized salt.

In the next six months, they plan to:

- Increase advocacy efforts.
- Notify all states of the ban on non-iodized salt.
- Intensify effort to create a demand for iodized salt.
- Establish a monitoring system from production to consumption level.

- Involve small producers.
- Increase access to iodized salt.

Over the following eighteen months, they plan to:

- Review progress
- Enact legislation to make iodization of salt for animals compulsory.
- Enact legislation to make powdering and packaging of salt compulsory.
- Establish regional labs.
- Undertake surveys for elimination of IDD on pilot basis.
- Create several databases of the salt requirements of industry.

Nepal

Nepal's strategy consists of focusing on:

i) A multisectoral approach.
ii) Enacting laws and enforcing them.
iii) Developing a family-size package as the norm.
iv) Increasing quality control.
v) Monitoring salt production.
vi) Raising awareness through the media and in schools.
vii) Stabilizing the price of iodized salt.

Their first steps will be to form a national coordinating committee, to work on advocacy, and to promote legislation.

In 1995, they will also work on stabilizing prices, increasing national coverage, improving logistic support, establishing an effective monitoring system, and ensuring continuous mass awareness.

The group anticipates barriers to accomplishing their objectives coming from:

- a lack of financial resources
- social practices and taboos (i.e.. washing salt)

- the country's mountainous terrain, which makes transportation and distribution difficult.

Pakistan

The delegation from Pakistan plans to develop a strategy which is multisectoral and which forges alliances between government, NGOs, and the private sector. They see the private sector as important in regulating the supply and demand of salt and in quality control. They will also look into incorporating material on IDD into educational curricula and the expansion of the existing programs to include other micronutrients.

They plan to foster the enactment of legislation, support national seminars on quality control and fortification, support the development of monitoring systems, and work on getting IDD into school curricula.

Sri Lanka

The action planning of the delegation from Sri Lanka focused on several objectives:

i) Clean, iodized, packaged salt.
ii) Quality control and monitoring.
iii) Law enforcement.
iv) IDD in school curricula.
v) Alliances between private sector, government, and NGOs.
vi) Provision of time on T.V./radio.
vii) Perpetual commitment at the highest political level from informed public pressure.

In the next six months, they plan to work on achieving:

- Clean, iodized salt packets (the first step).
- Enforcing existing laws.
- Time on both radio and T.V. to talk about IDD.

Over the next eighteen months, they will turn to other issues, such as:

- Quality control and monitoring.
- IDD in school curricula.
- Creation of an alliances between the private sector, government, and NGOs.
- Securing the continuing commitment at the highest political level.

They expect that roadblocks to achieving their objectives will come from:

- resistance of private sector salt manufacturers.
- difficulties with the transfer of technology.
- lack of public awareness of the seriousness of the issue.

International Agencies

They key elements of the strategies of the international agencies are:

i) Law enforcement.
ii) IDD in school curricula.
iii) Inclusion of the monitoring of IDD within other social monitoring programs.
iv) Quality control management.
v) Use of modern technology in communication and sharing information.
vi) Advocacy based on ethical considerations.

Immediately:

* UNICEF will go to New York to meet Ms Carol Bellamy to convince her that UNICEF should continue to give priority to USI.
* WHO will finalize documentation on the safety of iodized oil.

* Kiwanis plans to conduct IDD workshops in Japan.
* MI will finalize its IDD Asia monitoring project, script writing, and advocacy material for Beijing.
* CIDA will finalize its IDD Asia monitoring component.

In the next six months the agencies have set the following goals:

* UNICEF will try to make CRC part of the UNICEF mission statement.
* WHO will prepare and disseminate guidelines and technical advice in support of the initiative.
* Kiwanis will increase its focus on their IDD project.
* MI will insert IDD into the agenda of the Beijing Women's
* Conference and provide technical support for monitoring, regional training, and access to databases.
* CIDA will remove 'emergency food aid' from its definition of nutrition.

Over the next two years:

* UNICEF will try to make nutrition, in all its forms, a top priority for UNICEF.
* WHO will stabilize political and financial support for micronutrient programs in WHO regions.
* Kiwanis will start planning for their next project.
* MI will continue database networking, increase access to the database, monitoring and training support, and encourage industry collaboration.
* CIDA will make health and nutrition a top priority.

ICCIDD

ICCIDD will focus its efforts in the coming year on advocacy; in particular, working to obtain political commitment within countries and at the international level. They will build alliances with other groups, including Kiwanis, private food producers, educators, and communicators. They will work for the advancement of scientific research and the application of technology. They will provide technical assistance for monitoring iodization, establish an independent evaluation system, and will provide training, using modern technology.

In the next six months, those from ICCIDD plan to:

* Adapt ICCIDD to respond to these needs.
* Insert IDD messages in major international forums.
* Produce further translations of the key manual.
* Develop their training system.

Regional Plans

The last part of the action planning process at the conference was to look at the possibility for regional cooperation in the campaign to eliminate IDD. The entire group agreed that a cooperative regional approach was necessary for the successful elimination of IDD. There was interest in focusing on price control in South Asia. Banning all trade of non-iodized salt and developing uniform standards for salt quality and iodization were also suggested. There was also a desire to regionalize training about IDD. The group agreed that the fundamental issue is political - not financial. The respective Ministers of Finance need not be pressured on this issue. People wondered if adding IDD to the school curriculum could be done on a regional basis. They also believe that existing structures, rather than newly created organizations, should be used to raise awareness of the issue. The idea of developing a working group of people from WHO and UNICEF in each of the six countries with assistance from ICCIDD was positively received. The working group would review progress and pool resources.

Outcomes of the Conference

As one attempts to assess the impact of this conference, it is clear that a completely accurate appraisal will only be possible after some time has passed, once intents begin to translate themselves into action and further into a substantial reduction in the prevalence of IDD in all the South Asian countries.

Renewed Commitment

The first conference objective was to renew the commitment of the participants to the goal of eliminating IDD by 2000. Many participants reported that they were inspired by the conference and are once again fully committed to the campaign to eliminate IDD. Many expressed this point on their evaluations of the conference. Others expressed it with much feeling during the 'open floor' closing session. A high level of involvement was demonstrated by the excellent attendance at every session and by the extraordinarily high levels of energy maintained by the group over the three days.

Alliances, Networks, and Linkages

The second and third stated objectives of the conference were to forge new alliances and linkages, and to facilitate interdisciplinary and intersectoral networking that will help sustain the elimination of IDD. This was achieved within the country delegations, between the different stakeholder representatives who worked with each other for the first time ever. The broader sense of a community working towards the same goal in the same country was encouraged. Multiple new relationships were formed, including contacts between those in ICCIDD, who have a long term investment in these issues, and others, like salt producers, educators, and representatives from NGOs for whom eliminating IDD is only one of dozens of other priorities. Plans crystalized for all the country groups to continue working on the issue back home with the help of appointed coordinators to initiate meetings. Using this approach of exploring a network of allies that many never new existed in a participatory and level environment will serve as a model for further collaborative efforts in each country.

In addition, all the participants had the opportunity to work with others from different countries that shared similar backgrounds, but that had different perspectives to offer, within the stakeholder groups. Participants learned from each other, traded ideas and strategies, and have resolved to continue to communicate across country borders and stakeholder boundaries.

Strategies

The fourth objective of the conference was to develop strategies for eliminating IDD and sustaining its elimination. Not only were country and agency strategies developed, but stakeholder groups also explored different kinds of strategies that were appropriate to them. While not all the key decision-makers were present in any country delegation, the fact that certain strategies were commonly espoused by most countries and the extent of the 'Common Ground' indicates that there is a growing consensus about what needs to happen. This consensus will guide all those involved in working for the elimination of IDD.

A major result of the conference was increased clarity that eliminating IDD is not a scientific or technical issue. Political and social actions are needed. Although this might have been apparent prior to attending the conference, it was blatantly obvious throughout the conference. This clarity of understanding will shape every individuals' thinking and the day-to-day priorities in the near future.

Discovering Common Ground

Another result of the conference was the discovery that there is a large amount of agreement about the best pathway to eliminate IDD. Rather than differing or conflicting views, there is consensus and a shared understanding of the seriousness of the issue and priorities. Before the conference, individuals did not know that so many others held views similar to their own. Others who knew little about IDD before the conference received an education about IDD and what must be done. For example, all groups see a major strategy for eliminating IDD to be the development of curricula for schools.

Optimism

Finally, the conference rekindled optimism as well as commitment. The campaign to eliminate IDD has been a long and slow process. Some of those involved reported that they came to the conference discouraged and frustrated. Bringing people from a dozen countries together for three days with the sole purpose of thinking about IDD transformed attitudes. As one lady participant said, 'To witness the deep caring of so many others about this issue gave me new hope. I am going home with renewed energy.'

Individual Actions

At the closing session, participants were asked to say what action steps they were going to take as individuals. Comments ranged from 'Tell my boss what I have learned,' to 'Inform the other salt producers in my country about why it is important to iodize salt.' Change happens by small but continued actions and decisions made by individuals. We expect the efforts of this meeting will inspire thousands of individual actions and the ripples from the conference will continue for many years.

Conclusion

The strategy for management of sustained IDD elimination focuses on three essential issues:

* Ensuring a high quality product (i.e., iodized salt with appropriate iodine levels)

* Ensuring that the management process is in place

* Monitoring and tracking biological progress with respect to IDD status

If the Partnership to End Hidden Hunger Conference is an ocean, then these are its waves:

- Commitment from allies who are currently not involved to include sustaining the elimination of IDD as a priority in their operations.
- Creation of a nucleus of persons from each country from a range of professions which can build the national demand for sustainability.
- Demonstration of the efficacy of mutual support by private and public sector entities to a public health venture
- Expanded comprehension of the potential for fortification of different foodstuffs.
- Opportunity for creating alliances for the larger goal of micronutrient malnutrition.
- Creation of potential for increased technical and other exchanges between countries

(including trade in micronutrient fortified products)

Alan Kay, who used to work at Apple and who invented the mouse once said, 'The best way to predict the future is to invent it.' This Future Search Conference on Partnership to End Hidden

Hunger - Collaboration of Stakeholders in Sustaining the Elimination of Iodine Deficiency Disorders was truly an event where a group of people addressed a serious problem and invented a better future for themselves and all of South Asia.

Dreams into Action

The third part to the Partnership to End Hidden Hunger Conference (post-Dhaka meeting) will take place within each 'South Asian' country. The objective of this meeting will be to assess the commitments made at Dhaka and the activities that have since taken place to meet these commitments. Further regular meetings and activities will continue to be charted at this point to ensure the maintenance of networks.

At the time of publication of this report, many countries had voluntarily sent in progress up dates made with respect to the short term action planning goals of the conference. The efforts of Nepal, Sri Lanka, and Maldives are examples of how the conference has already motivated action. All the other countries are also well on track.

Nepal

The Nepal team that attended the Partnership to End Hidden Hunger workshop has initiated a number of activities since their return from the conference. A meeting was held at the National Planning Commission (NPC) in April 1995 where a draft USI plan of action was developed in conjunction with the National Planning Commission (NPC), National Nutrition Coordinating Committee (NNCC), and UNICEF. Special focus was given to the logistical aspect of salt iodization, proper packaging and distribution, social mobilization and communication, and monitoring and evaluation. A Task Force to see that the proposed plan of action will be implemented as planned includes stakeholders from the NPC, Ministry of Health, STC, UNICEF, Radio Nepal, and NTV.

The NNCC has prepared a report on the status of IDD problem in Nepal and UNICEF has made available all its reports on IDD and iodized salt. Draft legislation on salt iodization is being revised by NPC with input from copies of legislation from other South Asian countries and will go to Parliament as soon as possible.

A second meeting was held in May 1995 at the NPC where the problems of 22 remote and inaccessible districts were discussed, including poor road conditions, remoteness, lack of warehousing facilities, poor packing, high goitre endemic area, costly air transport, supply meeting only 7-25% of demand, and iodized oil injections. Draft booklets, flyers, and posters for policy makers, health workers, teachers, salt traders, and general public were also reviewed for input. Near future action proposed on iodized salt includes: increasing the iodine content in salt to 50 ppm, increasing availability and accessibility of iodized salt, improving iodized oil capsules and transport subsidy until 1997 when USI will be more effective. Long term strategies discussed include: improving transport subsidy, banning bargara rock salt and non-iodized salt, and building roads.

A third meeting was scheduled for early June 1995 at the NPC.

Sri Lanka

One month after the Partnership to End Hidden Hunger Conference, a meeting of all parties concerned with salt iodization, marketing, distribution, monitoring, information, education, and training was held by the Deputy Minister of Finance, Planning, Ethnic Affairs, and National Integration (MFPE & NI) and other senior officials. Of particular importance was the explicit commitment of the 280 private salt manufacturers to iodize their salt with the support of the Ministry of Industrial Development. After initial reluctance to iodize salt, representatives of the private salt producers were entrusted with a UNICEF-supported salt iodization plant and potassium iodate. Concessions to motivate Puttalam manufactures to produce iodized salt will be made.

On the communications front, the Sarvodya started the process of disseminating information to all staff on the insights gained from the Partnership to End Hidden Hunger Meeting and to heigthen their awareness on IDD control. The Ministry of Health trained 81 Public Health Inspectors and Divisional Directors of Health Services in April and May 1995 on IDD information booklet in three languages were distributed to Public Health Midwives and health staff.

The 'Ending Hidden Hunger' videotape is being distributed to all 23 regional Directors of Health Services for advocacy and training programmes. A comprehensive salt iodine monitoring scheme using both field test kits and titration analysis will be fully operational by the end of 1995.

Major tasks planned include: provision of supplies and equipment to the Salt Industry to improve quality control, training programmes for Public Health Professionals, launching IDD media campaign, and creating awareness at the village level through Sarvodya.

Maldives

Although Maldives was not directly represented at the conference, those recommendations made for all of South Asia helped to motivate action in this country. Initially, it was assumed that IDD was not a public health problem in Maldives, however, a very recent survey has proved otherwise. The Department of Public Health in association with UNICEF undertook a countrywide survey in June-July 1995 to assess the prevalence of IDD and estimate urinary iodine levels in a sub-sample of the population. The survey adopted the 'EPI-30 cluster' methodology with sampling 30 clusters chosen from 200 islands. A total of 2834 school children (aged 6 to 12 years) were examined and the total goitre prevalence rate was estimated to be 23.6% (Grade 1 = 22.5% and Grade 2 = 1.1%). The median iodine level was found to be 6.7 micrograms/decilitre. Maldives imports its total requirement of salt from India, Sri Lanka, Thailand, and Singapore and so it is feasible to introduce iodized salt in the country. The experience of other South Asian countries can be applied to introducing an IDD control programme and getting all the stakeholders in this country involved.

Acknowledgement

The organizers of the Meeting would like to say 'Thank you' to the following:
Canadian International Development Agency (CIDA), International Council for Control of Iodine Deficiency Disorders (ICCIDD), Micronutrient Initiative (MI), United Nations Children's Fund (UNICEF), World Health Organization (WHO), Government of Bangladesh, Unicef Regional Office, Kathmandu, Unicef Bangladesh, IBIS Consulting Group, Cambridge, USA, Communica, Dhaka, Centre for Community Medicine, All India Institute of Medical Sciences, New Delhi, Dhaka Sheraton, Dhaka

Reference

The major portion of this chapter is based on the report submitted by Dr Katharine Esty and Dr. Gilbert Steil of Ibis Consulting Group Cambridge, U.S.A. The authors would like to thank them for their contribution.

24

Progress Towards Elimination of IDD - Excerpts from Publications of International Agencies (UNICEF, WHO, World Bank) and International Conference on Nutrition (ICN)

UNICEF

- Excerpt from The State of the Worlds Children 1995 a UNICEF publication

Promise and Progress

At the 1990 World Summit for children, the international community agreed on a series of specific and measurable goals for the protection of the lives, the health and the normal growth and development of children. The goals included a halving of child malnutrition, control of major childhood diseases, the eradication of polio and dracunculiasis, the elimination of micronutrient deficiencies, a halving of maternal mortality, the achievement of primary school education by at least 80% of children, the provision of clean water and safe sanitation to all communities, and the universal ratification of the Convention on the Rights of the Child. It was subsequently agreed that a set of intermediate goals should be achieved by the end of 1995.

'Three quarters of a million fewer children each year will be disabled, blinded, crippled, or mentally retarded.'

'Iodine deficiency has condemned millions of children to

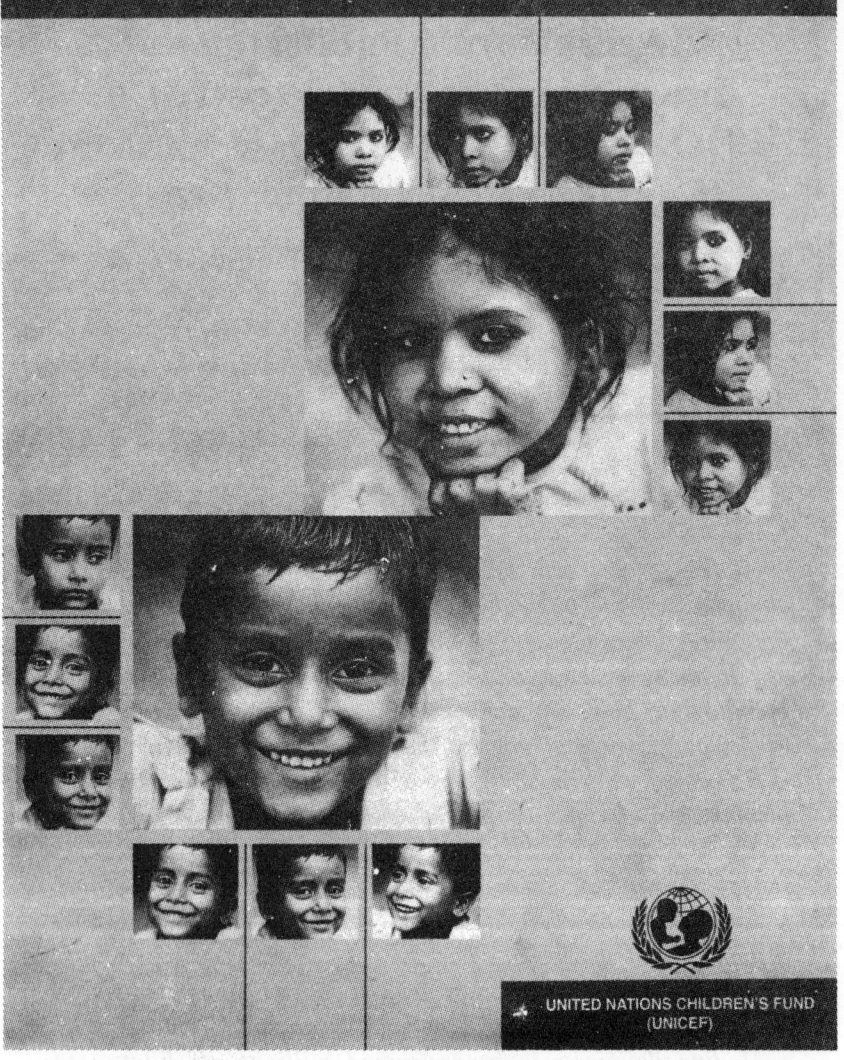

cretinism, tens of millions to mental retardation, and hundreds of millions to subtler degress of mental and physical impairment.'

'Today, as those children reach their fourth and fifth birthdays, their parents know only that their sons or daughters were born as cretins.'

In 1990, some 18 million women became pregnant while suffering from a little-known dietary disorder. In almost all cases those women did not know, and still do not know, what that problem was.

In approximately 60,000 cases, the damage caused was so severe that the foetus died or the infant survived for only a few hours.

For approximately 120,000 of those women, pregnancy and delivery proceed normally, and an apparently healthy baby was born. But in the first few months of life it became clear that all was not well. The infant was slow to respond to voices, and did not seem to recognize familiar faces. It was still possible to hope that there was nothing seriously wrong, but most of those mothers knew that a certain light that should have been there in the child's eyes is missing.

As these children reached the age of two, most had still not learned to walk. In some cases, the legs had never become fully extended, and the most the child could manage was a kind of awkward shuffle. Anxious comparisons were made with neighbours' children. Parent's tried to reassure each other by noting that some children develop more slowly that others. But with each passing day, the differences seemed less ignorable. Other family members started to make comments. Whispers began in the community.

Sometime in 1992 or 1993, when most of those children had still not learned to stand or to say their first words, the parents' fears were first mentioned to a health worker or doctor. Many were told to come back in three months. Others were referred to clinics or hospitals for tests. Many waited long months for the results.

All were eventually informed that their children were severely and permanently retarded.

Very few ever learned the cause - that a dietary deficiency in pregnancy had damaged the development of their child's central nervous system.

Today, as those children reach their fourth and fifth birthdays, their parents know only that their sons or daughters were born as cretins, and will remain so for the rest of their lives.

There are no statistics on the feelings experienced in those 120,000 homes on hearing this news. No records to capture the unwarranted shame of acknowledging the problem to husbands, parents, in-laws, neighbours. No figures to measure the courage with which those 120,000 families, almost all of them desperately poor, have set about coping with the practical and economic difficulties that severe mental retardation brings in its long wake.

The story does not end there. In approximately 1 million more of those pregnancies, early childhood appeared to proceed quite normally. But today, as those 1 million children reach school age, many are being found to have poor eye-hand coordination; others have become partially deaf, or have developed a bad squint, or a speech impediment, or other neuromuscular disorders.

In another 5 million or so cases, the parents may never know that there is anything specifically wrong. But if measurements could be taken as those children embark on their first year at primary school, all of them, even the brightest, would be found to have significantly lowered IQs. And in the years to come, they will merge into the estimated total of 75 million young people in the world today whose mental and physical development, and capacity for education, are impaired by the same problem—arising either from their own diets in childhood or from the diets of their mothers before and during pregnancy. Eventually they will be added to the estimated total of 150 million adults whose diminished mental alertness alertness and reduced physical aptitude mean that they are less able to meet their own and their families' needs./

Meanwhile, those most seriously affected, the 120,00 four- and five-year-old cretins born in 1990, will not be going to school at all. They will remain in the ranks of the dependent, eventually becoming part of the estimated 5.7 million people alive today who have been afflicted by cretinism from birth.[12]

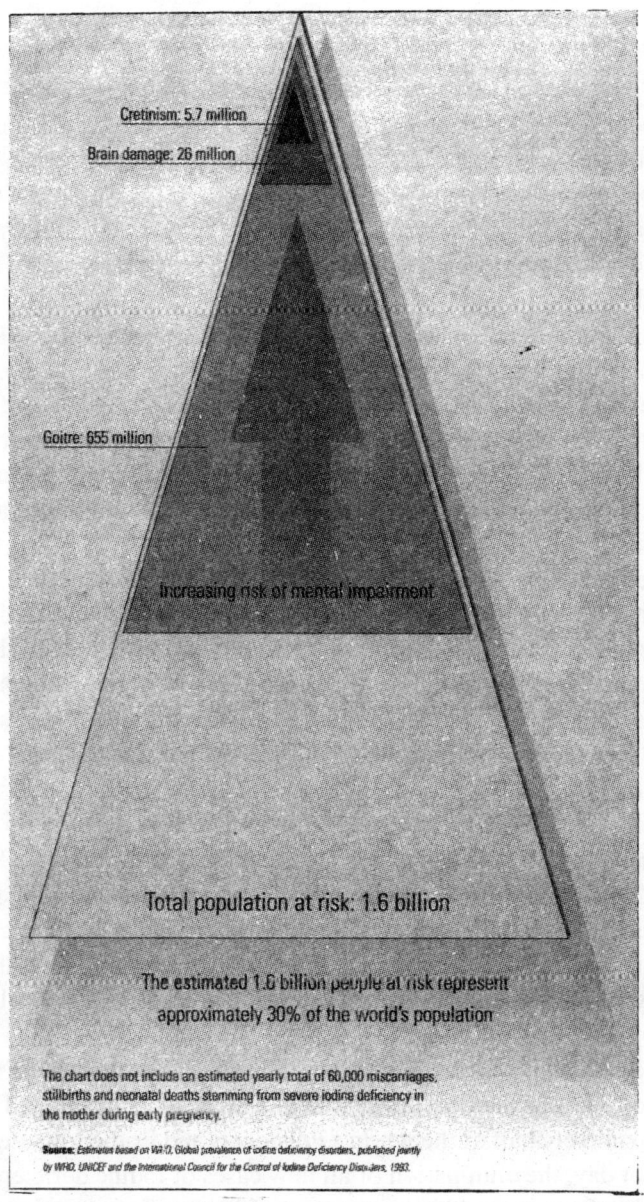

Fig. 24.1 The toll of iodine deficiency.
Estimated impact of iodine deficiency worldwide. Even mild goitre (thyroid gland enlargement) is associated with some degree of mental impairment.

Salt solution

The disorder which causes all of the above is the lack of minute amounts of iodine in the diet. The deficiency occurs mainly in hilly or flood-prone regions where iodine tends to be washed out of the soil, and the problems it gives rise to are collectively known as iodine deficiency disorders or IDD. In total, 1.6 billion people are at risk and 655 million suffer from goitre – the swelling of the thyroid gland at the throat which is the most obvious sign of IDD (fig.24.1.).

An inexpensive solution has been known for most of this century: iodine can be added to the one commodity that is consumed by all–common salt. That was how the problem was eradicated from most of the industrialized countries, led by Switzerland and the United States where edible salt supplies were iodized during the 1920s.

But in the developing world, the tragedy has been allowed to continue. And in the lifetime of most people reading this page, it has condemned millions of children to cretinism, tens of millions of mental retardation, and hundreds of millions to subtler degrees of metal and physical impairment.

The cost of salt iodization is approximately 5 US cents per person per year.

On 30 September 1990, the World Health Organization (WHO) and UNICEF confronted the world's political leaders with the challenge of salt iodization–along with several other equally powerful and equally inexpensive methods of preventing ill health, poor growth, and early death among many millions of the world's children.

The occasion was the World Summit for Children, held at the Headquarters of the United Nations in New York and attended by approximately half of the world's Presidents and Prime Ministers. On that day, the elimination of all new cases of iodine deficiency disorders by the year 2000 became one of 27 specific goals adopted by governments.[13]

To make that goal practicable, it was subsequently agreed that all countries would attempt the iodization of at least 95% of all salt supplies in each country by the end of 1995.

Just over four years later, what has been achieved?

Of the 94 countries with IDD problems, the great majority are now implementing national plans for the iodization of all salt and 58 are on track to achieve the goal of iodizing 95% of salt supplies by the end of 1995 (fig.24.2). Those 58 countries are home to almost 60% of the developing world's children. Another 32 countries could achieve the 1995 goal with an accelerated effort.

In the Middle East and North Africa, 10 out of 17 nations will have iodized all salt within the next 12 months. In Asia, 7 out of 20 countries (including Bangladesh and India) are within a year of universal iodization. In India, the legislation requiring iodization has been passed, a monitoring system is being set up in every state, the necessary equipment is in place in every major salt-works, and over 50% of all salt is already iodized. In Central and South America, all nations with the possible exception of Haiti are likely to iodize all salt by the end of 1995 (although an acceleration of progress will be required in Colombia, Paraguay, and Peru). Bolivia and Ecuador, the two South American countries with the worst history of IDD, are very close to eliminating the problem. Remarkably, salt iodization is also being achieved in 28 of the 39 affected nations is sub-Saharan Africa where all 16 nations of the Economic Community of West African States have also prohibited both the import and export of uniodized salt.

After taking such a toll on the mental and physical health of so many and for so long, the iodine problems is therefore now being forced to give ground. WHO and UNICEF have reasonable confidence that, in three or four years from now, the overall goal will be achived: no more infants will be born as cretins as a result of iodine deficiency; no more parents will suffer the long-drawn-out agony of discovering that their children are severely and permanently retarded; no more sons and daughters will be mentally and physically impaired by this age-old disorder.

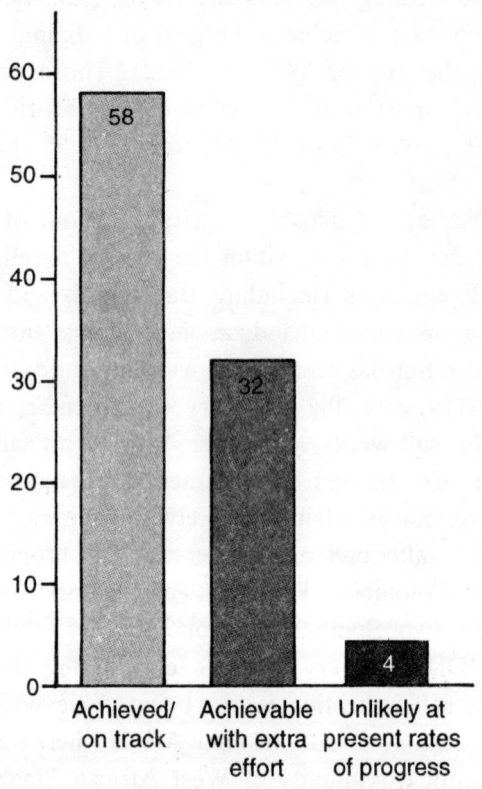

Source : *Country assessments by UNICEF field staff, for 94 countries, September 1994*

Fig. 24.2 Meeting the mid-decade goals.
Number of developing countries on track to achieve the mid-decade goal of iodizing at least 95% of salt in countries affected by iodine deficiency disorders.

Excerpts from The Progress of Nations, 1995 a UNICEF publication.

I welcome The Progress of Nations 1995 as a contribution to the cause of social development. This valuable publication records the practical progress being made by many States toward the goals that were established at the World Summit for Children, held at the United Nations in September, 1990. These impressive achievements are in large part the result of the commitments made on that occasion, and the subsequent sustained cooperation between Member States and the United Nations. In providing a detailed account of the deeds that have followed words, these pages provide an effective response to those who rightly ask for practical results from the convening of conferences and the setting of goals. They also show an aspect of the developing world– and of the work of the United Nations–which both needs and deserves wider acknowledgement.

Boutros Boutros-Ghali
Secretary-General of the United Nations

This is the third year in which UNICEF has issued this important document. It sets out for all to see the progress being made for children and women, in all regions of the world. Part of the record shows progress country by country, in relation to the goals agreed at the World Summit for Children held at the United Nations in 1940. Part relates to progress or set–backs in other areas of concern for child survival, protection and development. All is provided by UNICEF as a stimulus to us all–countries and communities, individuals and international organizations–to make the world a better place for all the world's children.

May I thank Peter Adamsoh, editor of The Progress of Nations, and his colleagues for once again providing UNICEF with a publication which brings into such sharp focus the advances and the set-backs in this struggle.

Carol Bellamy
Executive Director, UNICEF

THE PROGRESS OF NATIONS

The nations of the world ranked according to their achievements & in child health, nutrition, education, family planning, and progress for women

1995

Nutrition Achievement and Disparity

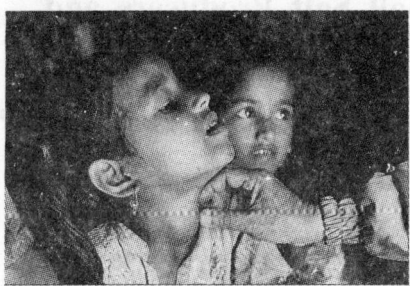

Bangladesh – swelling of the thyroid gland (goitre) is a visible sign of iodine deficiency

50 close on salt target

Lack of iodine in the diet has condemned millions of children to cretinism, tens of millions to mental retardation, and hundreds of millions to milder degrees of mental and physical impairment. In total, 1.6 billion people in over 100 countries are at some degree of risk. The solution – employed in Europe and North America since the 1920s – is to iodize all edible salt at a cost of about 5 cents per person per year.

At the beginning of the 1990s, most of the affected countries agreed to attempt the iodization of at least 90% of all edible salt by the end of 1995. With less than a year to go, about 50 countries have a realistic chance of reaching that goal. Many others will surpass the 80% mark – putting them in a good position to reach the year 2000 target of virtually eliminating iodine deficiency.

India, which produces over 5 million metric tons of salt a year, has made massive efforts in the 1990s and now iodizes about two thirds of its salt. Nigeria, Africa's most populous country, has reached the 90% target within the last 12 months.

Meanwhile, a recent analysis of 21 research studies has shown that moderate iodine deficiency is associated with an average reduction of over 13 IQ points.

The table to the right shows the percentages of domestic and imported salt iodized in countries affected by iodine deficiency.

The problem has not entirely disappeared from the industrialized nations. In Luxembourg, for example, average daily consumption of iodine is well below the recommended level, and a campaign is now under way to persuade all bakers in the Duchy to use iodized salt in bread.

Table salt
Iodine deficiency disorders can be eliminated by iodizing all salt.

	% salt iodized		% salt iodized
Sub-Saharan Africa			
Cameroon	100	Niger	1
Nigeria	96	Angola	0*
Kenya	95	Benin	0
Rwanda	90	Burkina Faso	0
Burundi	80	Côte d'Ivoire	0*
Zambia	50	Guinea-Bissau	0
Sierra Leone	43	Mali	0
Tanzania	32	Namibia	0*
C. African Rep.	20	Togo	0
Middle East and North Africa			
Iraq	91	Syria	18*
Libya	90	Jordan	2
Algeria	80	Egypt	1
Iran	70	Morocco	0
Turkey	31	Yemen	0
South Asia			
Bhutan	100	Nepal	18
India	65	Pakistan	11
Bangladesh	18	Sri Lanka	4
East Asia and Pacific			
Thailand	50*	Myanmar	7
Viet Nam	24	Mongolia	0
Philippines	17		
Latin America and Caribbean			
Panama	95*	Chile	76
El Salvador	92*	Honduras	67*
Bolivia	90	Venezuela	65*
Peru	90	Paraguay	48
Ecuador	85	Dominican Rep.	2*
Brazil	84	Cuba	0*
Guatemala	80*		
Countries in transition			
Macedonia	100	Kazakhstan	10*
Yugoslavia	80	Ukraine	4*
Croatia	75	Romania	0
Belarus	37*	Russian Fed.	0
Tajikistan	32*	Turkmenistan	0*
Hungary	10	Uzbekistan	0

*Figures for iodized salt may include salt which is imported.
Note: Only countries with salt iodization data not abstained.
Source: Updated from UNICEF Nutrition Section, Progress towards universal salt iodization, December 1994.

19 nations still have no salt legislation

As at March 1995, there are 19 countries which are known to have iodine deficiency problems but which still have no legislation on salt iodization.

In most countries that have defeated iodine deficiency disorders, legislation has been a necessary but not sufficient condition. Educating consumers to choose iodized salt, and regular checks on salt producers, are also needed.

As in health or schooling, the list again shows that the countries that lag furthest behind are often those that are or have been affected by armed conflict or political turmoil.

Several of the world's poorest countries, including Bhutan, Bolivia, Cameroon, Kenya and Nigeria, have succeeded in iodizing the majority of salt consumed.

No salt laws

Afghanistan	Liberia
Albania	Lithuania
Azerbaijan	Mali
Cambodia	Mauritania
Estonia	Moldova
Fiji	Mongolia
Georgia	Mozambique
Haiti	Niger
Kyrgyzstan	Togo
Latvia	

Source: Updated from UNICEF Nutrition Section, Progress towards universal salt iodization, December 1994.

Pakistan takes legal action

In the last few years, Pakistan has shown that it is possible for a large low-income country to move rapidly towards universal salt iodization.

Half of the nation's 130 million population are thought to be at risk. But in the severely affected north, consumption of iodized salt has jumped from 10% to 80% in less than a year.

A bill now before Parliament is expected to make salt iodization compulsory nationwide. "*The bill will have far-reaching effects on health and the quality of life,*" says the UNICEF office in Islamabad.

Even before the new law comes into effect, 468 salt producers have been identified, of which 232 have ordered the necessary machinery for adding iodine, and 157 are already producing iodized salt.

Consumers as well as producers are being targeted. Thousands of billboards, banners and posters are urging people to choose iodized salt – a message reinforced by mass media, health and immunization workers, schoolteachers, religious leaders, and local community organizations.

The new law is the result of many years of work by the Ministry of Health, WHO, UNICEF, the Programme Against Micronutrient Malnutrition, and the International Council for the Control of Iodine Deficiency Disorders.

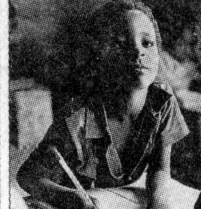

Without salt legislation, iodine deficiency can invisibly lower learning ability

Flow chart on strategies for small producers to iodize salt.
- Reproduced from Small Salt Producers and Universal Salt Iodisation a UNICEF Publication.

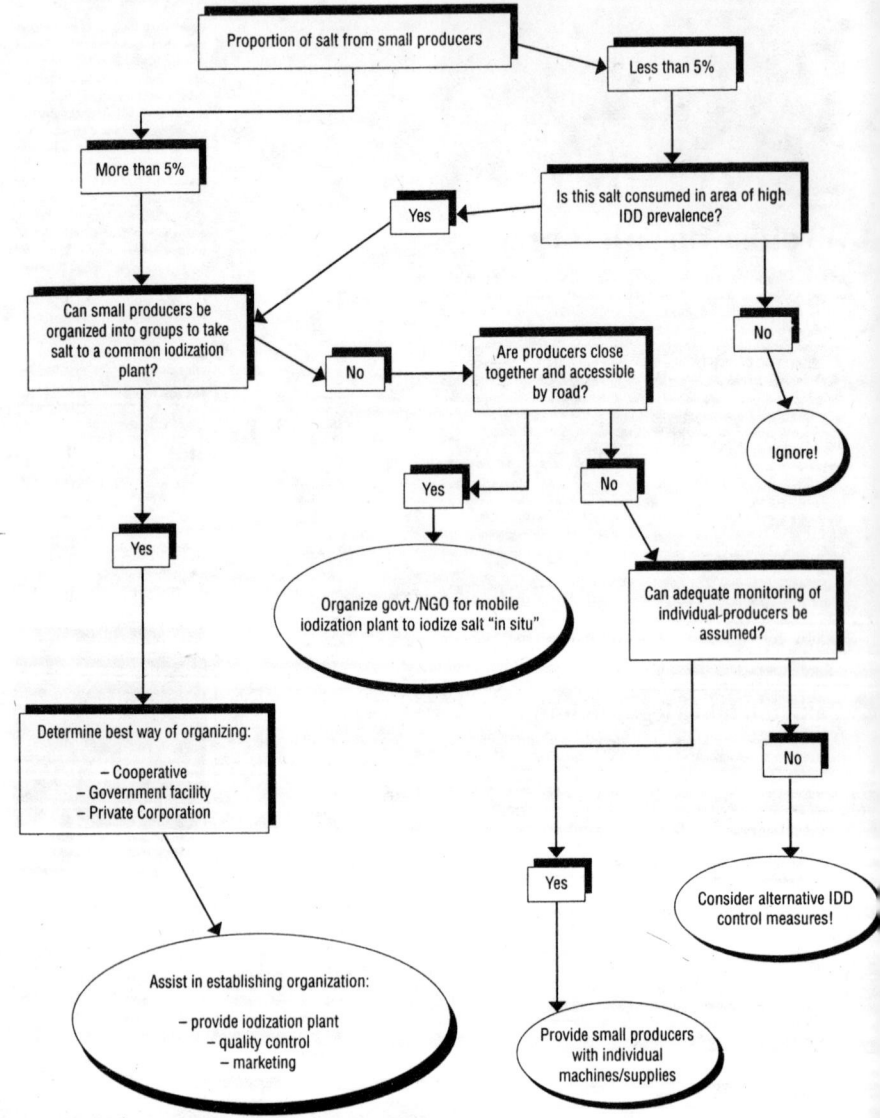

WHO

Forty-Third World Health Assembly
WHA 39.31

The Forty-third world Health Assembly,
Having considered the report of the Director-General on infant and young child nutrition, in particular regarding the progress achieved in preventing and controlling iodine deficiency disorders;
Recalling resolution WHA39.31 on the prevention and control of iodine deficiency disorders;

1. Commends governments, intergovernmental and bilateral agencies and nongovernmental organizations, in particular the International Council for Control of Iodine Deficiency Disorders:

(1) on their efforts to prevent and control iodine deficiency disorders and to support related national, regional and global initiatives;

(2) on the encouraging progress achieved since 1986, through joint activities in many countries, towards the elimination of iodine deficiency disorders as a major public health problem throughout the world;

2. Decides that, in view of the progress already achieved and the promising potential of current and planned national prevention and control programs, WHO shall aim at eliminating iodine deficiency disorders as a major public health problem in all countries by the year 2000;

3. Urges Member States to continue to give priority to the prevention and control of iodine deficiency disorders through appropriate nutrition programs as part of primary health care;

4. Requests that the Joint FAO/WHO Expert Committee on Food Additives verify the effectiveness and safety of the long-term use of potassium iodide and potassium iodate to fortify salt for the prevention and control of iodine deficiency disorders;

5. Requests the Director-General:

(1) to continue to monitor the incidence and prevalence of iodine deficiency disorders;

(2) to reinforce the technical support provided to Member States, on request, for assessing the most appropriate approaches to preventing and controlling iodine deficiency disorders;

(3) to mobilize additional technical and financial resources to permit those Member States in which iodine deficiency disorders are still a significant problem to develop or expand their programs for the prevention and control of these disorders;

(4) to report to the Health Assembly by 1996 on progress achieved in preventing and controlling iodine deficiency disorders.

Forty-Fifth World Health Assembly
WHA 45.33

National Strategies for Overcoming Micronutrient Malnutrition

The Forty-fifth World Health Assembly,

Having considered the report of the Director-General on national strategies for overcoming micronutrient malnutrition;

Recalling resolutions WHA39.31 and WHA43.2 on iodine deficiency, resolutions WHA22.29, WHA25.55, WHA28.54 and WHA37.18 on vitamin A deficiency and xerophthalmia, resolutions WHA38.27 and WHA40.27 relating to maternal anaemia, and resolution WHA44.33 recognizing the goals for the 1990s endorsed by the World Summit for Children, which include the virtual elimination of iodine deficiency disorders and vitamin A deficiency, and a substantial reduction in iron deficiency anaemia;

Recognizing the great human suffering and the important health and socioeconomic problems caused by micronutrient deficiencies, especially brain damage and mental retardation from iodine deficiency, childhood blindness and increased mortality from vitamin A deficiency, and retarded physical and mental development, low birth weight and maternal mortality from iron deficiency;

Concerned about the large numbers of people at risk, estimated at 1000 million for iodine deficiency, 190 million for vitamin A deficiency and over 2000 million for nutritional anaemia;

Aware of the success of strategies for overcoming micronutrient malnutrition which include dietary diversification and supplementation, food fortification, and specific public health measures for the control of related human infection and infestation with parasites;

Aware of the need to build on the experience of the past decade to accelerate and intensify specific activities and integrated approaches in regard to micronutrient malnutrition in order to achieve concrete results in countries in the short term,

1 URGES Member States:

(1) to strengthen the activities recommended in the report and integrate them in their national health and development programmes, taking into account any recommendations that may be made to this effect by the International Conference on Nutrition;

(2) to establish, where appropriate, a focal point and coordinating mechanism to promote and intergrate activities in common for the control of iodine deficiency disorders, vitamin A deficiency and nutritional anaemia;

(3) to establish, as part of the health and nutrition monitoring system, a micronutrient monitoring and evaluation system capable of assessing the magnitude and distribution of these micronutrient deficiency disorders, and monitoring the implementation and impact of control programmes, and to report as appropriate to WHO thereon;

(4) to mobilize the necessary human, technical and financial resources to ensure the successful implementation of national activities to overcome micronutrient malnutrition;

2 REQUESTS the Director-General:

(1) to prepare guidelines on national strategies for prevention and control of micronutrient deficiencies;

(2) to establish as part of the WHO nutrition data base a global micronutrient deficiency information system comprising data on iodine deficiency, vitamin A deficiency and nutritional anaemia;

(3) to encourage the establishment of regional mechanisms, such as task forces and working groups, for catalysing and providing technical support to national programmes, and promoting cooperation among countries;

(4) to encourage effective cooperation among the agencies concerned–international, bilateral and nongovernmental–and the scientific bodies of experts in the fields of iodine, vitamin A and iron deficiencies;

(5) to continue to disseminate information among countries and to provide technical support and training in the prevention and control of micronutrient malnutrition;

(6) to support operational research on integrated methods of assessing and combating micronutrient deficiencies;

(7) to mobilize additional technical and financial resources for intensified support to Member States.

Forty-Sixth World Health Assembly
WHA 46.7

International Conference on Nutrition: Follow-Up Action

The Forty-sixth World Health Assembly,

Having considered the report of the Director-General on the International Conference on Nutrition and the consequent proposed WHO strategy for supporting nutrition action at all levels;

Commending Member States, organizations of the United Nations system and other intergovernmental and nongovernmental organization concerned for their participation in the preparatory process and in the International Conference itself, and for their pledge to follow it up;

Commending the Director-General for his effective collaboration with other organizations of the United Nations system, especially

FAO, in organizing the International Conference and for according high priority to nutrition by allocating additional resources, in particular for those countries most in need,

1. ENDORSES in their entirety the World Declaration and Plan of Action for Nutrition adopted by the Conference;[1]

2. URGES Member States:

(1) by the year 2000, to strive to eliminate famine and famine-related deaths, starvation and nutritional deficiency diseases in communities affected by natural and man-made disasters, and in particular iodine and vitamin A deficiencies;

(2) by the year 2000, to reduce substantially the prevalence of starvation and widespread chronic hunger; undernutrition, especially among children, women and old people; iron deficiency anaemia; foodborne diseases; and social and other impediments to optimal breast-feeding; and to remedy inadequate sanitation and poor hygiene;

(3) to contain and reduce the rising prevalence of diet-related diseases and conditions related to them;

(4) to develop, or strengthen as appropriate, plans of action setting out national nutritional goals and how they are to be achieved in keeping with the objectives, major policy guidelines and nine action-oriented strategies that were elaborated in the Plan of Action adopted by the International Conference on Nutrition, which also endorsed the nutritional goals of the Fourth United Nations Development Decade and of the World Summit for Children;

(5) to ensure the implementation of plans of action which:

(a) incorporate nutrition objectives into national development policies and programmes;

(b) strengthen measures in various sectors to improve nutrition through governmental mechanisms at all levels, especially district development plans, and in collaboration with nongovernmental organizations and the private sector;

---

[1] International Conference on Nutrition. World Declaration and Plan of Action for Nutrition. Rome, December 1992, Food and Agriculture Organization of the United Nations and World Health Organization.

(c) include community-based measures, particularly through primary health care activities, for nutritional improvement that are crucial if full and sustainable benefits are to be obtained for all people;

(d) are sustainable in the long term and contribute to protection of the environment;

(e) enlist the cooperation of all groups concerned;

3. CALLS UPON organizations of the United Nations system, other intergovernmental and nongovernmental organizations and the international community as a whole:

(1) to renew their commitment to the achievement of the objectives and strategies set out in the World Declaration and Plan of Action for Nutrition including, to the extent that their mandates and resources allow, technical cooperation and financial support to recipient countries;

(2) to reinforce and foster concerted action at all levels for the establishment and implementation of national plans of action in nutrition with a view to attaining health and nutritional well-being for all;

4. REQUESTS the Director-General:

(1) to support Member States in establishing and implementing national plans of action for nutritional improvement that emphasize self-reliance and community-based action, especially as regards their health-related aspects;

(2) to reinforce WHO's capacity for food and nutrition action in all relevant programmes, so that increased emphasis can be given as a priority to maternal, infant and young child nutrition, including breast-feeding; micronutrient malnutrition; nutrition emergencies (particularly training in preparedness and management); monitoring of nutritional status; control of diet-related chronic diseases; food safety control and the prevention of foodborne diseases; and research and training in subjects related to food and nutrition, including health implications of the misuse of chemicals and hormones in agriculture;

(3) to give priority to least developed, low income, and drought-affected countries, and to provide support to Member States in

establishing national programmes, especially those concerned with nutritional well-being of vulnerable populations, including women and children, refugees and displaced persons;

(4) to stimulate regional exchange of ideas and plans;

(5) to report on progress in implementation by Member States of the World Declaration and Plan of Action for Nutrition to the Health Assembly in 1995 as stated in the Plan of Action

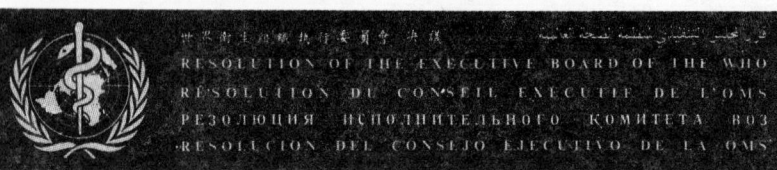

Ninety-third Session **EB93.R20**
Agenda items 23.1, 23.2 and 23.3 26 January 1994

Collaboration with nongovernmental organizations
Report of the Standing Committee on Nongovernmental Organizations

The Executive Board,

Having examined the reports of its Standing Committee on Nongovernmental Organizations,

1. DECIDES to establish official relations with the following nongovernmental organizations:
   International Commission on Non-ionizing Radiation Protection
   International Consultation on Urological Diseases
   International Council for Control of Iodine Deficiency Disorders
   International Occupational Hygiene Association
   International Society for Preventive Oncology
   International Society of Surgery

2. DECIDES to postpone consideration of the application of the International Association of Technicians for the Health Sciences for a period of one year during which working relations should continue, recommending further that when reapplying the Association should delineate clearly its activities and specific areas of competence;

3. DECIDES to postpone consideration of the application of the European Centre for Ecotoxicology and Toxicology of Chemicals and requests that working relations be continued for a further two-year period;

4. DECIDES to postpone consideration of the application of the World Federation of Chiropractic, working relations being continued for a further two-year period to enable a strengthening of collaboration, and recommends that when reapplying the Federation should clearly describe and demonstrate the extent and practical nature of its activites and their work for the ideals of WHO;

5. DECIDES to postpone consideration of the application of the Council on Health Research for Development, in the light of its recent establishment, working relations being continued for a further two-year period;

6. DECIDES that, while welcoming the interest shown by the organization in collaborating with WHO when viewed in the light of its aims and activities as contained in its application, it was not appropriate at this time to establish official relations with Public Services International;

7. DECIDES to readmit into official relations the World Medical Association.

Fourteenth meeting, 26 January, 1994
EB93/SR/14

World Bank

Excerpts from Development in Practice - Enriching Lives - Overcoming Vitamin and Mineral Malnutrition in Developing countries A World Bank Publication

Executive Summary

The control of vitamin and mineral deficiencies is one of the most extraordinary development-related scientific advances of recent years. Probably no other technology available today offers as large an opportunity to improve lives and accelerate development at such low cost and in such a short time.

Dietary deficiencies of vitamins and minerals–life–sustaining nutrients needed only in small quantities (hence,'micronutrients') –cause learning disabilities, mental retardation, poor health, low work capacity, blindness, and premature death. The result is a devastating public health problem: about 1 billion people, almost all in developing countries, are suffering the effects of these dietary deficiencies, and another billion are at risk of falling prey to them.

To grasp the enormous implications at the country level, consider a country of 50 million people with the levels of micronutrient deficiencies that exist today in South Asia. Such a country would suffer the following losses each year because of these deficiencies:

- 20,000 deaths
- 11,000 children born cretins or blinded as preschoolers
- 1.3 million person-years of work lost due to lethargy or more severe disability
- 360,000 student-years wasted (3 percent of total student body).

Enriching Lives

Overcoming Vitamin and Mineral Malnutrition in Developing Countries

> "No other technology offers as large an opportunity to improve lives... at such low cost and in such a short time..."

A WORLD BANK PUBLICATION

In terms of losses by type of deficiency, more than 13 million people suffer night blindness or total blindness for the lack of vitamin A. In areas without adequate iodine in the diet, five to ten offspring of every 1,000 pregnant women are dead upon birth or soon thereafter due to iodine deficiency. Severe iron deficiency causes as many as one in five maternal deaths, as well as the death of about 30 percent of children who enter the hospital with it and do not get a blood transfusion (those who do get the transfusion are exposed to other risks).

The World Bank's World Development Report 1993 found micronutrient programs to be among the most cost-effective of all health interventions. Most micronutrient programs cost less than $50 per disability-adjusted life-year (DALY) gained. Deficiencies of just vitamin A, iodine, and iron–the focus of this book–could waste as much as 5 percent of gross domestic product, but addressing them comprehensively and sustainably would cost less than 0.3 percent of gross domestic product (GDP).

The Need for a Comprehensive Approach

The alleviation of poverty and the strengthening of national care systems alone cannot solve the problem of micronutrient deficiencies. Because the micronutrient content of foods is a hidden property, consumers do not automatically demand micronutrient-rich foods with increased income. Thus, food and agriculture policies need to watch over not only the quantity but the nutritional quality of the food supply and promote the production, marketing and consumption of micronutrient-rich foods. Likewise, safety net programs, including refugee feeding, must respond to the total nutritional needs of target groups and not just to their calorie and protein needs.

An overall improvement in health system management will go a long way toward improving micronutrient malnutrition as long as programs train and monitor medical personnel for the prevention and management of micronutrient deficiencies, reach groups not currently using the health care system, and, through teaching and persuasion, transform consumers into a constituency for healthful diet.

Three Types of Approaches

Even with the most nutritionally enlightened economic development plan, developing countries must still take direct aim at micronutrient malnutrition through consumer education, aggressive distribution of pharmaceutical supplements, and the fortification of common foodstuffs or water.

Fortunately, all of these options are inexpensive and cost-effective. The particular mix of interventions chosen depends on country conditions. But the key constraints to achieving the summit goals are a lack of awareness and commitment of policymakers and consumers, a weak capacity to deliver supplements and education, and a lack of enforcement of industry compliance with fortification laws.

Social Mobilization

Policymakers must be motivated to take action against micronutrient malnutrition. They need persuasive information on the economic and social costs of micronutrient malnutrition and on the political salience and cost-effectiveness of micronutrient programs. Then, during implementation, good management information systems and public education programs designed into the overall initiative can make the public aware of the improvements resulting from the micronutrient programs and draw the connection to the responsible program managers and policymakers. That conection provides public support and reward for the initiative of the political leaders.

Beyond the immediate political feedback they provide, programs to educate, persuade, and change the behavior of consumers are essential to the long run elimination of micronutrient deficiencies. Subconscious consumer demand for micronutrients needs to be made conscious and directed to appropriate foods and pharmaceuticals. This demand will serve as a 'pull' factor to bring the target groups to distribution points for supplements, to overcome resistance, and, if necessary, to induce consumers to pay a little more for a better (that is, a fortified, although unfamiliar) diet. Social marketing of micronutrients and micronutrient-rich foods is necessary in virtually all developing countries, even where health service delivery is good and the food industry is well developed.

Pharmaceutical Supplementation

Two key problems in pharmaceutical supplementation have been poor coverage of at-risk groups and inadequate supply management. To overcome the coverage problem, the delivery of supplements must break out of a single-clinic-based track and employ every possible avenue of convenience and opportunity, including school visits, workplace programs, and nutritional safety net programs.

The goals of supply management are to procure effective supplements that look appealing, have helpful packaging and labelling, come in the right doses, and are affordable; to store and transport them for maximal quality and preservation; and to deliver them to well-selected distribution points in adequate numbers of doses at an appropriate frequency. Achieving these goals requires committed program leaders, motivated and well-trained workers, good monitoring and surveillance, and a demanding public. The private pharmaceuticals market may have an important role to play in developing new products and delivering supplements in a cost-effective manner at the community level.

Effective Regulation and Incentives for the Private Food Industry

The food industry responds to both positive and negative policy signals. Broad legislation, followed by technical regulations, should require micronutrient fortification of basic foodstuffs and support a fair and honest regulatory system that monitors compliance and punishes the noncompliant.

This legislation should be joined by financial and political inducements to industry. Some of the incentives used in effective fortification programs have been tax relief, import licenses, loans for equipment, subsidies on fortificants, and positive press coverage.

A third component of any successful food control system is consumer awareness and pressure for industry compliance. Consumers can be mobilized through social marketing and consumer organizations to demand effective fortification. Without confidence in both the industry and the regulatory apparatus, enlightened consumers will not be willing to buy new products.

Developing Nutritional Awareness and Habits

Political sustainability comes from monitoring and communications as well as satisfaction of consumer demands. One of the greatest advantages of micronutrient programs is that, because results are unambiguously attributable to specific interventions, policymakers can take credit for improvements.

Operational sustainability depends upon good management, continual overseeing, the retraining of personnel, and the supervision of delivery systems (particularly the health system and food industry).

Behavioral sustainability is a function of national and household ability to pay. Micronutrients are so inexpensive that, regardless of the form, they should ultimately be affordable by the intended beneficiaries. For equity reasons or in the sort term, some form of targeted subsidy may be necessary to reach the poorest and to form habits among the desired beneficiaries. In the long run, however, financial sustainability will depend sustainability will depend upon consumers' willingness to pay for the nutrients. It is the government's responsibility to choose the most cost-effective means of delivering micronutrients to the population.

The Need for External Start-up Support

Micronutrient interventions are among the most cost-effective investments in the health sector. Because fortification of water and foods is also extremely cost-effective, nontraditional sector involvement is desirable as well. Donors have a key role to play in assisting with program design and financing. Addressing micronutrient deficiencies globally will require an estimated $1 billion per year–about $1 per affected person (all dollar amounts are U.S. dollars). That figure is equivalent to the economic costs of endemic deficiencies of vitamin A, iodine, and iron in a single country of 50 million people. Most of these costs will ultimately be borne by consumers when purchasing food with higher nutritional quality.

In the short run, however, donors and governments may have to assume a major financial burden for project preparation, start-up costs, and recurrent costs in the early years. The economic and social payoffs from micronutrient programs reach as high as 84 times the program costs. Few other development programs offer such high social and economic payoffs.

INTERNATIONAL CONFERENCE ON NUTRITION

Rome, December 1992

WORLD DECLARATION AND PLAN OF ACTION FOR NUTRITION

Excerpts from The International Conference on Nutrition: (ICN) World Declaration and Plan of Action for Nutrition, Rome, December, 1992.

World Declaration on Nutrition (Paragraph 19)

19. As a basis for the plan of Action for Nutrition and guidance for formulation of national plans of action, including the development of measurable goals and objectives within frames, we pledge to make all efforts to eliminate before the end of this decade:

- famine and famine-related deaths;
- starvation and nutritional deficiency diseases in communities affected by natural and man-made disasters;
- iodine and vitamin A deficiencies.

We also pledge to reduce substantially within this decade:

- starvation and widespread chronic hunger;
- undernutrition especially among children, women and the aged;
- other important micronutrient deficiencies, including iron;
- diet-related communicable and non-communicable diseases;
- social and other impediments to optimal breast-feeding;
- inadequate sanitation and poor hygiene, including unsafe drinking-water.

References

Development in Practice Enriching Lives Overcoming Vitamin and Mineral Malnutrition in Developing Countries. 1994. A World Bank Publication.

Forty-Third World Health Assembly Resolution WHA43.2, May 1990.

Forty-Fifth World Health Assembly Resolution WHA45.33, Agenda item 21, Thirteenth Plenary meeting A45/VR/13, May 1992.

Forty-Sixth World Health Assembly Resolution WHA46.7, Agenda item 18.2, Eleventh Plenary meeting A46/VR/11, 1993.

International Conference on Nutrition. World Declaration and Plan of Action for Nutrition. Rome, December 1992, Food and Agriculture Organization of the United Nations and World Health Organization.

UNICEF, 1995. The Progress of Nations.

UNICEF, 1995. The State of the World's Children.

UNICEF New York, November 1994. Small Salt Producers and Universal Salt Iodisation, Nutrition Section.

Index

Africa, 4, 47, 52, 104, 117
assessment of IDD problem, 179-180
national programme for IDD in, 177-203
Africa, Eastern and Southern
IDD and its control programme in, 52, 235-55
IDD belt in, 238-9
see also specific countries in
Africa, Western and Central
IDD and its control programme, 242-48
see also Algeria, Cameroun, Mali, Zaire
African Task Force, 1, 178, 184
Afghanisthan, 259
Agencies (bilateral) for IDD programmes, 72-4
Algeria, 121, 242-44
All China Women's Association, 174
All India Institute of Medical Sciences, 195
Annals of Allergy, 361
Argentina, 325
See also Latin America
Ashgabad, 160
Asia, 4, 9-14, 104
goitre control in, 195-98
national programmes for IDD in, 190-98
see also South East Asia and specific countries in
Asian Congress of Nutrition
4th, 37
6th, 298
Association of South-East Asian Nations (ASEAN), 113
Australian, 32, 58, 72
Australian International Development Assistance
Azerbaijan, 259-60

Bureau (AIDAB), 37-8, 72-3, 298
Bangladesh, 6, 60, 104, 113-4, 193-4, 413-4
Bangladesh Small Industries Corporation, 114
Belgium, 58, 72
Bhutan, 69, 115, 116, 117, 130, 192, 194, 414-5
Bolivia, 11, 17, 69, 114, 115, 116, 117, 123, 126, 328-9
See also Latin America
Brazil, 115, 116, 330
See also Latin America
Bureau of Endemic Diseases Contorl, 299, 300

Cattle, 384
Cameroun, 47, 104, 244
See also Africa, Western and Central
Canada, 21, 32, 58, 73
Canadian International Development Agency (CIDA), 38, 274
Center for Diseases Control, 214
Central Leading Group for Endemic Diseases Control (China), 295-99
Child Survival and Safe Motherhood (CSSM), 191
Chernobyl, 363
China, 159

Index

cretinism in, 10, 23, 46, 104, 114
IDD in, 70, 72, 293-302
impact of iodine deficiecny in, 60
medical colleges dealing with IDD problem in, 296-9
Chinese Disabled Person's Federation, 60
CIDA, 401
Columbia, 327
Cretinism, 10-2, 23, 60, 92-3 251 in Europe, 12
see also names of specific countries
Cultural revolution, 296

Eastern, Central and Southern Africa (ECSA) Cooperation in Nutrition, 237
Ecuador, 11, 16, 23, 85, 94, 114, 115, 116, 117, 137-8, 173
and endemic goitre and IQ, 137-8
Educators, 410
Elimination of IDD, 156
Emory University School of Public Health, 214
endemic cretinism, 83, 179
areas with, 280
and control programmes (national), 278-80
countries free of,
in different countries, 136-45, 165-67, 177-80
in Europe, 23
see also names of specific countries
'Ending Hidden Hunger', 50, 64, 73, 152, 174, 209-10, 217, 232
Epidemiology, 303-6
Eritrea, 104

Ethiopia, 104, 115, 236
see also Africa, Eastern and Southern
Europe
assessment of the IDD problem in, 303-6
cretinism studies in, 23
IDD in Europe, 303-19
see also names of specific countries

FAO, 58
foetus, 10-4
food goitrogens, 251

Germany, 58, 125
economic costs of IDD in, 21
Ghana, 104
Global Verification Commission, 353
goitre, 34, 36, 44-5, 121, 177, 285-7
call for elimination of, 35-8
classification of, 83-5
cost and benefits of, 137
development of, 9-10
endemic, *see under* endemic cretinism in Himalayan Range, 278-80
histroy of, 4-5
and iodized salt, *see under* iodized salt rate assessment,
and ultra sinography, 85
and USA, 35
see also names of specific countries and endemic Cretinism, IDD
Goitre and Cretinism Eradication Project (GCEP), 191
goitre fixation, 296
'goitrogens' 9, 12

Index

Goitre and Cretinism Eradication Porject, 287-8
goitre control
administrative infrastructure, 196
in Asia, 190-8
requirements for success, 195-98
Government, 409
Goats, 387-8

Himalayas, the, 278-80
Holland, 58, 73
Horses, 386
hypothyroidism, 17-8, 21, 26, 90, 121
cerebral, 24, 26
in different cities, 15-6
in Zaire, 104

Immunization, expanded programme of, 55
Indain Council of Medical Research, 278-80
India, 6, 10, 17, 46, 60, 121, 138-41, 278-82, 415-6
goitre affected areas, 279-80
goitre and IQ, in, 138-40
iodized salt in, 60, 391-3
see also South East Asia
Indonesia, 10, 23, 46, 60
Infact feeding practies in India, 172
International Bank for Reconstruction and Development (IBRD), 70
International Council for control of Iodine Deficiency Disorders (ICCIDD), 27, 32, 38-44, 48-54, 57-8, 65-6, 70-5, 96, 206-8, 214, 219, 232, 283, 236-7, 244, 299-301, 348, 350, 353, 419-20
in Delhi, 37, 216
and different agencies, 72-4
and different countries, 39-41, 57
global activities of, 41-4
meetings with UN agencies, 42-3
office bearers and board members, 40
and salt industry, 74-5
International Conference on Nutrition, 36, 64, 209-10, 217
International Thyroid Congress, tenth,
International Training and Support Programme for Control of IDD (IPCIDD), 214
International Union of Nutritional Sciences, 208
International Working Group on IDD Control for China (IWGIDD), 300
iodide, 105
iodine, 277
cycle in nature, 5-7
excretion of, 96
direct supply of, 126-7, 349
fortifying food with, 126-7
intervention, effects of, on human and livestock, 134-5, 139-40
recommended level of, in salt, 227
urinary excretion of, 86-8
iodine toxicity, 395
iodine induced thyrotoxicosis, 369
iodine deficiency
in adults, 10, 18
in animals, 19-20
in Asia, 5-10
in Childhood, 10-1, 16-7
in Europe, 7
control programme, *see under* IDD elimination control programme

(international and national),
see under IDD elimination
costs of, 20-3
ecology of, 5-7
foetus, 10-4
and mental deficiency, 3
in neonats, 11, 14-6
Iodine Deficiency Disorders (IDD), 23-5
and the affected countries, 58-62
see also under specific countries,
ancillary signals of, 93
assessment of problems,
causes of, 99-100
communication, 194
and communication to the masses, 165-72
detection of, 81-2
various techniques of, 82-94
also see under individual techniques, e.g. palpitation of thyroid, ultrasonography urinary excretion thyroglobulin, TSH, thyroid hormone, radioiodine
elimination, not eradication of, 214-5
extent of Studies by WHO, 24-5
in Europe, 303-19
and global Verification Commission, 66
govts of the affected countries, 57-62
history of, 325
and inadequate communication, 185-7
in Latin America, 200-3, 325-35
measurement of, 82, 350
as a public health problem, 57-62
result of geographical conditions, 100-1
and WHA, 31
and World Summit for Children, 31
IDD Control, 31-55, 62, 64, 79-97, 129-45, 342-3
and awareness among people, 60, 165-72, 175, 350
benefits of, 129-45, 139-42
in China, 54
see also China
cost of national programme for, 44-7, 57, 62-5, 174-5, 182
and regional support for, 47-8, 57-8
and sub-regional working group, 179
in Columbia, 54
in different countries, 135-43
see also under specific countries
economic evaluation of, 130-1, 143
types of, 131-5
in Equador, 129
grand alliances for, 173
in Guatemala, 54
in Latin America, 52, 325-35
monitoring and verification of, 347-53
national programme for, in Africa, 177-89
in Andean Colony, 200
in Asia, 190-99
in Latin America, 200-3
national policy on, 252
progress towards, 51-5
proposed guidelines for, 348-50
in Switzerland, 32-4
in USA, 35

Index

ICN, 429, 457
IDD Control in South East Asia :
in Bangladesh, 272-5
in Bhutan, 275-7
in DPR, 138-41, 277-8
in India, 278-82
in Indonesia, 282-3
in Mongolia, 284-5
in Myanmar, 285-7
in Nepal, 121, 287-9
in Sikkim, 141-2
in Sri Lanka, 289-90
in Thailand, 290-1

IDD endemia, 93-4
iodine supplements, see under iodized salt
iodized oil, 26, 45, 94, 130, 207, 220
iodized oil in pregnancy, 366-8
compared with iodized salt, 123
injection of, 13, 121, 273, 277, 287
in Latin and Central America, 200-3
oral administration of, 121, 123
in Papua New Guinea, 12, 130
target groups for use of, 130
iodized salt, 27, 34, 35, 45, 94-5, 206-7, 220-1, 278, 325
in African countries, 180-3, 210-1
best means of meeting iodine deficiency, 101-3
and change of social behaviour, 60
and China, 18-9
cost of, 102
for elimination of IDD, 99-118, 345
and goitre, 34-5
historical background of, 103-5
history of introducing, 103-5
production and distribution of, 286
programme for, adequacy of, 228
reasons for introducing, 101-2
in SAARC Countries, 210-1
and Switzerland, 32-4
and USA, 35, 125, 126
see also salt, salt iodization
iodized tea, 127
iodized water, 124-5, 128
IQ, 17
Iran, 260
Italy, 58, 73
IDD in Livestock, 375
ecology and economics,
Iodine Content of water, soil, and plants, 378-80

Japan, 75
Joint Committee on Health Policy (JCHP), 206

Kazakhstan, 261
Kiwani Clubs, 78, 174
Kiwani International, 27, 229-32
and World Service Project, 27, 57 79
and UNICEF 57-8
Korea, 75
Kyrgyzstan, 261

Latin America, 4, 11, 325-35
history, 325
IDD as health problem in, 200-3
IDD in, 325-35
salt iodization programme in 325, 331
poor progress of IDD control

in, 327
see also specific country
Lipidol, 120, 121, 123
see also iodized oil

Malawai, 104
Maldives, 427
Malaysia, 125
Mali, 245-6
Medical Research Centre, Nairobi, 177
Mexico, see Latin America
Miconutrient DIS, 222
Middle East, 45
Mimosine, 382
Mindmap,405-6
IDD in, 337-44
Mozambique, 104
myxoedematous cretinism

Namibia, 104
National IDD Commission, 349
National Iodine Deficiency Disorders Control Programme, 280
National Centre for IDD Control, 299
National Goitre Control Project, 138-41, 278-82
National Advocacy Meeting, 153-61
Nepal, 121, 130, 191-92, 298, 416-7, 425-6
and ORT, 173
New Zealand, 32
nervous endemic cretinism, see endemic cretinism
NGOs, 402, 409-10
Nigeria, 104
Cretinism in, 251
IDD situations in, 251
national policy on IDD in, 252-3

requirements of IDD elimination in, 254-5

Opportunities for Micronutrients Initiatives (OMNI), 73
Oceania Thyroid Congress, 36
Organization for African Unity (OAU), 113
Oriodol, 121, 124
Other iodine antagonists, 382-3

Pakistan, 262, 337-8, 417
Parasitic infection, 383
Pan American Health Organization, 36
Papua New Guinea, 12, 13, 120
iodine deficiency in foetus in, 36
People's Republic of China, see China
Peru, 11, 121, 328, 329-30
see also Latin America
Philippines 104, 113
pituitary gland, 9
Pigs, 388
Poultry, 388
Policy Makers, 408
Policy Conference on Micronutrient Malnutrition, 64
Productivity, 388-9
Produs and Sorries, 406-8
Programme Aganist Micronutrient Malnutrition (PAMM), 74, 158, 214, 300

radioactive iodine, 18
radioiodine, 7, 92
Red Barna, 290
Review if social Development, 149-53
Regional Plans, 420

Index

Salt, 51, 105, 128, 325
iodine level in, 116
iodization process of, 105-7
iodization programme :
supporting measure, 110-12
iodization programme :
characteristics of, 112-17
manufacturing and trading
community, 113-14
industry and IOD elimination,
  117-18
salt, iodization of, 51, 105, 325
intervention with, 251-2
see also salt and iodized salt
Salt Iodization Committee, 251
salt industry, 58, 74-5, 78, 409
Senegal, 104
Sheep, 386
Sicliy, 125
Sikkim, 141-3
smallpox, eradication of, 67
South America, 4, 11
see also Latin America and
specific countries in
South Asia Association for
Regional Cooperation (SAARC),
  65
SAARC, 151
child and the law,
child and health,
child and nutrition,
child and learning,
child and its environment,
Social communicators, 151
South-East Asia, 47
for specific countries see
under IDD control in South
East Asia
Sri Lanka, 113, 271-91, 417-8,
  426-7
Sub-Sahara Africa, see Africa and
names of specific countries in

Sudan, 104
Sweden, 58-73
Swedish International
Development Agency, 73

Tadjikistan, 262-3
TSH see thyorid stimulating
hormone (TSH)
T_3 see triodothyronine
T_4 see thyroxine
Taiwan, 75
table salt, 94-6
see also iodized salt
Tanzania, 85, 114, 235
Tanzania Food and Nutrition
Centre, 237
Task Force for Child Survival and
Development of the President
Carter Centre, 214
tetraiodothyronine, see thyroxine
(T_4)
Thailand, 123
thiocynates, 9
thyroglobulin, 9
measuement of, 88-9
and Papua New Guinea, 13
Thyroid Association of different
countries,
thyroid gland,
effects of ID on, 7-9
importance of, 4
iodine metabolism of, 96
palpation of, 83, 96
thyroid hormone
measurement of, 91-2
importance of, 4
replacement therapy of, 10
Thyroid stimulating hormone
(TSH), 9, 45, 89-91, 96
thyrotoxicosis see
hyperthyroidism
triodothyronine (T_3), 9

Tibet, 50
Turkmenistan, 160, 263-4

UNDP, 65, 69, 114
UNCEF, 27, 32, 37-9, 42, 47, 49-51, 57-8, 65, 66, 67-8, 71-6, 96, 114, 148, 178, 205-15, 237, 245, 281, 284, 290, 298, 300, 350, 352-3, 401, 429-40
history of, 67-8
and iodized oil and salt, 207-8
its role in IDD control, 205-15
see also ICCIDD, IDD Control, Kiwani International, and specific countries
United Nations Agencies, 65-9
see also UNICEF, WHO, ICCIDD, and other agencies
USA, 32, 58, 73, 75, 103, 125-8
US Agency for International Development (USAID), 73
Uzbekistan, 264-5

WFP, 58, 68-9
Water iodized, see iodized water
World Bank, 429, 447-53
World Food Conference, 177
World Food Council, 35, 177
World Health Assembly (WHA) 31, 42, 50, 64, 67, 68, 283

World Health Organization (WHO),
3, 24-5, 27, 43, 47, 48, 49, 51, 58, 65, 66, 70-1, 96, 178, 181, 205, 206, 237, 245, 251, 300, 337, 338, 339, 353, 358, 401, 429, 434, 441-47,
action by regional offices, 341-2
development history, 216-8
functions of, 65-7, 218-21
and iodized oil and salt, 220-1
its monitoring, evaluation or information systems, 221-5
and other Working partners in this field, 225-6
its three-dimensional programme, 216-8
WHO Committee for South-East Asia, 35
WHO Regional Office for the Eastern Mediterranean, 338-9
WHO Safety of Iodized Salt and Iodized Oil, 357
World Summit for Children, 31, 42, 64, 100, 174, 209, 210, 232, 283

Young Childten : Priority One, 231

Zaire, 11, 12, 14, 16, 104, 123, 130, 178, 246-8
Zimbabwe, 73, 104, 126

8 p126 p.8 Requirement = ? 30mg per month.
29 mg iodine a month =
1 drop Lugols iodine = 6mg ∴ 5 drops per month
Usual iodine sold for wounds.   n a glass of water

? Can you overdose — isn't it like vitamins?
                                 excess excreted.